Frontiers in Natural Product Chemistry

(Volume 10)

Edited by

Atta-ur-Rahman, *FRS*
Honorary Life Fellow
Kings College
University of Cambridge
Cambridge
UK

Frontiers in Natural Product Chemistry

Volume # 10

Editor: Prof. Atta-ur-Rahman, *FRS*

ISSN (Online): 2212-3997

ISSN (Print): 1574-0897

ISBN (Online): 978-981-5040-76-0

ISBN (Print): 978-981-5040-77-7

ISBN (Paperback): 978-981-5040-78-4

Published by Bentham Science Publishers Pte. Ltd. Singapore. All Rights Reserved.

need for a court order if at any point you breach any terms of this License Agreement. In no event will any delay or failure by Bentham Science Publishers in enforcing your compliance with this License Agreement constitute a waiver of any of its rights.

3. You acknowledge that you have read this License Agreement, and agree to be bound by its terms and conditions. To the extent that any other terms and conditions presented on any website of Bentham Science Publishers conflict with, or are inconsistent with, the terms and conditions set out in this License Agreement, you acknowledge that the terms and conditions set out in this License Agreement shall prevail.

Bentham Science Publishers Pte. Ltd.
80 Robinson Road #02-00
Singapore 068898
Singapore
Email: subscriptions@benthamscience.net

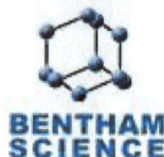

BENTHAM SCIENCE

CONTENTS

PREFACE

Frontiers in Natural Product Chemistry presents recent advances in the chemistry and biochemistry of naturally occurring compounds. It covers a range of topics including important researches on natural substances. The book is a valuable resource for pharmaceutical scientists and postgraduate students seeking updated and critically important information on bioactive natural products.

The chapters in this volume are written by eminent authorities in the field. In chapter 1, Mastino *et al.*, discuss the traditional usage and the biological and pharmacological properties of various *Cistus* species, with particular emphasis on *Cistus* species growing in Sardinia. Yuan *et al.*, in the second chapter, summarize the current knowledge regarding the phytohormone abscisic acid (ABA) in the regulation of fruit development and ripening, as well as in responses to environmental stresses. Gorai *et al.*, in chapter 3 present the progress in the research on naturally occurring biflavonoids. Victório *et al.*, in the next chapter of the book review the protective effects of plant metabolites on cell injury caused by radiation therapy against cancer and high doses of radiation exposure. Mammen in the last chapter presents a detailed overview of chemical perspective and drawbacks in flavonoid estimation assays that how plant metabolites may protect human cells against radiation-associated damage.

I hope that the readers will find these reviews valuable and thought-provoking so that they may trigger further research in the quest for new and novel therapies against various diseases. I am grateful for the timely efforts made by the editorial personnel, especially Mr. Mahmood Alam (Director Publications), Mr. Obaid Sadiq (In-charge Books Department) and Miss Asma Ahmed (Senior Manager Publications) at Bentham Science Publishers.

Atta-ur-Rahman, *FRS*
Honorary Life Fellow
Kings College
University of Cambridge
Cambridge
UK

List of Contributors

Alexander Machado Cardoso	Western Rio Janeiro State University - UEZO, Avenida Manuel Caldeira de Alvarenga, 1203, Rio de Janeiro - RJ, 23070200, Brazil
Bing Yuan	Environment, University of Melbourne, Melbourne, VIC 3010, Australia
Claudia Juliano	Dipartimento di Chimica e Farmacia, Università degli Studi di Sassari, *via* Muroni 23/A, I-07100 Sassari, Italy
Cristiane Pimentel Victório	Western Rio Janeiro State University - UEZO, Avenida Manuel Caldeira de Alvarenga, 1203, Rio de Janeiro - RJ, 23070200, Brazil
Debasish Kundu	Department of Chemistry, Govt. Degree College, Mangalkote, Burdwan - 713132, West Bengal, India
Denni Mammen	Division of Chemistry, School of Science, Navrachana University, Vasana-Bhayli Road, Vadodara, India
Dilip Gorai	Department of Chemistry, Bolpur College, Bolpur, Birbhum - 731204, West Bengal, India
Edmilson Monteiro de Souza	Western Rio Janeiro State University - UEZO, Avenida Manuel Caldeira de Alvarenga, 1203, Rio de Janeiro - RJ, 23070200, Brazil
Fernanda Marques Peixoto	Western Rio Janeiro State University - UEZO, Avenida Manuel Caldeira de Alvarenga, 1203, Rio de Janeiro - RJ, 23070200, Brazil
João Bosco de Salles	Western Rio Janeiro State University - UEZO, Avenida Manuel Caldeira de Alvarenga, 1203, Rio de Janeiro - RJ, 23070200, Brazil
Marchetti Mauro	C.N.R. - Istituto di Chimica Biomolecolare, traversa La Crucca 3, I-07040 Sassari, Italy
Maria Cristina de Assis	Western Rio Janeiro State University - UEZO, Avenida Manuel Caldeira de Alvarenga, 1203, Rio de Janeiro - RJ, 23070200, Brazil
Marianna Usai	Dipartimento di Chimica e Farmacia, Università degli Studi di Sassari, *via* Muroni 23/A, I-07100 Sassari, Italy
Patrizia M. Mastino	Dipartimento di Chimica e Farmacia, Università degli Studi di Sassari, *via* Muroni 23/A, I-07100 Sassari, Italy
Ping Leng	College of Horticulture, China Agricultural University, Beijing 100193, P. R., China
Qian Li	College of Horticulture, China Agricultural University, Beijing 100193, P. R., China
Shyamal K. Jash	Department of Chemistry, Krishna Chandra College, Hetampur, Birbhum - 731124, West Bengal, India
Yandan Xu	College of Horticulture, China Agricultural University, Beijing 100193, P. R., China

An Overview of *Cistus* Species Growing in Sardinia: A Source of Bioactive Compounds

Patrizia M. Mastino[*, 1], **Marchetti Mauro**[2], **Claudia Juliano**[3] and **Marianna Usai**[4]

[1] *Dipartimento di Chimica e Farmacia, Università degli Studi di Sassari, via Muroni 23/A, I-07100 Sassari, Italy*

[2] *C.N.R. - Istituto di Chimica Biomolecolare, traversa La Crucca 3, I-07040 Sassari, Italy*

[3] *Dipartimento di Chimica e Farmacia, Università degli Studi di Sassari, via Muroni 23/A, I-07100 Sassari, Italy*

[4] *Dipartimento di Chimica e Farmacia, Università degli Studi di Sassari, via Muroni 23/A, I-07100 Sassari, Italy*

Abstract: Extracts obtained from many plants have recently gained popularity and scientific interest for their antibacterial, antifungal and antioxidant activity. Many results have been reported on the antimicrobial properties of plant extracts containing essential oils and different classes of phenolic compounds. In this chapter, we will discuss the traditional usage and the biological and pharmacological properties of various *Cistus* species, with particular emphasis on *Cistus* species growing in Sardinia. *Cistaceae* family is widespread in the Mediterranean region with several species, and it is known as a traditional natural remedy. *Cistus* genus grows in Sardinia with populations of *C.monspeliensis, C.salvifolius, C. albidus* and *C. creticus subspecies: C.creticus* subsp. *creticus, C.creticus* subsp. *corsicus,* and *C.creticus* subsp. *eriocephalus.* Despite being widespread, only a few phytochemical research has been reported for *Cistus* species growing in Sardinia. Moreover, *C.creticus* subsp. *eriocephalus* (Viv) Greuter & Burdet growing in Sardinia is characterized by an important polymorphism due to hybridization and occurrence of various ecotypes based on intermediate morphological characters. The recent studies have shown that the extracts of *Cistus* species may be used as therapeutic agents in a wide range of human diseases. The use of plant extracts for controlling postharvest fungal pathogens can enhance healthy fruit production. Further knowledge regarding the bioactivity of Sardinian *Cistus* species will be useful to verify their potential as profitable sources of functional ingredients in applications, such as food preservation, cosmetic, hygiene or medical device.

[*] **Corresponding author Patrizia Monica Mastino:** Dipartimento di Chimica e Farmacia, Università degli Studi di Sassari, *via* Muroni 23/A, I-07100 Sassari, Italy; E-mail monicamastino@gmail.com

Keywords: Antifungal activities, Antioxidant activities, *C. albidus*, *Cistaceae*, *C.creticus* subsp. *creticus*, *C.creticus* subsp. *corsicus*, *C.creticus* subsp. *eriocephalus*, *C.monspeliensis*, *C.salvifolius*, Essential oil, Microbiological activities, Polyphenols, Sardinia, Taxonomy.

INTRODUCTION

Plants have always been a source of nourishment and care for living beings. Their twofold task of producing nutrients and medicines has played a key role in the evolution (and co-evolution) of herbivorous and omnivorous organisms.

Plants have the characteristic of being much richer in their biochemical diversity than animals. This phenomenon is probably because the plants are constrained to the ground and must evolve a multiplicity of adaptation mechanisms more than necessary for the animals, which have other means for their survival (for example, the move to search for food or escape for defense). The biologically active substances potentially usable in nutraceutical, phytotherapy, or as additives food are to be found among the secondary metabolites of plants or the products of metabolism that is not essential for the simple growth, development, or reproduction of the plant, such as mucilage, gums, glycosides, tannins, alkaloids, saponins, anthraquinones, flavonoids, essential oils, and others.

These compounds are molecules with well-defined functional roles aimed to defend the plants against abiotic stress (temperature, light, water availability, *etc.*) and biotic stress (herbivores, fungi, bacteria, and viruses' attacks) [1].

In fact, although most of the latest drugs in the market are of synthetic origin, the natural substances, in particular, secondary metabolites, isolated and characterized by a large and varied number of species, have had a fundamental role in the research and development of new drugs.

The chemical diversity that characterizes natural molecules makes the exploration of their biological characteristics not just one of the main sources of potential new compounds usable for the new drugs' realization but also a useful tool for the discovery of new mechanisms of action and the identification of plant species with the chemotaxonomy study.

Therefore, phytochemical studies are in constant evolution and continuous progress, especially due to new techniques that have allowed us to achieve the desired objectives more easily and in less time; at the same time, studies of botany, ethnobotany, pharmacology, and medicine have endured an increment and today, due to this interdisciplinarity, it is possible to have much more information on medicinal plants and their rational use in medicine [1].

The Mediterranean area is a peculiar geomorphologic, climatic and social environment in which the islands play a predominant role due to their characteristic by heavy changes in different seasons (from moderate to high temperatures and humidity). For this reason, the islands promote vegetal biodiversity and biological adaptation to this seasonal variability. In this context, the plants produce peculiar chemical compounds as secondary metabolites and therefore have been used in the past for medical purposes. Extracts obtained from many plants have recently gained popularity and scientific interest for their antibacterial and antifungal activity [2 - 4]. Many results have been reported on the antimicrobial properties of plant extracts containing different classes of phenolic compounds [5]. These compounds represent a rich source of biocides and preservatives, and many studies have pointed out the antimicrobial efficacy of certain classes of phenolic compounds, such as hydroxybenzoic acid derivatives [6], coumaric and caffeic acid derivatives [7, 8], flavonoids, and coumarins [9 - 11], catechin, epicatechin, proanthocyanidins, and tannins [12 - 14]. Moreover, some authors have studied the relationship between molecular structure and antimicrobial activity of some phenolic compounds [15, 16]. The antimicrobial properties of certain classes of polyphenols have been proposed either to develop new food preservatives [17] due to the increasing consumer pressure on the food industry to avoid synthetic preservatives or to develop innovative therapies for the treatment of various microbial infections [18, 19], considering the increase in microbial resistance against conventional antibiotic therapy. The antimicrobial activity of polyphenols occurring in vegetable foods and medicinal plants has been extensively investigated against a wide range of microorganisms. Among polyphenols, flavan-3-ols, flavonols, and tannins received the most attention due to their wide spectrum and higher antimicrobial activity in comparison with other polyphenols and to the fact that most of them can suppress several microbial virulence factors (such as inhibition of biofilm formation, reduction of host ligands adhesion, and neutralization of bacterial toxins) and show synergism with antibiotics [1].

Many biological activities from secondary metabolites of plants can also be attributed to, Essential Oils (EO), which have been long recognized for their antibacterial, antifungal, antiviral, insecticidal, and antioxidant properties. They are widely used in medicine and the food industry for these purposes. The increased interest in alternative natural substances is driving the research community to find new uses and applications for these substances, as will be broadly described below.

HISTORICAL BIOGEOGRAPHY OF SARDINIA

Sardinia is an eco-region of the central Mediterranean with a biodiversity wealth unique in Europe, with over 2300 estimated spontaneous vascular plants. Nine hundred of them are known in various ways and used for the most disparate purpose, and 300 are endemic species [20].

The first studies on the Sardinian flora dated back to the second half of the 1700s, but in the first years of the 1800s, a systematic investigation began throughout the Island territory due to Piedmont Doctor, Giuseppe Giacinto Moris. His work, entitled "Flora Sardoa", although incomplete, was fundamental for the knowledge of the plant heritage of the Island and starting point for further and more detailed research. From that moment, the contribution of numerous botanists has allowed defining the state of the current knowledge of the Sardinian flora, as reported by Arrigoni [20].

There are several factors that have contributed to characterize and differentiate the natural vegetal landscape of the island from other geographically close ones. For the first, the favor geographical position of Sardinia in the middle Mediterranean, and especially the conditions of isolation in which the island is found starting from the Miocene and that they have determined the genetic differentiation of species that are therefore unique. Another element that has decisively influenced the Sardinian floristic composition is the climate, given by the alternation of two seasons, a hot-arid and a cold-humid. The summer water deficit is the main limiting factor and forces the flora to a series of structural and functional adaptations.

The conditions of prolonged isolation due to the presence of geographic, ecological or biological barriers that prevent the dispersion and the diffusion of a given species have determined for many entities (especially the most polymorphic ones) morphological and genetic differentiation in response to environmental conditions, such as to produce speciation phenomena.

The greater floristic affinities are shared with Corsica, with which until about 10.000 years ago constituted a single geographic entity, forming a great block that has often been considered as a microplate or microcontinent.

Thirty million years ago, these land blocks began to move away from the European plate, from Provence, turning counterclockwise. Subsequently, the isolation was briefly interrupted by phenomena related to the closure of the Strait of Gibraltar (5.6 million years ago) and glaciations (the last glacial maximum dates to about 15,000 years ago), encouraging the development of indigenous species evolutions and entire biocenosis. Therefore, the Island is today characterized by typically Sardinian endemic species, and others shared with the nearby Corsica with which it constitutes the Sardinian-Corsican floristic Dominion (*e.g.: Genista corsica, Crocus minimus, Colchicum corsicum, Silene velutina, Helleborus argutifolius, Cistus creticus corsicus*).

In Sardinia, the presence of a rich contingent of plant species with potential pharmaceutical interest has been highlighted: well over 390 species are recognized as medicinal [21, 22], and 20 are included in the XI Edition of the F.U.I. (Official Italian Pharmacopoeia) as they are recognized as officinal *sensu stricto*.

In particular, the plants that constitute the "Mediterranean maquis" have been the subject of attention by researchers from quite different fields from each other, ranging from systematic botany to naturalistic engineering, phytochemicals, agronomy, ethnobotany, diet, and linguistics. Unfortunately, despite the presence of these species, the Mediterranean maquis nowadays is still considered invasive by the local populations. Knowledge of the biological, agronomic, and productive characteristics of these plants is an important step to allow the exploitation of their potential.

The Mediterranean maquis is a type of woody vegetal formation, typical of the Mediterranean climate (littoral and sublittoral zone), mainly formed by shrubs usually evergreen and sclerophyllic, associated with liana plants also mainly xerophytic and often spinescent. Herbaceous plants, on the other hand, vegetate in clearings that are reduced in the closed or continuous scrub and more extensive in the discontinuous or open scrub. The shrubby species that make the Mediterranean maquis are about 150, but the main mass consists of only about forty of them [23].

The Mediterranean scrub covers a substantial part of the Sardinian territory, and this ensures that the use of these plants are, and more over has been, of interest for a large part of the island's population and that have covered all aspects of traditional uses constituting a wealth of knowledge maintained thanks to the knowledge handed down orally by the elderly population [24, 25].

For all these reasons, the valorization of the Mediterranean maquis of Sardinia must be seen in a framework that considers the tradition and their potential for use in many fields. The research could range from environmental protection to sustainable exploitation of resources, from high-quality products (food and non-food) to new discoveries for human health. Of all the shrubs that deserve some attention stand out *Cistus* genus for his ethnobotanical use and for the wide availability of biomass.

BOTANICAL STUDY

Cistaceae Family

The *Cistaceae* family belongs to the order of the *Parietales* or *Cistales* that includes shrub, sub-shrubs, or herbs both perennial and annual. They have simple leaves with entire margin, commonly opposite especially in the lower part of the stem, less frequently scattered; they can be stipulated or not, but in this case the petiole is dilated in the shape of a sheath and are mostly characterized by a tomentose garment of starry trichomes. Arrington and Kubitzki (2003) [26], report that there is different combination of hair types on calyx, stem, and leaf. Characteristic of the family glandular hairs (multicellular and capitate or elongate-uniseriate, rarely peltate scales) or no glandular (simple, tufted, stellate). Leaves of *Cistaceae* often possess cystoliths. Stomates are anomocytic, on one or both leaf surfaces. In the minor leaf veins, phloem transfer cells are present (*e.g.*, *Helianthemum*) or absent (*e.g.*, *Cistus*). Flowers are solitary or grouped in unilateral, scorpioid, or symmetrical cymose inflorescences. Flowers usually open only in full sunlight for a few hours, and the petals are typically ephemeral. Most flowers are pentamers and hermaphrodites. The fruit is a coriaceous or woody capsule, loculicid, surrounded by the persistent calyx with numerous, small, angular seeds.

It is known that *Cistaceae* seeds have extremely hard seed coat that minimizes water loss and water uptake, this makes these seeds dormancy externally but endowed to a high viability. Moreover, Arrington and Kubitzki (2003) [26] cited other authors [27, 28], whom affirm that these properties have been interpreted as an adaptation to summer-dry and fire-prone Mediterranean climatic conditions.

Some species of *Cistus* may lead environmental problems in wildfires because they are rich in resins [29]. Over the years, the classification of *Cistaceae* family has undergone remarkable modifications by many researchers, due to the polymorphism of the numerous species belonging to it and to their possibility of interspecific and intergenic hybridization.

Currently, the division into 7 genera (Fig. **1**), made by the German botanist Grosser [30] is accepted: *Cistus, Fumana, Helianthemum, Tuberaria, Halimium, Hudsoni* and *Lechea* within which some AA. next distinguishes the genus *Crocanthemum* for American species.

These plants are mainly diffused in the Mediterranean basin and mainly prefer arid, sunny environments and, some species, have a marked predilection for the calcareous soils. However, they are present throughout the rest of Europe, North America, North Africa and West Asia.

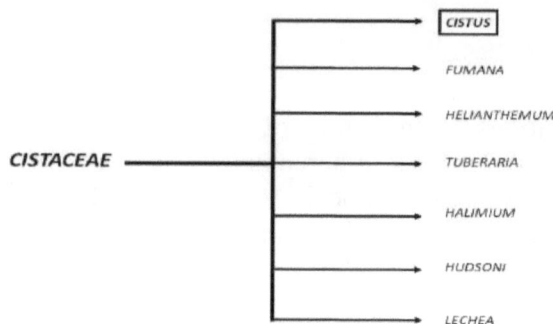

Fig. (1). Classification of *Cistaceae* family according to Grosser.

Cistus Genus

Cistus L. (from the Greek κίστοσ), known also as rock rose, is a genus of perennial ever green shrub with hard leaves growing wild also in stony and infertile soils. *Cistus* genus is indigenous of the Mediterranean region, and it is considered a pioneer genus. Impenetrable masses of *Cistus* plants are formed as early successional stages following woodland disturbances such as fire and soil overturning.

Morphological and physiological variation exists between populations of some Mediterranean species, both along large climate gradients [31]. *Cistus* species have a great ability to modify the structure and function on their leaves in the mid-term to cope with changing environmental conditions [31].

In some species, seasonal dimorphism is observed, enabling the plants adaptation to drought conditions, which induces leaves to decrease in size and grow more hair [32]. The adaptation of the genus in Mediterranean environments is evident from ecological characteristics such as fire-dependent seed germination, insect-dependent pollination, flower-dependent reproduction and "spring-dependent phenology". A long history of human activities has favored distribution and abundance of *Cistus* species in the Mediterranean [32]. According to Guzman and Vargas (2005) co-occurring species of *Cistus* are frequent, particularly in mountain ranges composed by both acidic and basic soil [33]. Environmental specificity referring to substrate confers additional value to acidophilous and basophiles species as predictable indicators of woodland disturbance. In marked contrast to the detailed knowledge of ecological characteristic, understanding of the evolution of morphological characters and phylogenetic relationship within the genus is extremely limited [33]. Lo Bianco *et al.* (2017) reported that even if *Cistus* is a relatively small genus, includes several species distributed in the warm-arid and temperate Mediterranean regions (Fig. **2**), it is complex because it shows significant morphological diversification, caused by polymorphism of many species and hybridization between related species [34].

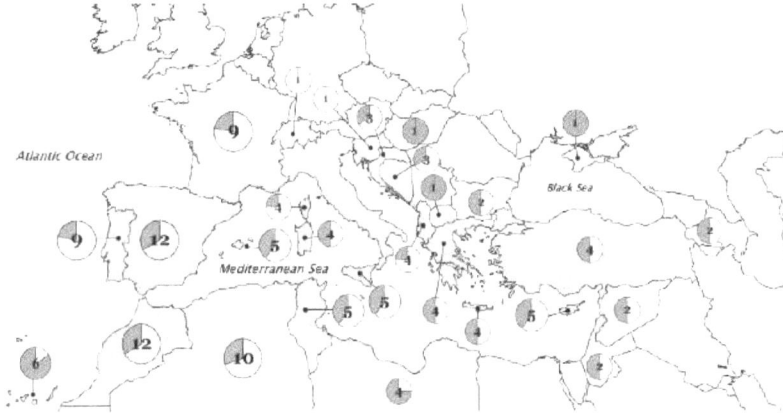

Fig. (2). Distribution map and number of Cistus species. Pie diagrams include proportions of white-flowers (white) and purple-flowers (dark grey) species in every country. Notice the highest species diversity in the western Mediterranean. The Mediterranean region shown in grey [33].

Lo Bianco *et al.* (2017), reported that "indeed, hybridization has been reported to be an active process in the *Cistus* genus and many hybrid combinations within and among pink or white flowered species have been recorded based on intermediate morphological characters [34]. The taxonomy of *Cistus* has been traditionally based on vegetative (never number, shape and airiness of leaves) and reproductive (sepal number, petal color, style length and number of fruit valves) characters, although evolutionary mechanism responsible for the morphological diversity within the genus remains poorly understood.

Several studies on the anatomical and morphological leaf traits of *Cistus* species have been published but there are few precedents of such studies for taxonomic purpose". In this study [34], the authors have evaluated the intraspecific phenotypic differentiation of *Cistus creticus* L. subspecies and the interpopulation variability among five *Cistus* subsp. *eriocephalus* population based on seed character measurements from image analysis. The results of this work have demonstrated the capability of the image analysis system as highly diagnostic for systematic purpose and confirm that seeds in the genus *Cistus* have important diagnostic value.

Systematics of Cistus Genus

In a review, Papaefthimiou *et al* (2014) [32], have reported that "taxonomic classification of *Cistus* was formed prior to 1800, but the first integrated separation was implemented in 1824 by Dunal, who described 28 species divided in 2 sections, *Erythrocistus* and *Ledonia*. Shortly thereafter, described 33 species also divided into *Erythrocistus* and *Ledonia,* where 3 additional species in section *Erythrocistus* and 7 species in section *Ledonia* were included. Spach separated them in 5 genera, named *Ladanium, Rhodocistus, Stephanocarpus, Ledonia* and *Cistus,* further divided into sections *Rhodopsis, Eucistus,* and *Ledonella*. The plant species divided in subgenera *Erythrocistus* and *Ledonia* were further separated into 7 sections: *Macrostylia, Brachystylia,* and *Astylia* in subgenus *Erythrocistus* and *Stephanocarpus, Ledonia, Ladanium,* and *Halimioides* in subgenus *Leucocistus*. Grosser, described 3 groups distributed into 16 species in 7 sections: Group A contained *Rhodocistus, Eucistus,* and *Ledonella* while Groups B and C, respectively, made up of *Stephanocarpus* and *Ledonia,* and *Ladanium* and *Halimioides*. Dansereau classified the species in subgenera *Erythrocistus* and *Ledonia,* according to Willkomm, and then separated them in 8 sections, with naming *Macrostylia, Erythrocistus,* and *Ledonella* for sections of subgenus *Erythrocistus,* and *Stephanocarpoidea, Stephanocarpus, Ledonia, Ladanium,* and *Halimioides* for sections of subgenus *Leucocistus* [32]. Demoly and Montserrat (1993), described the distribution of 12 species of genus *Cistus* that grow in Iberia. In this approach, 3 subgenera were classified: I. subgenus *Cistus,* containing *C. albidus, C.creticus, C. crispus,* and *C. heterophyllus*; II. subgenus *Leucocistus,* containing *Ledonia* with species *C.monspeliensis, C. salviifolius, C. psilosepalus,* and *C. populifolius,* and section *Ladanium* with *C. ladanifer* and *C. laurifolius*; and III. subgenus *Halimioides* containing *C. clusii* and *C. libanotis*. From this study, it became apparent that most *Cistus* species grow in western Mediterranean [35].

A recent classification of *Cistaceae* [33], is based on combined nuclear (ncpGS, ITS) and plastidic (trnL-trnF, trnK-matK, trnStrnG, rbcL) DNA sequence comparisons, divides *Cistus* into 3 subgenera: the purple flowered subgenus *Cistus* and the white flowered subgenera *Leucocistus* and *Halimioides*" (Fig. **3**).

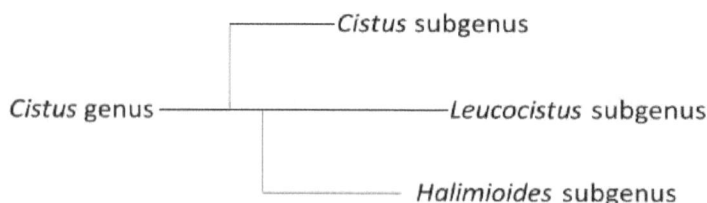

Fig. (3). Classification of three subgenus of *Cistus* genus based on analysis of tmF, maK and ITS sequences and plastid rbcL and tmL-tmF sequences.

Camarda and Valsecchi (2008) [36], described the distribution of four species of genus *Cistus* that grow in Sardinia. This include large population of *C.salvifolius* L., *C.monspeliensis* L. (white flowers), *C. albidus* L. and *C.creticus* L. (purple flowers), this last includes three different subspecies, namely subsp. *eriocephalus* (Viv.) Greuter et Burdet., subsp. *creticus* L. and subsp. *corsicus* (Loisel.) Greuter et Burdet (the latter endemic in Sardinia and Corsica) [36].

C.salvifolius (Fig. **4**) is the most widely spread species of the genus *Cistus* around the Mediterranean basin. At least three intercontinental colonization are responsible for its wide distribution, leading to little geographical isolation with high genetic diversity within populations, but no genetic differentiation between the different populations of *C.salvifolius* [32]. The factors that caused the dispersion of *C.salvifolius* around the Mediterranean were mostly ecological, such as the climate and the soil.

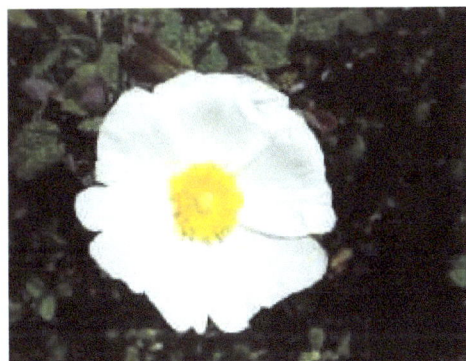

Fig. (4). *C. salvivolius* growing wild in Sardinia.

It grows in siliceous and calcareous soils and occurs on sandy soils of a wide range of habitats, while it is often located within the understory in wooded areas [32]. In Sardinia it is present in most of the island except for the higher crests of the Gennargentu Mountain [36].

C.monspeliensis (Fig. **5**), also known as the Montpelier rockrose, is characterized by its aromatic leaves and its small white flowers. It also exhibits seasonal leaf dimorphism with alternating wide and thin late autumn/early winter and thicker late spring/early summer leaves with larger trichome density, while both types coexist on the same plant during early spring. Summer leaves have high leaf mass area and tissue density, low leaf surface area and thick adaxial cuticle, traits that contribute to plants endurance to drought conditions and resistance to fire. As expected, long-term experimental drought conditions during the transition to summer leaves can have significant effect on leaf functioning. In a relevant study, over-imposed drought resulted in early leaf litter and a reduction of spring-leaf lifespan, thus a shorter vegetative season, which can have a negative effect on *C.monspeliensis* survival in Mediterranean shrubland [36]. *C.monspeliensis* is spread from the western Mediterranean to the Canary Islands and Madeira where it seems to have occurred naturally without any human interferences. *C.monspeliensis* is dominant in evergreen garrigue vegetation, inhabiting acidic, limestone, silicolous and calcareous hills and colonizing areas that are rich in *Quercus* and *Pinus* trees compost or have been disturbed by fire. It has also been demonstrated to be a non-strict calcifuge [36].

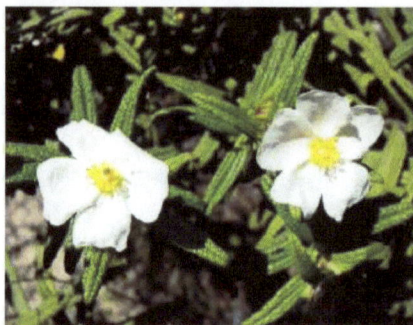

Fig. (5). *C.monspeliensis* growing wild in Sardinia.

In Sardinia, *C.monspeliensis* lives on arid, sterile, stony, sandy soils, extending from the coastal zones to the mountain ones, up to about 1200 m of altitude. It is a species which prefers the siliceous substrata and only very rarely extends on the calcareous soil.

C. albidus (Fig. **6**) has bright purple flowers (June to August), it displays ecotypic differentiation, at least when growing in semi-arid climates, being able to adapt the growth of its branches and leaf dimensions, acquiring the greatest growth under plentiful water availability, while slowing growth and tending to phenotypically converge under drier environments. *C. albidus* grows in evergreen shrublands, is partially drought deciduous and a non-strict calcicole that prefers calcareous and basic soils and woodlands with plenty *Pinus* and *Quercus* compost, in dry areas with altitude up to 1200 m. Phylogenetic studies have shown that it is closely related to the endemic species forming the Canarian *Cistus* lineage, while still forming a monophyletic group with two other purple-flowered species exclusive in the Mediterranean basin, *C.creticus* and *C. heterophyllus* [36].

In Sardinia *Cistus albidus* is present in the center of the Island, in the middle-mountain areas of Ortobene Mount, the mountains of Orune and of the Plateau of Bitti-Budduso, of Lerno Mount, where it forms extensive cistetus.

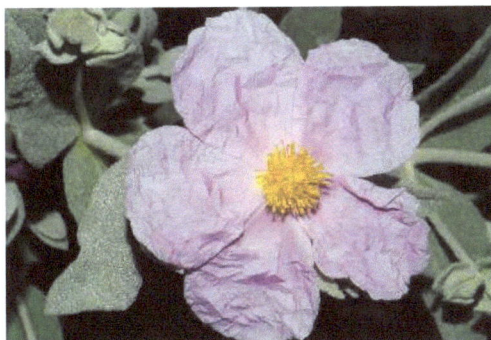

Fig. (6). *Cistus albidus* growing wild in Sardinia.

Among the Sardinian *Cistus*, *C. albidus* appears as the most mesophilic species; it lives in the stony zones from the sea level up to over the 1000 m of altitude, on the substrata preferably of siliceous nature, in sunny locations.

Cistus creticus (Cretan rock rose) it is a small tree about a meter high; flowering occurs at the end of spring and its pink petals are creased. The leaves exhibit the phenomenon of seasonal dimorphism, as an adjustment mechanism for acclimatization to the Mediterranean climate. During summertime, when water is limited, brachyblasts are developed that have leaves five-times shorter than the ones in winter, with stomata located abaxially inside crypts. During wintertime, the newly developed dolichoblasts are fourteen times longer, bearing a bigger number of leaves with stomata distributed across the lower surface.

Among the three *C.creticus* subspecies identified, subsp. *corsicus* (Fig. **7**) is limited to the islands of Corsica and Sardinia [36].

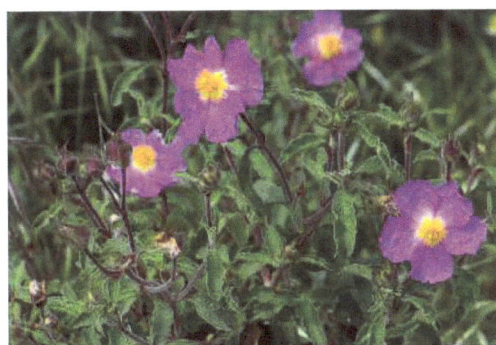

Fig. (7). *C.creticus* subsp. *corsicus* growing wild in Sardinia.

It is a Sardinian-Corsican endemism, in Sardinia is present in the schistose areas around Baratz Lake, in the north-western part of the Island.

More than twenty-five populations of *C.creticus* subsp. *creticus* (Fig. **8**) are endemic to the coastal areas of Crete (Greece) [36], whereas, the areal of *Cistus creticus* is centralized mainly on the eastern Mediterranean, and the Sardinian-Corsican system would represent the western limit of its diffusion area [22, 57]. In Italy it is present in the southern regions and in Sicily, whilst in Sardinia it has been reported in the coastal calcareous areas of the central-eastern part.

Subspecies *eriocephalus* (Fig. **9**), where the young branches, the floral peduncles and sepals are covered by long silky white hairs, is exclusive to the Mediterranean area mainly located on the islands of Corsica, Sardinia, and Crete [36]. Indifferent to the pedological substratum, it lives on any type of soil, from the sea level to over the 1000 m. It spreads in the zones with hot-arid climate and becomes part of the formations of the coastal or hilly spots and of the coastal garrigues, where it forms low felt tufts. In relation to the different environments, it has a great variability in the shape of the leaves, in the abundance of the hairy coating.

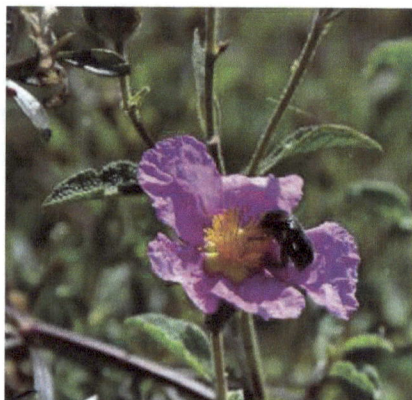

Fig. (8). *C.creticus* subsp. *creticus* growing wild in Sardinia.

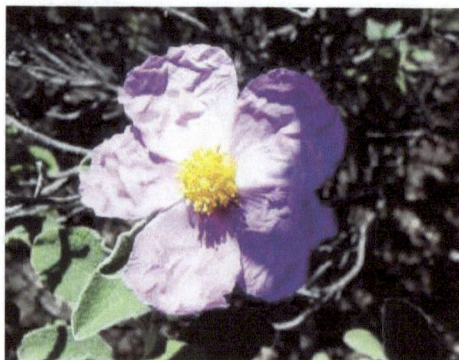

Fig. (9). *C.creticus* subsp. *eriocephalus* growing wild in Sardinia.

BIOLOGICAL ACTIVITIES

Modern scientific research has focused on the isolation and identification of compounds present in extracts, and resins from various species of *Cistus*. Studies have also analyzed their biological and pharmacological activity, which elicit healing properties. Phytochemical studies using chromatographic and spectroscopic techniques have shown that *Cistus* is a source of bioactive compounds, mainly phenylpropanoids (flavonoids, polyphenols) and terpenoids. These compounds determine the medicinal properties of *Cistus* such as anti-inflammatory, antibacterial, antifungal, antiviral, anti-allergic and strengthening the body's resistance and an analgesic effect which allows their use as therapeutic agents in a wide range of diseases [37].

According to Bouamama *et. al.* (2006) [38], we report in a recent paper, that the ancient ethnobotanical uses reveal that *Cistus* plants extracts are an excellent remedy for various microbial infections and are also well known and used as anti-inflammatory and antiulcerogenic, wound healing and vasodilator remedies [38, 39].

The inhibition of low-density lipoprotein (LDL) [40] and the possible protection against coronary heart diseases and strokes have also been described [41].

Several studies carried out using different *Cistus* species extracts demonstrated many pharmacological activities, such as: gastroprotective effect (*Cistus creticus* subsp. *eriocephalus* (Viv.) Greuter & Burdet and *Cistus laurifolius*); anti-inflammatory activity (*Cistus creticus* subsp. *eriocephalus* (Viv.) Greuter & Burdet); protective effect on DNA cleavage and dose-dependent free-radical scavenging capacity for (*Cistus creticus* subsp. *eriocephalus* (Viv.) Greuter & Burdet and *Cistus monspeliensis*); cytotoxic activity against several human leukemic cell lines *in vitro* (*Cistus creticus* L. subsp. *Creticus* and *Cistus monspeliensis*) and anticarcinogenic activities [42].

Currently, numerous manufacturers offer in the market some *Cistus* infusions ("*Cistus* tea") as useful antioxidant supplements to prevent chronic diseases [39].

Some researchers point out that extracts of various *Cistus* species are a source of compounds with high antioxidant potential and can be used in therapy for many diseases caused by oxidative stress and can be useful in the prevention and treatment of Alzheimer's disease [37]. For example quercetin, with its antioxidant activity, improve memory impairment that accompany Alzheimer's disease. Furthermore, the use of *Cistus* tea as a biological antibacterial mouth rinse, contributed to the prevention of biofilm induced diseases in the oral cavity by decreasing the number of bacteria and reducing the initial bacterial adhesion [42].

The aqueous extracts of *C.salvifolius* (L.) and *C.monspeliensis* (L.) have antinflammatory and both central and peripheral analgesical properties, supporting the traditional use of those plants in the treatment of inflammatory ailments [43]. In addition, was investigated the capacity of *C.salvifolius* and *C.monspeliensis* extracts to inhibit α-glucosidase enzyme and their significant inhibition of α-amylase indicate that they may be effective therapeutic agents for controlling hyperglycemia [44].

Scientific research indicates and confirms in many plants, including *Cistus* sp., the presence of compounds with anticancer properties. The anti-cancer compounds cause changes in the cancer cell cycle invoking a mechanism in the cell whose main element is the apoptotic pathway [45, 46]. The observed changes are a decrease in the proliferation index (cytostatic effect), and a decrease in cell survival resulting from the induction of apoptosis (cytotoxic effect) [37]. Moreover, Papaefthimiou *et al.* in the article published in 2014 [32], cited other authors [47, 48], whom affirm that cytotoxic activity of shoot extracts from *C.creticus* subsp. *creticus* shoot, in an *in vitro* culture of human HeLa cells, was shown. Shoot extracts (rich in labdane diterpenes) were able to exert cytotoxic activity on HeLa (cervix), MDA-MD-453 (breast), and FemX (melanoma) cancer cells. The labdane-type diterpene sclareol, which is used today as a certified drug, has antitumor activity against human breast cancer cell lines and enhances the activity of known anti-cancer drugs. Three flavonoids were also tested against eleven leukemic cell lines. Myricetin had no activity while a myricetin ether, that was isolated from the hexane extract of *C.monspeliensis*, exhibited significant cytostatic and cytotoxic activities while its 3′,5-diacetyl derivative (synthesized), had lower cytotoxic activity.

Research indicates that *Cistus* purified extracts can complement human cancer treatment. However, this assertion requires further research to understand its effects and its interaction with the recommended drugs [37].

The results of a recent study [49] showed that the use of *Cistus* extracts to controlling postharvest fungal pathogens can enhance healthy fruit production to avoid diseases caused from chemical residues used in storage.

Several studies have been carried out on the possible use of various *Cistus* species in phytoremediation [50, 51]. Some species showed variable accumulation patterns for metals at different soil concentration. This difference was also noted between parts of the same plant suggesting that whole plant–soil interactions should be considered when choosing plant species for developing and utilizing phytoremediation methods [52]. It is known that *C. albidus* displayed strong tolerance to Pb and accumulated large quantities of Pb and Cd in its roots; *C.*

libanotis accumulated large quantities of Pb and Cd in its above ground parts and for this reason was classified as a Pb and Cd accumulator species. The studies result showed that *C. albidus* is suitable for phytostabilization of Pb-contaminated soils, while *C. libanotis* can be used for phytoextraction of both Pb and Cd [53].

ESSENTIAL OILS

Among the secondary metabolites of plant, the most known are the essential oils. They are usually volatile and fragrant substances with an oily consistency mostly liquid at room temperature but few of them may be solid or resinous. They are synthesized in all plant organs and stored in special cells, cavities, canals, epidermal cells or glandular trichomes. Several techniques are used to extract EO but the most known is extraction using water or steam distillation.

All *Cistus* species secrete essential oils in different amounts that are mostly composed of monoterpene, sesquiterpene, and diterpene compounds, but not all of them are fully characterized [39].

For example, Paolini *et. al.* (2008) reports the complete characterization of the essential oil of *C. albidus*, which showed a high content of sesquiterpenes bearing the bisabolene and cadinene skeleton [54].

As already reported in our previous work. [39] "various reports have demonstrated the strength and effectiveness of the antimicrobial activity of *Cistus* essential oils. The antimicrobial activity of the essential oil of *C.salvifolius*, of *C.creticus*, and of *C. ladanifer* has been fully documented and scientifically proven. The responsible for the antimicrobial capacity of *Cistus* EO, seems to be mostly terpenes [55]. *Cistus* essential oil is now officially approved by the Food & Drugs Administration (USA) and by European Commission as a food additive and flavorings agent. *C. ladanifer* L. essential oil is hypothesized could be used as an herbicide because the oil showed herbicidal activity in *in vitro* bioassays. Research by Loizzo *et al.* (2013), indicated that EO of the species *C.creticus*, *C.salvifolius*, *C. libanotis*, *C.monspeliensis* and *C. villosus* exhibit antioxidant properties. Particularly *C.monspeliensis* and *C. libanotis* EO, have been shown the greatest antioxidant activity [56].

Here following we report the results obtained in our study, Mastino *et al.* (2016), carried out on EO deriving from all *Cistus* species growing in Sardinia. All EOs have been analyzed and has been characterized many constituents [39].

In this study are reported the differences found in six different profiles of EOs characteristic of each species and subspecies. Sardinian *C.salvifolius* showed a high quantity of norisoprenoids, absent in the other analyzed *Cistus* Eos. The most important components were ionones and β-damascenone with the presence also of cistodiol and clerodane diterpene [39]. The main component of this oil was manoyl oxide. The concentration of diterpenes is also very significant in the Eos of *C.salvifolius* growing in Tunisia and Sicily [56].

In Cretan *C.salvifolius* Eos the most abundant constituents were cis-ferruginol, manoyl oxide, and 13-epi manoyl oxide [56, 57] and sesquiterpenes hydrocarbons were well represented. In Eos of *C.salvifolius* growing at Aeolian Islands (Sicily) it is possible to find a high concentration of sesquiterpenes (hydrocarbons 12.5% and oxygenated 31.5%) close to that detected in Cretan population.[56] Leaves and flowers of *C.salvifolius* from Jordan give an oil reach in esters and in oxygenated and hydrocarbon diterpenes, the major components were *E*-ethyl cinnamate, *Z*-ethyl cinnamate, and manoyl oxide [58]. Finally, the essential oils of *Cistus salvifolius* from a polluted area of Elba Island showed different profiles in comparison with those from not polluted area. Ambroxide and ambrial were the most important compounds in the essential oil from *C.salvifolius* harvested in a polluted area of Elba Island while nonanal and tridecanal were the main compounds in Eos from non-polluted area [59].

In Eos of *C.monspeliensis* growing wild in Sardinia have been identified a total of 40 constituents [39]. The main fraction of the oil was represented by linear hydrocarbons, and heneicosane was the principal compound. Several hydrocarbons such as: heptacosane, nonacosane, pentacosane, and tricosane were also found in Eos from *C.monspeliensis* growing in the South of France, Greece, and Tunisia [56, 60 - 62]. The monoterpene α-terpineol is the only isolated in small quantities from Sardinian *C.monspeliensis*. While carvacrol was a major constituent of Tunisian *C.monspeliensis* leaves and essential oils [60, 63]. Moreover, carvacrol and α-terpineol were the only monoterpenes isolated from leaf essential oil of *C.monspeliensis* plants found in Crete (Greece) [62, 64]. In Tunisian and French plants the major components of essential oils of *C.monspeliensis* were hydrocarbons and oxygenated monoterpenes [56, 60, 65]. Sesquiterpenes are also present in good amount in Sardinian *C.monspeliensis* [39], so that in Tunisia has been found an accountable amounts of oxygenated sesquiterpenes and sesquiterpene hydrocarbons [56]. Also in *C.monspeliensis* growing wild in France and Greece were isolated several sesquiterpenes [61, 65]. It is noteworthy that in essential oils from aerial parts of *C.monspeliensis* grown in Greece has been revealed several clerodanes [62, 66 - 68].

In the essential oils produced by French, Greek and Tunisian *C.monspeliensis*, the norisoprenoids (*E*)-β-damascenone and ionones, were identified [56, 57, 60 - 64]. Several other carbonylic compounds as epi-13-manoyl oxide, kaur-16-ene and nonanal were the principal constituents of *C.monspeliensis* EO from Algeria [69], while *C.monspeliensis* EO from Croatia is characterized by the dominance of labdane-type diterpenes [70].

Essential oil composition of *C. albidus* growing in Sardinia showed high content of sesquiterpenes where β-caryophyllene, β-bourbonene, ar-curcumene are the major constituents. Moreover, several oxygenated sesquiterpenes were also identified; *cis*-cadin-4-en-7-ol and T-cadinol were the principal ones [39]. *C. albidus* essential oils from North-eastern Spain, France and Italian peninsula showed high content of sesquiterpenes, as β-sesquiphellandrene, β-caryophyllene, β-bourbonene, α-zingiberene, and germacrene D [54, 61, 71, 72]. Ormeño *et al.* (2007), observed that in *C. albidus* growing in competition with other wild Mediterranean species "germacrene D, ar-curcumene and allo-aromadendrene constitute the highest content of emissions from leaves". [73] The principal compound of *C. albidus* collected in Spain, was zingiberene [74], also essential oil of *C. albidus* obtained from Provence (France) is characterized by a high content of sesquiterpenes as α-zingiberene [64, 71]. In *Cistus* genus α-Zingiberene is present only in *Cistus albidus* therefore this compound may be considered characteristic for this species [75]. The presence of several monoterpenes, including α-pinene and limonene, was observed in *C. albidus* grown in Catalonia, Spain [72]. Only a small proportion of oxygenated monoterpenes but no monoterpene hydrocarbons, was identified in *C. albidus* leaves growing wild in France [54]. Diterpenes were found only in *C. albidus* plants collected in South France and Spain [54, 57], the largest concentration was measured for the labdane-type compound 13-epi-manoyl oxide [49]. In *C. albidus* collected from southern Catalonia, Spain are present docosane, octacosane, and tetracosane [72]. Linear hydrocarbons including n-tetradecane and n-hexadecane, were identified exclusively in essential oil extracted from the of *C. albidus* growing in Italy in late spring [71], as well as aliphatic aldehydes including octanal, nonanal, decanal and the keton 6-methyl-5-hepten-2-one were identified only in the pollen [71]. Nonanal, decanal, undecanal, and dodecanal were detected also in the essential oil of *C. albidus* plants growing wild in France [54].

Twenty components were identified in essential oil of *C.creticus* subsp. *creticus* grown in Sardinia [39], representing 99.26% of the total oil. Labdane-type diterpenes were a significant fraction of metabolites identified with manool and manoyl oxide being the most abundant [39]. Small concentration of monoterpenes were detected in essential oil of Cretan *C.creticus* subsp. *creticus* [76, 77]. studies conducted on Cretan plants revealed the presence of several sesquiterpenes and oxygenated sesquiterpenes and labdane-type diterpenes produced in *Cistus* by trichome- specific [78]. Similar chemical composition was reported from *C.creticus* subsp. *creticus* collected in Croatia [70]. Abu-Orabi *et al.* (2020), described that there are differences in chemical composition between the two organs, leaves, and flower buds in plants from Jourdan: oil extracted from leaves is characterized by oxygenated diterpenes and diterpenes hydrocarbon whereas the oil extracted from flowers shows an high content of oxygenated diterpenes [58].

Mastino *et al.* (2016) studied the essential oil of *C.creticus* subsp. *corsicus* (37 components, amounting to 94.6% of the total composition of the oil) that is the only Sardo-Corse endemic species [39]. the principal components are diterpenes which are present in good quantity, several hydrocarbon sesquiterpenes and oxygenated sesquiterpenes were identified; T-cadinol being the most abundant [39]. The essential oils distilled from of *C.creticus* subsp. *corsicus* from Corsica were qualitatively similar, but different in the percentages of major components [79]. In the study of Mastino *et al.* (2016) was also carried out an analysis of principal components (PCA) In (Fig. **10**) are reported the score plot (a) and the loading plot (b). The Score plot shows a cluster formed by the three *C.creticus* subspecies. *C.salvifolius* remains very close to that cluster [39]. These results suggest possible hybrid origin of *C.creticus* subsp. *eriocephalus* with *C. salvifolius*. In the loading plot is noteworthy the distribution of the essential oils' components that are in mostly agreement with the position of the *Cistus* species in the score plot (Fig. **11b**).

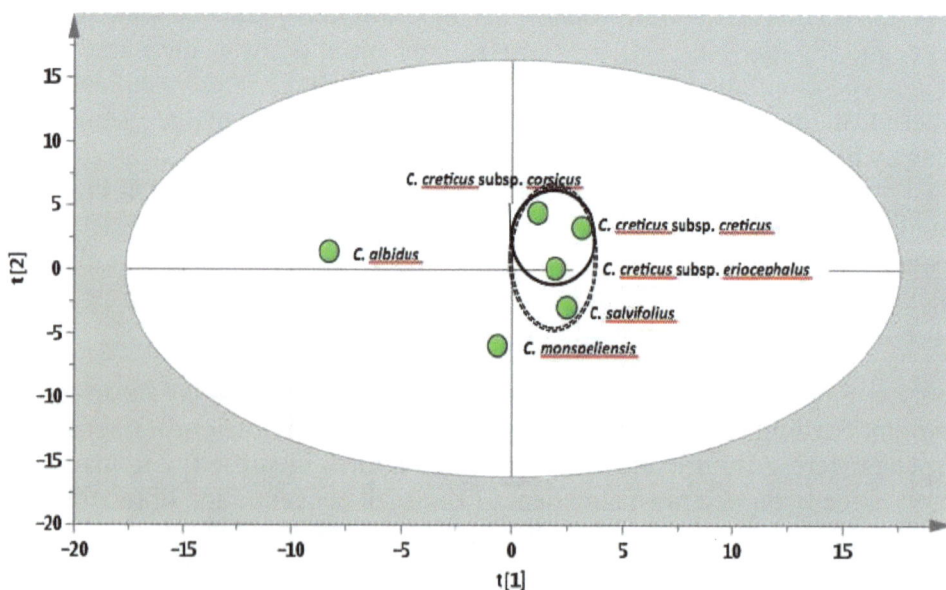

Score plot of PCA (a)

(Fig. 10) contd.....

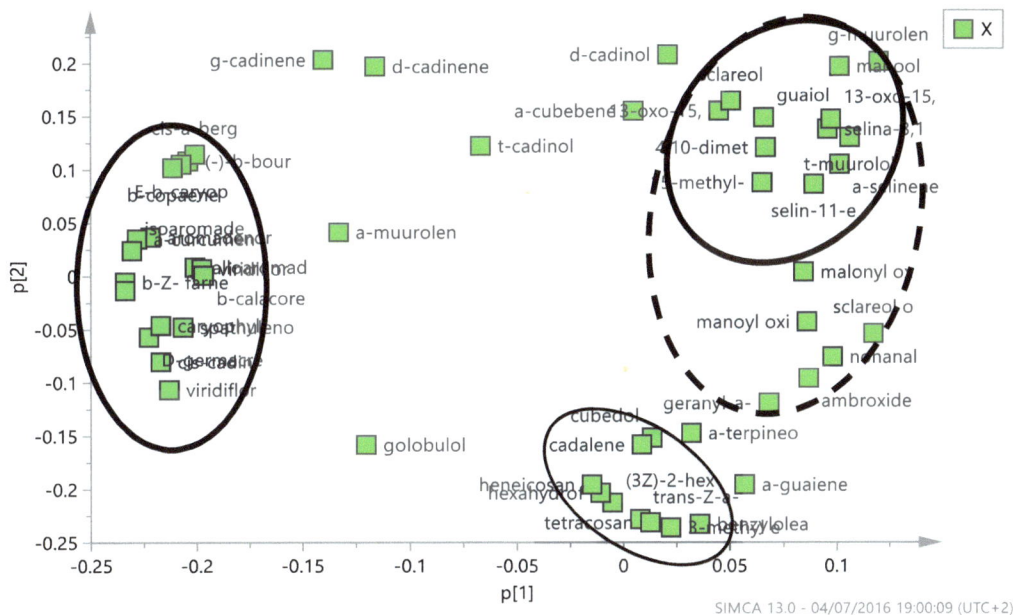

Loading Plot of PCA (b)

Fig. (10). PCA of essential oil of *Cistus* species grown in Sardinia [72].

In essential oil of Sardinian *C.creticus* subsp. *eriocephalus,* studied by Mastino *et al.* (2016) [39], where identified thirty-seven constituents, representing 94.15% of the total. Characteristic of this essential oil is the presence of a consistent quantity of labdane-type diterpenes as manoyl oxide, which represent the most abundant component that is considered chemotaxonomic markers and were found abundant also in *C.creticus* subsp. *Corsicus* [79]. In Cretan *C.creticus* subsp. *eriocephalus* leaf extract high concentration of labdane-type compounds manoyl oxide and 13-epi manoyl oxide was observed. The sesquiterpene fraction was the largest in the essential oils of *C.creticus* subsp. *eriocephalus* endemic in the Cretan flora in Greece [76]. Maggi *et al.* (2016) have found these compounds only in scant amounts [80]. Paolini *et al.* (2009) reported that no essential oil was obtained from the samples of *C.creticus* subsp. *eriocephalus* from different regions of Corsica and North Sardinia. This subspecies differs from *C.creticus* subsp. *creticus* and *C.creticus* subsp. *corsicus* for the absence or poorness of glandular trichomes This could be the reason why it does not produce any essential oil [79]. On the other hand, in our study [72] essential oil was obtained from a sample collected in the Central Eastern Sardinian region. Maggi *et al.* (2016), analyzed the essential oil obtained from the aerial parts of *C.creticus* subsp. *eriocephalus* collected in central Italy (Umbria and Marche Apennines) [80].

The sample showed a very low essential oil yield (0.03%), which was consistent with that reported for Greek populations [76].

The absence or the essential oil in *C.creticus* subsp. *eriocephalus* reported by Paolini *et al.* (2009) was not in accordance with our results, for this reason we thought necessary to enlarge the study on more stations of *C.creticus* subsp. *eriocephalus* growing wild representative of all Sardinia Island [81]. For this reason, we carried out a study on representative shrubs of *C.creticus* subsp. *eriocephalus* growing in seven sites differing in altitude and soil (Fig. **11**).

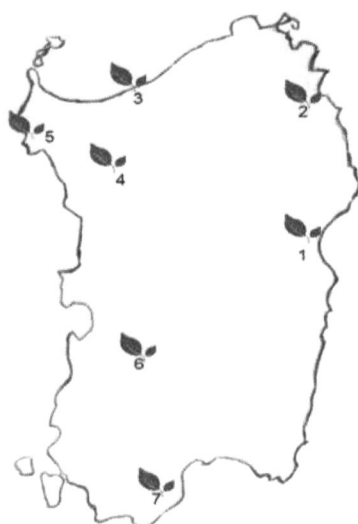

N°	Location
1 CG	Calagonone
2 MN	Monte Nieddu
3 CP	Costa Paradiso
4 BN	Bonnanaro
5 MD	Monte Doglia
6 MA	Monte Arci
7 PM	Pixinamanna

Fig. (11). Collection station for *C. creticus* subsp. *eriocephalus* [81].

The essential oils ranging from 5.05 mg/100 g to 128.70 mg/100 g of the fresh weight. No essential oil was obtained from the sample collected in Bonnanaro [81]. The different yields in essential oil may be due to different ecological and geographic factors. Carrying out an analysis of principal components (PCA), on the analytical data derived from essential oil, we demonstrated the existence of a high interpopulation variability within the essential oils of *C.creticus* subsp. *eriocephalus* growing in Sardinia (Fig. **12**) [81]. Sardinian population showed appreciable variations in their chemical composition, rather than well-defined different chemotypes. Very interesting is the population of *C.creticus* subsp. *eriocephalus* of Bonnanaro, where no essential oil was detected. The plants grew totally isolated from other species belonging to the same genus, consequently, the hybridization with other *Cistus* species was not possible. For this reason, we suppose that this station (Bonnanaro) represents the place, where was possible to find the putative progenitor of *C.creticus* subsp. *eriocephalus,* this observation suggests that the data related to the samples collected in the other Sardinian stations would be the results of hybridizations [81], however, our fieldwork in Sardinia does not reveal relevant morphological variability within the studied populations.

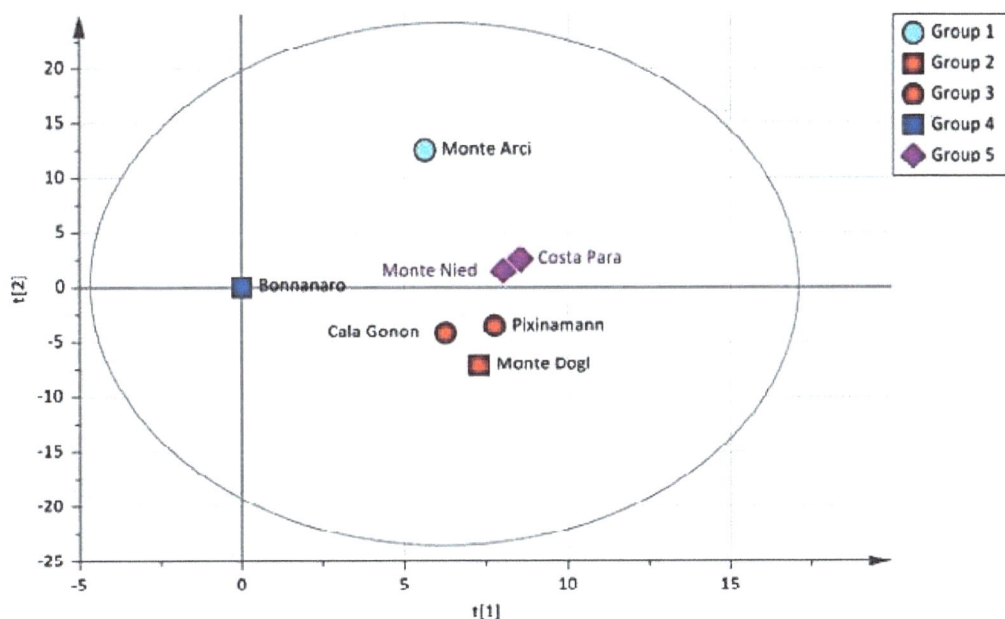

Fig. (12). PCA analysis of PCA of essential oil of studied populations [81].

Our data suggest that the basis of variation in the volatile composition of seven *C.creticus* subsp. *eriocephalus* populations depends more on the genetic background and less on geographical factor as demonstrated by the samples of groups 2 and 3 (Fig. **12**), which were qualitatively rather similar in chemical composition, also if the geographic places are far off [81].

PHENOLIC COMPOUNDS

Daglia (2012) [83] reports that "polyphenols are secondary metabolites ubiquitously distributed in all higher plants, which have important roles as defense against plant pathogens and animal herbivore aggression and as response to various abiotic stress conditions, such as rainfall and ultraviolet radiation. Over the course of the last years, polyphenols have been studied for their potential involvement in the prevention of chronic diseases, such as cardiovascular diseases, cancer, osteoporosis, diabetes mellitus, and neurodegenerative diseases" [82]. The phenolic fraction of *Cistaceae* is very important for its antioxidant and antibacterial characteristics as described in some publications [52, 83 - 85]. Several studies suggest that the principal components of *Cistus* species are phenolic compounds [86]. Particularly, Danne *et al.* (1994) report the presence of monomeric flavonoids belonging to the flavan-3-ols [87], whereas Santagati *et al.* (2008), note the presence of catechins family (catechin, gallocatechin, gallocatechin-3-gallate) together with oligomeric procyanidin B1 and B3. Several flavonoids, including quercetin, myricetin, kaempferol, apigenin and their derivatives, were isolated from leaves and resin of Cretan *C.creticus* subsp. *creticus* (*C.c.creticus*) [86]. The same compounds were also detected in aerial parts of Spanish *C.salvifolius* (*C.s.*) [32]. The antioxidant polyphenolic flavonoids catechin, gallocatechin and several of their derivatives, as well as other flavonols, flavanols, flavonoid glycosides and proanthocyanidin compounds have been identified in *C. albidus* (*C.a.*) leaves [32].

Studies on *Cistus* species leaves shown the presence of different flavonoid aglycones and glycosides belonging to the flavonols family, with proanthocyanidins and biogenetically related dihydroflavonols, as well as shikimic acid, epicatechin-(4→6)-catechin, dimeric prodelfinidins and further polyphenols [87, 88]. In several parts of *Cistus incanus* (*C.i.*) has been reported that the existence of monomeric and polymeric flavanols, gallic acid, rutin and diterpenes [89]. Polyphenols due to their potential beneficial health effects are of considerable interest. Loizzo *et al.* (2013), cited by Stępien *et al.* (2018), indicated that the leaves extract of *C.s.* (was characterized by a high inhibitory activity against the AChE enzyme. This activity is probably due to the high content of anthocyanins in the *C.s.* leaves extract that may have a significant effect on the inhibition of this enzyme [37, 56].

Mastino *et. al.* (2018, 2021), with the aim to characterize polyphenolic composition studied all the Sardinian *Cistus* species and subspecies [42, 86]. The polyphenolic compounds of *C.c.* subspecies growing wild in Sardinia were very similar among them. As shown in Fig. (**13**) *C.c.corsicus* and *C.creticus* subsp. *eriocephalus* (*C.c.e*) have many compounds in common, even though the relative percentages are different [42]. According to our data, we can affirm that some differences are evident between the chemical profile of polyphenols in the *C.c.creticus* and the other two subspecies; these data can be used to support the botanic classification in subspecies [42]. (Fig. **14**) reports a score plot deriving from a Principal Component Analysis (PCA) where it is clearly shown differences between the studied *Cistus* subspecies[140].

Mastino *et. al.* (2021), to complete their research also characterized the polyphenolic fraction of *C.s., C.m.* and *C.a.* that are the other three species growing wild in Sardinia [86]. In Fig. (**15**) are reported data on these analyses, it is possible to note that *C.s.* is the richest in polyphenolic compounds with respect to the other Sardinian *Cistus* species and subspecies, moreover an interesting point it is the presence of some bioactive compounds, such as oleuropein, olivil 9-O-E-D-xyloside and salvianolic acid G, which are not present in the other studied species and subspecies [86]. *C.a.* has the less quantities of phenolic compounds found also in the other studied species [86].

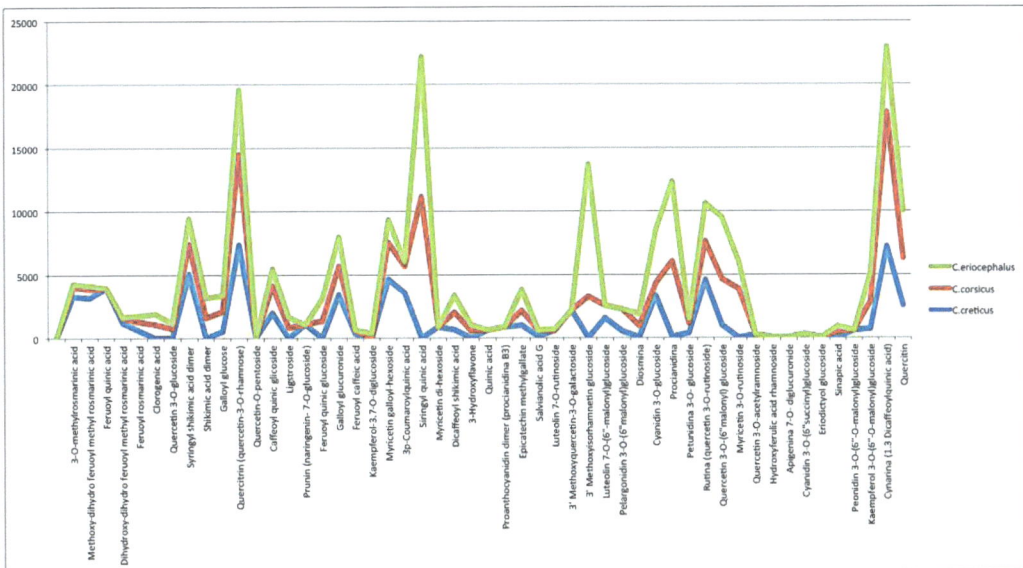

Fig. (13). *Cistus creticus* subspecies: polyphenols composition.

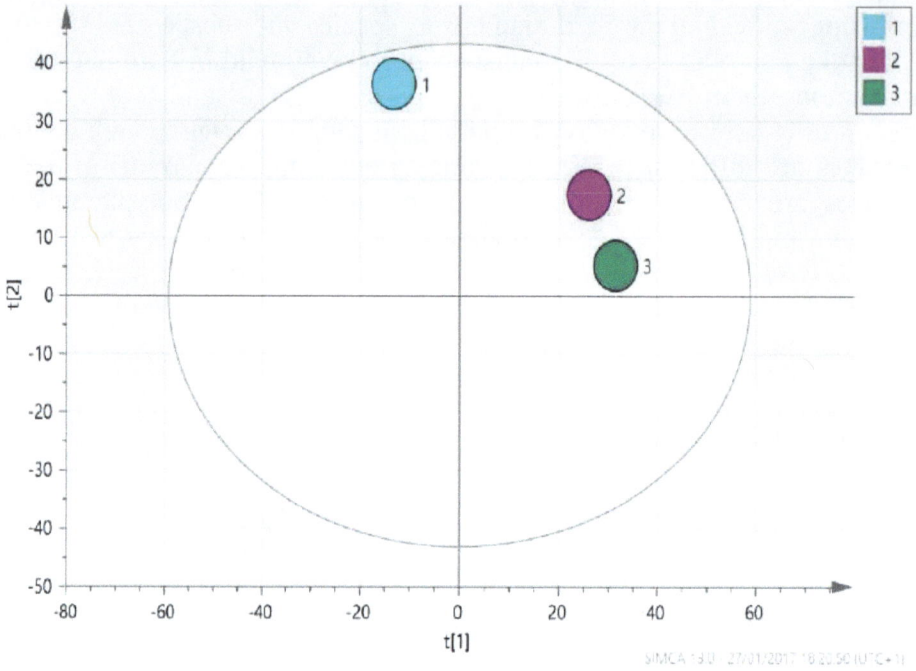

Fig. (14). Score plot from PCA statistical analyses of polyphenol compounds in the three different *Cistus creticus* subspecies [42].

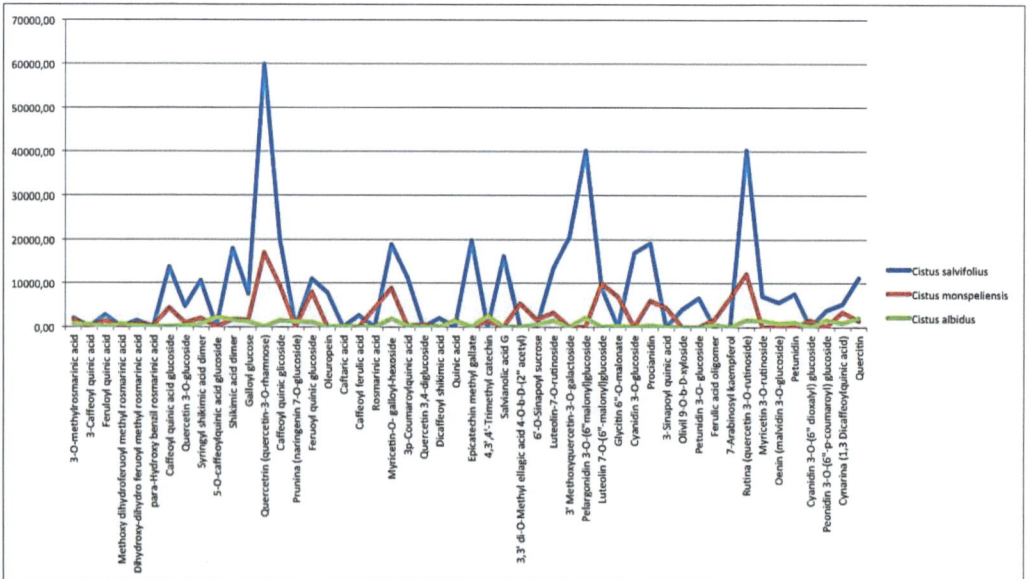

Fig. (15). *Cistus salvifolius, Cistus monspeliensis* and *Cistus albidus:* polyphenols composition.

All the studied species, even in their diversity, are characterized by a high content of phenolic acids and their glycosidic derivatives. Rosmarinic acid and its derivatives, and dicaffeoyl quinic acid are present in great quantity, as well as flavonols, including quercetin and derivatives are present in good quantities. *C.s.* is the richest in polyphenols with respect to the other Sardinian *Cistus* species and subspecies. Some components of the catechin family were detected in all species and subspecies of Sardinian *Cistus* but not in significant amount compared with previous studies on *Cistus* species collected in other Mediterranean areas [42, 86].

ANTIMICROBIAL ACTIVITY

Previous pharmacological investigations showed that *Cistus* leaf extracts possess significant antimicrobial properties against many bacteria and fungi responsible of human infections [38]. The study that have conducted by Mahmoudi *et al.* (2016), and Rebaya *et al.* (2016), carried out on different *Cistus* species, evidenced antibacterial and antifungal activities for *C.s.* and *C.m.* from Tunisia [84, 85]. Karim *et al.* (2017) and Talibi *et al.* (2012), have reported that the aqueous extracts of *C.m.* growing in Morocco, inhibited the fungal growth of *Geotrichum candidum* (*G.c.*) [49, 92] Other works report the effectiveness of ethanol extract of *C.s.* growing in Spain and found effects against *E. coli* and *S. aureus* (*E.c.; S.a.*) [93]. Bouamama *et al.* (2006) in their study determined that organic and aqueous leaf extracts of *C.m.*, and *C.v.* (*=incanus*), growing naturally in Morocco and Tunisia, inhibits the growth of *S.a.*, *Enterococcus hirae* (*E.h.*) *Pseudomonas aeruginosa* (*P.a.*), and the yeast *Candida glabrata* (*G.g.*) [38]. As reported by Sassi *et al.* (2007), "flower extracts of *C.m.* were active against gram-positive bacteria species of genus *Staphylococcus* and had significant growth-inhibitory effects on *S. epidermis* (*S.e.*) [94]. The available literature reports chemical studies on the composition of extracts of *Cistus* species, obtained by different solvents. Catechin related compounds were identified on the aqueous extracts of *C.m.* In *C. ladanifer (C.l.)*, the most abundant group was ellagic acid derivatives with punicalagin gallate being the most abundant phenolic compounds. These compounds (*i.e.*, ellagitannins) could be related to the strong inhibition of *C.a.*, *C.g.* and *C. parapsilosis* (*C.p.*) growth [84].

Extracts obtained from many plants have recently gained popularity and scientific interest for their antibacterial and antifungal activities [86]. The use of antimicrobials derived from plants is increasingly replacing the use of chemical products not only in the pharmaceutical field but also in food, cosmetic and hygiene industries. These naturally occurring compounds are considered a therapeutic alternative to the use of synthetic antibiotics, entailing a low risk of microbial resistance occurrence. Important advantages related to environmental impact are also offered using plant-derived compounds [43]. Many studies have been reported on the antimicrobial properties of plant extracts containing different classes of phenolic compounds [86]. Moreover, the antimicrobial activity of polyphenols occurring in vegetable foods and medicinal plants has been extensively investigated against a wide range of microorganisms. Among polyphenols, flavan-3-ols, flavonols, and tannins received most attention due to their wide spectrum and higher antimicrobial activity in comparison with other polyphenols, and to the fact that most of them are able to suppress a number of microbial virulence factors (such as inhibition of biofilm formation, reduction of host ligands adhesion, and neutralization of bacterial toxins) and show synergism with antibiotics [81]. The antimicrobial properties of certain classes of polyphenols, due to the increasing consumer pressure on the food industry to avoid synthetic preservatives, have been proposed either to develop new food preservatives [90] or to develop innovative therapies for the treatment of various microbial infections [19, 91] considering the increase in microbial resistance against conventional antibiotic therapy [86].

Phenolic compounds present in extracts from *C.l.* aerial tissues displayed antifungal activity against *Candida* species in a dose-dependent manner. Strong antimicrobial activity against gram-positive bacteria was also demonstrated for *C.l.*, and against gram-negative bacteria for *C. populifolius (C.p.)* [32].

We carried out a study to obtain preliminary information on antibacterial, antifungal and antioxidant activity of *Cistus* species growing wild in Sardinia to verify its potential in applications such as food preservation, cosmetics, hygiene or phytoterapeutic [42, 86]. The antimicrobial activity, using either EOs and polyphenolic extracts, was measured using two different bacterial strains, which are widely used as models for Gram-positive and Gram-negative bacteria such as *S.a.* and *E.c.*, and four different *Candida* species for the antifungal activity. All the used oils didn't show antibacterial or bacteriostatic activity (data not reported), while, using the polyphenolic extracts interesting data were obtained.

Regarding *C.c.* subsp., the obtained results revealed that all extracts showed similar antibacterial and antifungal activity with specific differences, according to the plant extract and the test microbial strain. The Minimum Inhibitory Concentration (M.I.C.) values ranged between 1.25 to 24.8 mg/mL. In more detail, butanol extracts showed the highest antimicrobial activity essentially against *S.a.* (M.I.C. 1.25 mg/mL). Also, ethyl acetate extracts showed the highest inhibition activity against *S.a.* (M.I.C. 1.25 mg/mL and 2.5 mg/mL for *C.c.corsicus* and *C.c.e.*). As far as *E.c.* is concerned, *C.c.corsicus* showed the lowest MIC (1.25 mg/mL), whereas *C.c.creticus* and *C.c.e.* showed the highest M.I.C. (5 mg/mL). In the case of *Candida* species, growth inhibition was only observed for the highest tested concentration (5 mg/mL), confirming the low susceptibility of these species to *Cistus* extracts. Finally, aqueous extracts of all *C.c.* subspecies showed the highest M.I.C. values against *E.c.* (M.I.C. 24.8 mg/mL) and *Candida* species (M.I.C. 24.8 mg/mL), proving to be less active in terms of the examined extracts; these results were also confirmed by the tests performed on *P.a.* (data not reported). Due to this low activity of aqueous extracts, their M.I.C. values against *S. aureus* were relatively high (6.2 mg/mL). As already explained in our previous work [86], the extracts obtained from *C.s.*, *C.m.*, and *C.a.* showed different antibacterial and antifungal activities depending on the evaluated plant species and microbial strain. For instance, the MIC values of the butanol extracts of *C.s.* and *C.m.* showed the highest antimicrobial activities against *S.a.* (MIC 1.25 mg/mL), while that of *C.a.* was less but still high (2.5 mg/mL). For the ethyl acetate extracts, the three plants showed the strongest activity against *S.a.* (MIC 1.25 mg/mL). *E.c.* was inhibited by the *C.a.* (MIC 1.25 mg/mL) and *C.s.* (MIC 2.5 mg/mL) ethyl acetate extracts, while the MIC was not significant for the *C.m.* extracts (>5 mg/mL). The butanol and ethyl acetate extracts were not effective against the *Candida* strains, with MICs ranging from 5 to 10 mg/mL. No interesting inhibitory effects were observed for the aqueous extracts against the investigated bacterial strains and fungal species. We only observed a low activity against *S.a.* using the water fraction (WF) of extracts of *C.m.* and *C.s.* (MIC 6.2 mg/mL). Among the procedures utilized, methanol acidified extraction followed by repartition in ethyl acetate led to the most effective extract, which showed inhibitory effects against *S.a.* and *E.c.* The results obtained, in agreement with the previous studies [95, 96], revealed that Gram-positive bacteria are more sensitive to the plant extracts than Gram-negative bacteria, which is due to the presence of hydrophobic lipopolysaccharides in the outer Gram-negative membrane (which provides protection against several agents).

Comparing the antimicrobial data of our *Cistus* extracts we found that aqueous extracts of *C.i.* and *C.m.* clearly differed in their antimicrobial activities. In particular, *C.v.* extracts exhibited stronger activity compared to *C.m.* when tested on *S.a.* (M.I.C. 0.8 mg/mL) and *C.g.* (M.I.C. 0.2 mg/mL) [42]. Moreover a study reported antimicrobial activity against *S.a.* and *E.c.* of *C.l.* (M.I.C. 0.154 mg/mL and 0.9 mg/mL, respectively) and *C. populifolius* (*C.p.*) (M.I.C. 0.344 mg/mL and 0.123 mg/mL, respectively) aqueous extracts [89]. A research on *C.s.* and *C.m.* revealed that the ethanol extracts tested showed the strongest activity against *S.a.* (M.I.C. 1.562 mg/mL) whereas the M.I.C. values against *E.c.* were found to be 12.5 mg/mL [85]. Finally, M.I.C. values are reported of *C.s.* and *C.m.* ranging from 3.1-25.0 mg/mL and 6.3- 12.5 mg/mL respectively [84].

Concerning plant extracts, their activity is significant if the M.I.C. values are below 100 µg/mL for crude extract and moderate when M.I.C values range between 100 and 625 µg/mL [31]. Therefore, the activity recorded in our experiments with butanol and ethyl acetate extracts can be considered moderate for all *Cistus* species. Aligiannis *et al.* (2001), proposed a classification for plant extracts effects against *Candida* species based on the M.I.C. values obtained: strong inhibitors (M.I.C. up to 0.5 mg/mL); moderate inhibitors (M.I.C. between 0.6 and 1.5 mg/mL); and weak inhibitors (M.I.C. above 1.6 mg/mL). According to that distribution, all our extracts failed to inhibit *Candida* species [97].

These antibacterial and antifungal activities of the *Cistus* extracts may be indicative of the presence of a broad spectrum of antibiotic compounds [98] and may be attributable to the presence of phenolic compounds as previously explained. Moreover, the preliminary microbial activity of Sardinian *Cistaceae* extracts observed in our study deserves further investigation to determine the compounds or combinations of compounds that are mainly responsible, as well as the potential mechanisms and their activities against other bacterial strains.

ANTIOXIDANT ACTIVITY

Potential sources of antioxidant compounds have been searched in several types of plant materials such as vegetables, fruits, leaves, oilseeds, cereal crops, barks and roots, spices and herbs, and crude plant drugs [99]. To understand the several positive and negative effects of antioxidants a definition of these compounds is necessary. Plant-derived antioxidants are molecules, which donate electrons or hydrogen atoms. These compounds can form less reactive antioxidant-derived radicals, which are efficiently quenched by other electron or hydrogen sources to prevent cellular damage. Furthermore, plant-derived antioxidants are hypothesized to be protective against oxidative stress events [63]. Phenols are antioxidants with redox properties, which allow them to act as reducing agents, hydrogen donators, and singlet oxygen quenchers [100]. They also have metal chelation properties [95]. Flavonoids and other plant phenols, such as phenolic acids, stilbenes, tannins, lignans, and lignin, are especially common in leaves, flowering tissues, and woody parts [99]. They are important in the plant for normal growth development and defense against infection and injury. *Cistus* species are a rich source of natural compounds with antioxidant properties, mainly flavonoids [32]. In one review Stępien [37] was confirmed that *C. laurifolius (C.Lau.)*is characterized by antioxidant properties. In the extract from leaves and small branches of *C.lau.* was determined the presence of 16 bioactive compounds by 1 H and 13C NMR techniques and EI-MS mass spectrometry. The following compounds from *C.lau.* have shown the ability to capture free radicals: 3---methyl quercetin, 3,7-O-dimethyl quercetin, ellagic acid, quercetin 3-O-α-rhamnoside, 1-(4-hydroxy-3-methoxyphenyl)-2-[4-(3-α-L-rhamnopyranoxy propyl)-2methoxyphenoxy]-1,3-propanediol, olivil 9-O-β-D-xyloside, berchemol

9-O-rhamnoside and (7S,8R)-dihydrodehydrodiconiferyl alcohol 9'-O--L-rhamnoside (major isomer) [101]. Extracts of *C.i.* and *C. parv.* shown high activity of scavenging free toxic radicals [102], as well as *Cl.*, and *C.pop.* which has higher antioxidant activity than *C.l.* because of its higher phenolic contents [89, 103].

C.i. and *C.m.* contain numerous compounds potentially antioxidant, among polyphenols [104]. This antioxidant activity is due to the presence of phenols, flavonoids and tannins of the obtained ethanol, hexane and water extracts from the leaves. The highest antioxidant activity was found for ethanol extracts from both *Cistus* species.

Research on *Cistus* EOs carried out by Loizzo *et al.* (2013), analyzed the acetylcholinesterase and butyrylcholinesterase (BChE) inhibitory activity of *C.c.*, *C.s.*, *C. libanotis*, *C.m.* and *C.v. C.s.* was characterized by the highest activity against AChE [56], while *C.lib.*, *C.c.*, *C.s.* had good inhibitory activity against BChE. *C.c.* is one with the most extensive accumulation of phenolic compounds in its leaves [105].

Recently, we compared the polyphenol composition and antioxidant properties of all *Cistus* growing wild in Sardinia [86]. To investigate the antioxidant activity of the extracts, we compared three complementary assays (DPPH, ABTS, and FRAP).

In our research [86], the results showed that "the extracts derived from *C.s.* showed the highest antioxidant activity. The EC_{50} values from the DPPH radical scavenging assay were 3.233 $\mu g_{d.w.}$/mL for the butanol fraction, 7.083 $\mu g_{d.w.}$/mL for the ethyl acetate fraction, and 14.866 $\mu g_{d.w.}$/mL for the water fraction. In contrast, the extracts derived from *C.a.* showed lower antioxidant activities, with DPPH assay EC_{50} values of 31.93 $\mu g_{d.w.}$/mL for the butanol fraction, $\mu g_{d.w.}$/mL for the ethyl acetate fraction, and 33.235 $\mu g_{d.w.}$/mL for the water fraction. In general, the DPPH EC_{50} values were in the range of 3–33 $\mu g_{d.w.}$/mL, and those for the ABTS assay were in the range of 13–108 $\mu g_{d.w.}$/mL. The ability to reduce Fe^{3+} as determined by the FRAP assay ranged from 0.312 to 1.654 $mmol_{Fe2+}/g_{d.w.}$.

To adequately measure the antioxidant potential, the ABTS and DPPH assays were considered the most appropriate as they were in good agreement with the concentrations of phenolic derivative. The results of the DPPH antioxidant activity experiments are shown in Fig. (**16**).

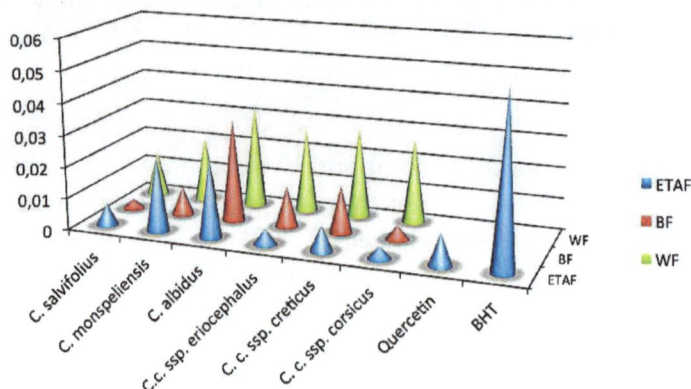

Fig. (16). DPPH test on extracts from Sardinian *Cistus* species (ETAF= Ethylacetate; BF = Butanol; WF = Water).

The results showed that all fractions are likely to exhibit excellent activity. In all cases, the *Cistus* fractions exhibited significant DPPH radical scavenging activities higher than that of BHT and sometimes higher than that of quercetin (0.054 and 0.01 mg/mL, respectively). The highest antioxidant activity, three times higher than that of quercetin and eighteen times that of BHT, was observed in the *C.s.* fractions. As shown in Figs. (**17 - 19**), the different distributions of polyphenols strongly influence the antioxidant capability of the extracts. The water partitions were not very efficient due to their minor contents of flavonoids and cyanidins, with only *C.s.* showing good antioxidant efficiency in the water. The ethyl acetate and butanol fractions, on the other hand, were highly effective.

The potential of compounds contained in the different fractions of *Cistus* extracts suggests a possibility to use they, in the food industry to make more appealing food and to increase shelf life by inhibiting oxidation. We think that the best extracts are that coming from C.s. fractions.

STATISTICAL ELABORATION OF DATA

Using multivariate statistical techniques and principal component analysis (PCA), we elaborated [86] on the data for all *Cistus* species vegetating in Sardinia. We collected analytical data related to metabolomics in the last several years [42, 81, 86] and combined them with the polyphenol data to find relationships between the different species of *Cistus* growing in Sardinia and their biological activities.

Fig. (17). EC$_{50}$ in DPPH test and HPLC profile of butanolic partitions (BF) of *Cistus* species vegetating in Sardinia (1 = *Cistus creticus creticus*; 2 = *Cistus creticus corsicus*; 3 = *Cistus creticus eriocephalus*; 4 = *Cistus salvifolius*; 5 = *Cistus monspeliensis*; 6 = *Cistus albidus*).

Fig. (18). EC$_{50}$ in DPPH test and HPLC profile of Ethyl acetate partitions (ETAF) of *Cistus* specie vegetating in Sardinia (1 = *Cistus creticus creticus*; 2 = *Cistus creticus corsicus*; 3 = *Cistus creticus eriocephalus*; 4 = *Cistus salvifolius*; 5 = *Cistus monspeliensis*; 6 = *Cistus albidus*).

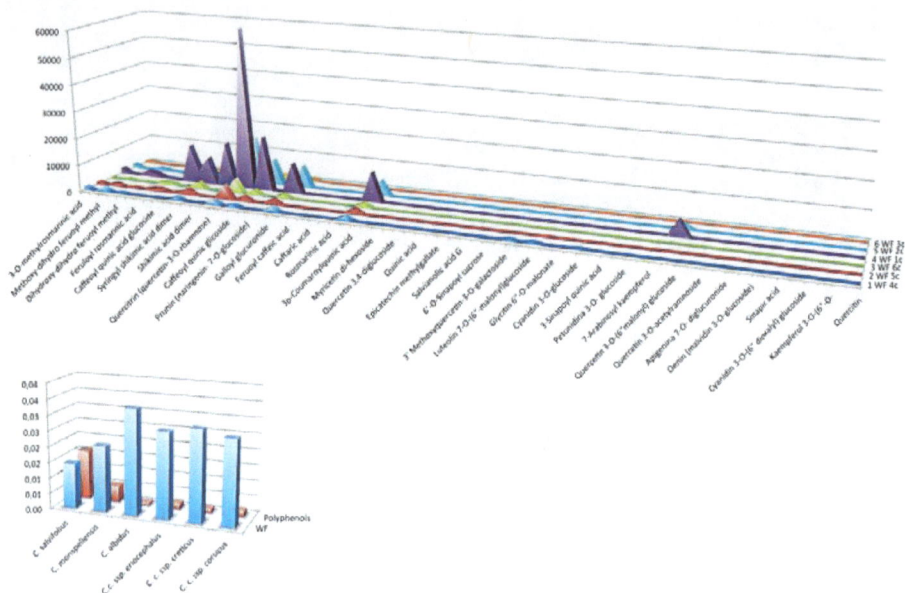

Fig. (19). EC_{50} in DPPH test and HPLC profile of Water partitions (WF) of *Cistus* species vegetating in Sardinia (1 = *Cistus creticus creticus*; 2 = *Cistus creticus corsicus*; 3 = *Cistus creticus eriocephalus*; 4 = *Cistus salvifolius*; 5 = *Cistus monspeliensis*; 6 = *Cistus albidus*).

The score plot (Fig. **20**) shows the correlation between the secondary metabolites in the investigated plants and their antioxidant properties. Considering the harmonic mean of the EC_{50} values corresponding to the antioxidant capacity of all fractions of the *Cistus* species growing in Sardinia, the PCA assembles the species into two distinct groups: one with EC_{50} below 0.006 mg/mL and one with EC_{50} higher than 0.02 mg/mL, except for *C.c.* (EC_{50} 0.008 mg/mL). On this basis, a model can be established to act as a guide to choose between the different species for use as antioxidants. Furthermore, in the score plot, the three subspecies of *C.c.* are positioned in the right quadrant, while the other species are in the left quadrant. Notably, *C.s.* remains close to the subspecies of *C.c.*, particularly *C.c.e.* Therefore, the statistical results derived from the secondary metabolite contents support the results reported by Vogt *et al.* (1987), who suggested a possible hybrid origin of *C.c.e.* with *C.s* [107].

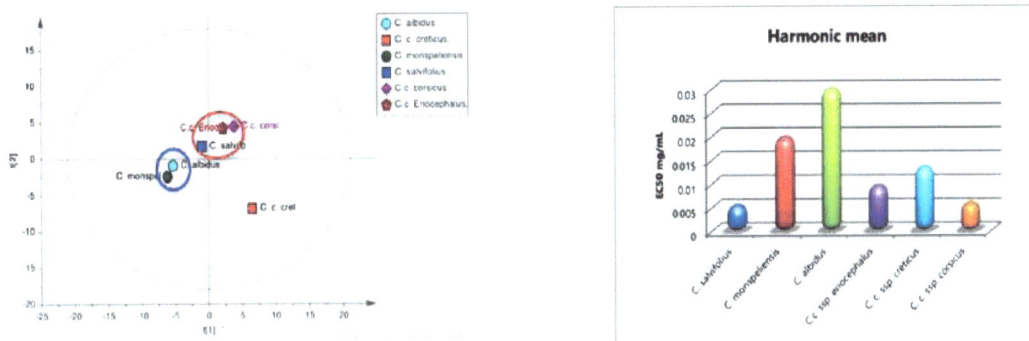

Fig. (20). PCA score plot of *Cistus* species secondary metabolites and graphic variation of the harmonic mean of DPPH antioxidant capabilities.

CONCLUDING REMARKS

Species of the genus *Cistus* exhibit several medicinal properties due to the presence of compounds with biological activity. These compounds represent a rich source of biocides and preservatives, and many studies have pointed out the antimicrobial efficacy of phenolic compounds, which are generally involved in oxidative stress prevention. The antimicrobial properties of polyphenols have been proposed to develop new food preservatives that can be utilized in innovative therapies for the treatment of various microbial infections. Several studies carried out on different *Cistus* species have shown effectiveness in health care, exhibiting gastroprotective effects, anti-inflammatory activity, protective effect on DNA cleavage, dose-dependent free-radical scavenging capacity, and cytotoxic activity against several leukemic cell lines *in vitro*.

This draws attention to the possibility of using extracts and biologically active compounds isolated from *Cistus* in the treatment of several diseases, like senescence, Alzheimer's disease, cardiosclerosis, stenocardia, and cancer. In Sardinia, *Cistus* is traditionally used as a natural remedy in folk medicine. The results of our research on the Sardinian *Cistus* species indicated that these plants possess antioxidant, antibacterial, and antifungal properties.

CONSENT FOR PUBLICATION

Not Applicable

CONFLICT OF INTEREST

The author declares no conflict of interest, financial or otherwise.

ACKNOWLEDGEMENTS

Declared none.

DISCLOSURE

Part of this article has previously been published in:

"Mastino, P.M.; Marchetti, M.; Costa, J.; Juliano, C.; Usai, M. Analytical Profiling of Phenolic Compounds in Extracts of Three Cistus Species from Sardinia and Their Potential Antimicrobial and Antioxidant Activity, Chemistry & Biodiversity, Vol. 18, No. 6, 2021, e2100053".

REFERENCES

[1] Maffei, M. *Molecole bioattive delle piante. Libro pubblicato dall'autore*; , **2015**.

[2] Lee, S.H.; Su, M.S.; Huang, Y.S.; Yang, H.D. Effect of Chinese medicinal plants extract on five different fungi. *Food Control,* **2007**, *18*(12), 1547-1554.
[http://dx.doi.org/10.1016/j.foodcont.2006.12.005]

[3] Verástegui, A.; Verde, J.; García, S.; Heredia, N.; Oranday, A.; Rivas, C. Species of agave with antimicrobial activity against selected pathogenic bacteria and fungi. *World J. Microbiol. Biotechnol.,* **2008**, *24*(7), 1249-1252.
[http://dx.doi.org/10.1007/s11274-007-9563-8]

[4] Santas, J.; Almaiano, M.P.; Carbo, R. Antimicrobial and antioxidant activity of crude onion (*Allium cepa*) extracts. *Int. J. Food Sci. Technol.,* **2010**, *45*(2), 403-409.
[http://dx.doi.org/10.1111/j.1365-2621.2009.02169.x]

[5] Al-Zoreky, N.S. Antimicrobial activity of pomegranate (*Punica granatum L.*) fruit peels. *Int. J. Food Microbiol.,* **2009**, *134*(3), 244-248.
[http://dx.doi.org/10.1016/j.ijfoodmicro.2009.07.002] [PMID: 19632734]

[6] R.; Marín-Martínez, R.; Veoz-Rodríguez, R.; Rodríguez-Guerra, R.; Torres-Pacheco, I.; Gonzáles-Chavira, M.M.; Anaya-López, J.L.; Guevara-Olvera, L.; Feregrino-Pérez, A.A.; Loarca-Piña, G.; Guevara-Gonzáles, R.G. Antimicrobial activities of cascalote (*Caesalpina cacalaco*) phenolics-containing extracts against fungus *Colleotrichum lindemunthianum. Ind. Crops Prod.,* **2010**, *31*, 134-138.

[7] Zhu, X.; Zhang, H.; Lo, R. Phenolic compounds from the leaf extract of artichoke (Cynara scolymus L.) and their antimicrobial activities. *J. Agric. Food Chem.,* **2004**, *52*(24), 7272-7278.
[http://dx.doi.org/10.1021/jf0490192] [PMID: 15563206]

[8] Karukluogu, M.; Sahan, Y.; Yigit, A. Antifungal properties of olive leaf extracts and their phenolic compounds. *J. Food Saf.,* **2008**, *28*(1), 76-87.
[http://dx.doi.org/10.1111/j.1745-4565.2007.00096.x]

[9] Ojala, T.; Remes, S.; Haansuu, P.; Vuorela, H.; Hiltunen, R.; Haahtela, K.; Vuorela, P. Antimicrobial activity of some coumarin containing herbal plants growing in Finland. *J. Ethnopharmacol.,* **2000**, *73*(1-2), 299-305.
[http://dx.doi.org/10.1016/S0378-8741(00)00279-8] [PMID: 11025169]

[10] Ortuño, A.; Báidez, A.; Gómez, P.; Arcas, M.C.; Porras, I.; García-Lidón, A.; del Río, J.A. *Citrus paradisi* and *Citrus sinensis* flavonoids: their influence in the defense mechanism against *Penicillum digitatum. Food Chem.,* **2006**, *98*(2), 351-358.
[http://dx.doi.org/10.1016/j.foodchem.2005.06.017]

[11]   Sanzani, S.M.; De Girolamo, A.; Schena, L.; Solfrizzo, M.; Ippolito, A.; Visconti, A. Control of *Penicillium expansum* and patulin accumulation on apples by quercetin and umbelliferone. *Eur. Food Res. Technol.,* **2009**, *228*(3), 381-189.
       [http://dx.doi.org/10.1007/s00217-008-0944-5]

[12]   Terry, L.A.; Joyce, D.C.; Adikaram, N.K.B.; Khabay, B.P.S. Preformed antifungal compounds in strawberry fruit and flower tissues. *Postharvest Biol. Technol.,* **2004**, *31*(2), 201-2012.
       [http://dx.doi.org/10.1016/j.postharvbio.2003.08.003]

[13]   Engels, C.; Knödler, M.; Zhao, Y.Y.; Carle, R.; Gänzle, M.G.; Schieber, A. Antimicrobial activity of gallotannins isolated from mango (Mangifera indica L.) kernels. *J. Agric. Food Chem.,* **2009**, *57*(17), 7712-7718.
       [http://dx.doi.org/10.1021/jf901621m] [PMID: 19655802]

[14]   Parashar, A.; Gupta, C.; Gupta, S.K.; Kumar, A. Antimicrobial ellagitannin from pomegranate (*Punica granatum*) fruits. *Int. J. Fruit Sci.,* **2009**, *9*(3), 226-231.
       [http://dx.doi.org/10.1080/15538360903241286]

[15]   Amborabé, B.E.; Fleurat-Lessard, P.; Chollet, J.F.; Roblin, G. Antifungal effects of salicylic acid and other benzoic acid derivatives towards *Eutypa lata*: structure- activity relationship. *Plant Physiol. Biochem.,* **2002**, *40*(12), 1051-1060.
       [http://dx.doi.org/10.1016/S0981-9428(02)01470-5]

[16]   Bisogno, F.; Mascoti, L.; Sanchez, C.; Garibotto, F.; Giannini, F.; Kurina-Sanz, M.; Enriz, R. Structure-antifungal activity relationship of cinnamic acid derivatives. *J. Agric. Food Chem.,* **2007**, *55*(26), 10635-10640.
       [http://dx.doi.org/10.1021/jf0729098] [PMID: 18038998]

[17]   Rodríguez Vaquero, M.J.; Aredes Fernández, P.A.; Manca de Nadra, M.C.; Strasser de Saad, A.M. Phenolic compound combinations on Escherichia coli viability in a meat system. *J. Agric. Food Chem.,* **2010**, *58*(10), 6048-6052.
       [http://dx.doi.org/10.1021/jf903966p] [PMID: 20438131]

[18]   Jayaraman, P.; Sakharkar, M.K.; Lim, C.S.; Tang, T.H.; Sakharkar, K.R. Activity and interactions of antibiotic and phytochemical combinations against Pseudomonas aeruginosa *in vitro. Int. J. Biol. Sci.,* **2010**, *6*(6), 556-568.
       [http://dx.doi.org/10.7150/ijbs.6.556] [PMID: 20941374]

[19]   Saavedra, M.J.; Borges, A.; Dias, C.; Aires, A.; Bennett, R.N.; Rosa, E.S.; Simões, M. Antimicrobial activity of phenolics and glucosinolate hydrolysis products and their synergy with streptomycin against pathogenic bacteria. *Med. Chem.,* **2010**, *6*(3), 174-183.
       [http://dx.doi.org/10.2174/1573406411006030174] [PMID: 20632977]

[20]   Arrigoni, P.V. *Flora dell'Isola di Sardegna*; Carlo Delfino Editore: Sassari, **2010**.

[21]   Camarda, I.; Satta, V. Piante officinali di interesse economico nella comunità della Baronie. *Gal Barbagia-Baronie, Dip. Di Botanica ed Ecol. Veg., Università di Sassari,* **1996**.

[22]   Atzei, A.D. *Le piante nella tradizione popolare della Sardegna*; Carlo Delfino Editore, **2003**.

[23]   Atzei, A.D.; Camarda, I.; Piras, G.; Satta, V. Usi tradizionali e prospettive future delle specie della macchia mediterranea in Sardegna. *Italus Hortus,* **2004**, *11*(4) [luglio-agosto.].

[24]   Angioni, G. *I pascoli erranti: antropologia del pastore in Sardegna*; Liguori Editore: Napoli, **1989**.

[25]   Camarda, I. Ricerche etnobotaniche nel Comune di Dorgali. *Boll. Soc. Sarda Sci. Nat.,* **1990**, *27*, 147-204.

[26]   Arrington, J.M.; Kubitzki, K. Cistaceae.*The families and genera of vascular plants. V. Flowering plants. Dicotyledons. Malvales, Capparales and Non-betalain Caryophyllales*; Kubitzki, K.; Bayer, C., Eds.; Springer: Berlin, Heidelberg, New York, **2003**, pp. 62-70.

[27]   Gonzalez-Rabanal, F.; Casal, M. Effect of high temperature and ash on germination of ten species

from gorse shrubland. *Vegetatio,* **1995**, *116*, 123-131.
[http://dx.doi.org/10.1007/BF00045303]

[28] Perez-Garcia, F.; Iriondo, J.M.; Gonzalez-Benito, M.E.; Carnes, L.F.; Tapia, J.; Prieto, C.; Plaza, R.; Perez, C. Germination studies in endemic plant species of the Iberian Peninsula. *Isr. J. Plant Sci.,* **1995**, *43*(3), 239-247.
[http://dx.doi.org/10.1080/07929978.1995.10676608]

[29] Henaoui, S. El-A.; Bouazza, M.; Amara, M. The fire risk of the plant groupings with *Cistus* in the area of Tlemcen (Western Algeria). *Eur. Sci. J.,* **2013**, *9*, 84-103.

[30] Grosser, W.H.C. Cistaceae.*Das Pflanzenreich 14 (IV.193)*; Engler, A., Ed.; W.Engelmann: Leipzig, **1903**, pp. 61-63.

[31] Puglielli, G.; Cuevas Román, F.J.; Catoni, R.; Moreno Rojas, J.M.; Gratani, L.; Varone, L. Provenance effect on carbon assimilation, photochemistry and leaf morphology in Mediterranean *Cistus* species under chilling stress. *Plant Biol.,* **2017**, *19*(4), 660-670.
[http://dx.doi.org/10.1111/plb.12574] [PMID: 28419758]

[32] Papaefthimiou, D.; Papanikolaou, A.; Falara, V.; Givanoudi, S.; Kostas, S.; Kanellis, A.K. Genus Cistus: a model for exploring labdane-type diterpenes' biosynthesis and a natural source of high value products with biological, aromatic, and pharmacological properties. *Front Chem.,* **2014**, *2*, 35.
[http://dx.doi.org/10.3389/fchem.2014.00035] [PMID: 24967222]

[33] Guzmán, B.; Vargas, P. Systematics, character evolution, and biogeography of Cistus L. (Cistaceae) based on ITS, trnL-trnF, and matK sequences. *Mol. Phylogenet. Evol.,* **2005**, *37*(3), 644-660.
[http://dx.doi.org/10.1016/j.ympev.2005.04.026] [PMID: 16055353]

[34] Lo Bianco, M.; Grillo, O.; Cañadas, E.; Venora, G.; Bacchetta, G. Inter- and intraspecific diversity in *Cistus* (*Cistaceae*) seeds, analyzed with computer vision techniques. *Plant Biol.,* **2017**, 19. [and references therein].

[35] Demoly, J.P.; Montserrat, P. *"Cistus," in LXVI. CISTACEAE Flora Iberica*; Castroviejo, S.; Aedo, C.; Cirujano, S.; Laínz, M.; Montserrat, P.; Morales, R.; Muñoz-Garmendia, F.; Navarro, C.; Paiva, J.; Soriano, C., Eds.; Consejo Superior de Investigaciones Científicas: Madrid, **1993**, pp. 319-337.

[36] Camarda, I.; Valsecchi, F. *Alberi e arbusti spontanei della Sardegna*; Carlo Delfino Editore: Sassari, **2008**.

[37] Stępien, A.; Aebisher, D.; Bartusik-Aebisher, D. Biological Properties of *Cistus* species. *European Journal Clinical and Experimental Medicine,* **2018**, *16*(2), 127-132.
[http://dx.doi.org/10.15584/ejcem.2018.2.8]

[38] Bouamama, H.; Noël, T.; Villard, J.; Benharref, A.; Jana, M. Antimicrobial activities of the leaf extracts of two Moroccan Cistus L. species. *J. Ethnopharmacol.,* **2006**, *104*(1-2), 104-107.
[http://dx.doi.org/10.1016/j.jep.2005.08.062] [PMID: 16213684]

[39] Mastino, P.M.; Marchetti, M.; Costa, J.; Usai, M. Comparison of essential oils from *Cistus* species growing in Sardinia. *Nat. Prod. Res.,* **2017**, *31*(3), 299-307.
[http://dx.doi.org/10.1080/14786419.2016.1236095] [PMID: 27681295]

[40] de Whalley, C.V.; Rankin, S.M.; Hoult, J.R.; Jessup, W.; Leake, D.S. Flavonoids inhibit the oxidative modification of low density lipoproteins by macrophages. *Biochem. Pharmacol.,* **1990**, *39*(11), 1743-1750.
[http://dx.doi.org/10.1016/0006-2952(90)90120-A] [PMID: 2344371]

[41] Hertog, M.G.; Kromhout, D.; Aravanis, C.; Blackburn, H.; Buzina, R.; Fidanza, F.; Giampaoli, S.; Jansen, A.; Menotti, A.; Nedeljkovic, S. Flavonoid intake and long-term risk of coronary heart disease and cancer in the seven countries study. *Arch. Intern. Med.,* **1995**, *155*(4), 381-386.
[http://dx.doi.org/10.1001/archinte.1995.00430040053006] [PMID: 7848021]

[42] Mastino, P.M.; Marchetti, M.; Costa, J.; Juliano, C.; Usai, M. Analysis and potential antimicrobial activity of phenolic compounds in extracts of *Cistus creticus* subspecies from Sardinia. *Nat. Prod. J.,*

2018, *8*(3), 1-9. [and references therein].
[http://dx.doi.org/10.2174/2210315508666180327151318]

[43]   Sayah, K.; Marmouzi, I.; El Jemli, M.; Cherrah, Y.; El Abbes Faouzi, M. In vivo anti-inflammatory and analgesic activities of *Cistus salvifolius (L.)* and *Cistus monspeliensis (L.)* aqueous extracts. *S. Afr. J. Bot.,* **2017**, *113*, 160-163.
[http://dx.doi.org/10.1016/j.sajb.2017.08.015]

[44]   Sayah, K.; Marmouzi, I.; Naceiri Mrabti, H.; Cherrah, Y.; Faouzi, M.E. Antioxidant Activity and Inhibitory Potential of *Cistus salviifolius* (L.) and *Cistus monspeliensis* (L.) Aerial Parts Extracts against Key Enzymes Linked to Hyperglycemia. *BioMed Res. Int.,* **2017**, *2017*, 2789482.
[http://dx.doi.org/10.1155/2017/2789482] [PMID: 28116307]

[45]   Guy, M.; John, H.A. Apoptosis and cancer chemotherapy. *Cell Tissue Res.,* **2000**, *65*, 290-295.

[46]   Ghobrial, I.M.; Witzig, T.E.; Adjei, A.A. Targeting apoptosis pathways in cancer therapy. *CA Cancer J. Clin.,* **2005**, *55*(3), 178-194.
[http://dx.doi.org/10.3322/canjclin.55.3.178] [PMID: 15890640]

[47]   Dimas, K.; Demetzos, C.; Angelopoulou, D.; Kolokouris, A.; Mavromoustakos, T. Biological activity of myricetin and its derivatives against human leukemic cell lines *in vitro. Pharmacol. Res.,* **2000**, *42*(5), 475-478.
[http://dx.doi.org/10.1006/phrs.2000.0716] [PMID: 11023711]

[48]   Dimas, K.; Papadaki, M.; Tsimplouli, C.; Hatziantoniou, S.; Alevizopoulos, K.; Pantazis, P.; Demetzos, C. Labd-14-ene-8,13-diol (sclareol) induces cell cycle arrest and apoptosis in human breast cancer cells and enhances the activity of anticancer drugs. *Biomed. Pharmacother.,* **2006**, *60*(3), 127-133.
[http://dx.doi.org/10.1016/j.biopha.2006.01.003] [PMID: 16527443]

[49]   Karim, H.; Boubaker, H.; Askarne, L.; Cherifi, K.; Lakhtar, H.; Msanda, F.; Boudyach, E.H.; Ait Ben Aoumar, A. Use of Cistus aqueous extracts as botanical fungicides in the control of Citrus sour rot. *Microb. Pathog.,* **2017**, *104*, 263-267.
[http://dx.doi.org/10.1016/j.micpath.2017.01.041] [PMID: 28131951]

[50]   Barbafieri, M.; Dadea, C.; Tassi, E.; Bretzel, F.; Fanfani, L. Uptake of heavy metals by native species growing in a mining area in Sardinia, Italy: discovering native flora for phytoremediation. *Int. J. Phytoremediation,* **2011**, *13*(10), 985-997.
[http://dx.doi.org/10.1080/15226514.2010.549858] [PMID: 21972566]

[51]   Jiménez, M.N.; Bacchetta, G.; Casti, M.; Navarro, F.B.; Lallena, A.M.; Fernández-Ondono, E. Potential use in phytoremediation of three plant species growing on contaminated mine-tailing soils in Sardinia. *Ecol. Eng.,* **2011**, *37*(2), 392-398.
[http://dx.doi.org/10.1016/j.ecoleng.2010.11.030]

[52]   Pratas, J.; Favas, P.J.C.; D'Souza, R.; Varun, M.; Paul, M.S. Phytoremedial assessment of flora tolerant to heavy metals in the contaminated soils of an abandoned Pb mine in Central Portugal. *Chemosphere,* **2013**, *90*(8), 2216-2225.
[http://dx.doi.org/10.1016/j.chemosphere.2012.09.079] [PMID: 23098582]

[53]   El Mamoun, I.; Mouna, F.; Mohammed, A.; Najib, B.; Zine-El Abidine, T.; Abdelkarim, G.; Didier, B.; Laurent, L.; Smouni Abdelaziz, S. Zinc, lead, and cadmium tolerance and accumulation in *Cistus libanotis, Cistus albidus*, and *Cistus salviifolius*: Perspectives on phytoremediation. *Rem. J.,* **2020**, *30*(2), 73-80.
[http://dx.doi.org/10.1002/rem.21638]

[54]   Paolini, J.; Tomi, P.; Bernardini, A.F.; Bradesi, P.; Casanova, J.; Kaloustian, J. Detailed analysis of the essential oil from *Cistus albidus* L. by combination of GC/RI, GC/MS and 13C-NMR spectroscopy. *Nat. Prod. Res.,* **2008**, *22*(14), 1270-1278.
[http://dx.doi.org/10.1080/14786410701766083] [PMID: 18932091]

[55]   Barrajón-Catalán, E.; Fernández-Arroyo, S.; Roldán, C.; Guillén, E.; Saura, D.; Segura-Carretero, A.;

Micol, V. A systematic study of the polyphenolic composition of aqueous extracts deriving from several *Cistus* genus species: evolutionary relationship. *Phytochem. Anal.,* **2011**, *22*(4), 303-312.
[http://dx.doi.org/10.1002/pca.1281] [PMID: 21259376]

[56]   Loizzo, M.R.; Ben Jemia, M.; Senatore, F.; Bruno, M.; Menichini, F.; Tundis, R. Chemistry and functional properties in prevention of neurodegenerative disorders of five Cistus species essential oils. *Food Chem. Toxicol.,* **2013**, *59*, 586-594.
[http://dx.doi.org/10.1016/j.fct.2013.06.040] [PMID: 23831310]

[57]   Demetzos, C.; Angelopoulou, D.; Perdetzoglou, D. A comparative study of the essential oil of *Cistus salviifolius* in several populations of Crete (Greece). *Biochem. Syst. Ecol.,* **2002**, *30*(7), 651-665.
[http://dx.doi.org/10.1016/S0305-1978(01)00145-4]

[58]   Abu-Orabi, S.T.; Al-Qudah, M.A.; Saleh, N.R.; Bataineh, T.T.; Obeidat, S.M.; Al-Sheraideh, M.S.; Al-Jaber, H.I.; Tashtoush, H.I.; Lahham, J.N. Antioxidant activity of crude extracts and essential oils from flower buds and leaves of *Cistus creticus* and *Cistus salviifolius*. *Arab. J. Chem.,* **2020**, *13*(7), 6256-6266.
[http://dx.doi.org/10.1016/j.arabjc.2020.05.043]

[59]   Pistelli, L.; Bandeira Reidel, R.V.; Parri, F.; Morelli, E.; Pistelli, L. Chemical composition of essential oil from plants of abandoned mining site of Elba island. *Nat. Prod. Res.,* **2019**, *33*(1), 143-147.
[http://dx.doi.org/10.1080/14786419.2018.1437430] [PMID: 29417841]

[60]   Ben Jemia, M.; Kchouk, M.E.; Senatore, F.; Autore, G.; Marzocco, S.; De Feo, V.; Bruno, M. Antiproliferative activity of hexane extract from Tunisian Cistus libanotis, Cistus monspeliensis and Cistus villosus. *Chem. Cent. J.,* **2013**, *7*(1), 47.
[http://dx.doi.org/10.1186/1752-153X-7-47] [PMID: 23497569]

[61]   Robles, C.; Garzino, S. Infraspecific variability in the essential oil composition of *Cistus monspeliensis* leaves. *Phytochemistry,* **2000**, *53*(1), 71-75.
[http://dx.doi.org/10.1016/S0031-9422(99)00460-4] [PMID: 10656410]

[62]   Angelopoulou, D.; Demetzos, C.; Dimas, C.; Perdetzoglou, D.; Loukis, A. Essential oils and hexane extracts from leaves and fruits of *Cistus monspeliensis*. Cytotoxic activity of ent-13-epi-manoyl oxide and its isomers. *Planta Med.,* **2001**, *67*(2), 168-171.
[http://dx.doi.org/10.1055/s-2001-11497] [PMID: 11301869]

[63]   Riehle, P.; Vollmer, M.; Rohn, S. Phenolic compounds in *Cistus incanus* herbal infusions — Antioxidant capacity and thermal stability during the brewing process. *Food Res. Int.,* **2013**, *53*(2), 891-899.
[http://dx.doi.org/10.1016/j.foodres.2012.09.020]

[64]   Angelopoulou, D.; Demetzos, C.; Perdetzoglou, D. Diurnal and seasonal variation of the essential oil labdanes and clerodanes fron *Cistus monspeliensis* L. leaves. *Biochem. Syst. Ecol.,* **2002**, *30*(3), 189-203.
[http://dx.doi.org/10.1016/S0305-1978(01)00074-6]

[65]   Rivoal, A.; Fernandez, C.; Lavoir, A.V.; Olivier, R.; Lecareux, C.; Greff, S.; Roche, P.; Vila, B. Environmental control of terpene emissions from *Cistus monspeliensis* L. in natural Mediterranean shrublands. *Chemosphere,* **2010**, *78*(8), 942-949.
[http://dx.doi.org/10.1016/j.chemosphere.2009.12.047] [PMID: 20092868]

[66]   Berti, G.; Livi, O.; Segnini, D. Cistodiol and cistodioic acid, diterpenoids with a cis-fused clerodane skeleton. *Tetrahedron Lett.,* **1970**, *11*(17), 1401-1404.
[http://dx.doi.org/10.1016/S0040-4039(01)97980-8]

[67]   Kalpoutzakis, E.; Aligiannis, N.; Skaltsounis, A.L.; Mitakou, S. cis-Clerodane type diterpenes from *Cistus monspeliensis. J. Nat. Prod.,* **2003**, *66*(2), 316-319.
[http://dx.doi.org/10.1021/np0204388] [PMID: 12608877]

[68]   Yeşilada, E.; Gürbüz, I.; Ergun, E. Effects of Cistus laurifolius L. flowers on gastric and duodenal lesions. *J. Ethnopharmacol.,* **1997**, *55*(3), 201-211.

[http://dx.doi.org/10.1016/S0378-8741(96)01502-4] [PMID: 9080341]

[69]   Bechlaghem, K.; Allali, H.; Benmehdi, H.; Aissaoui, N.; Flamini, G. Chemical Analysis of the Essential Oils of Three *Cistus* Species Growing in North-West of Algeria. *ACS Agric. Conspec. Sci.,* **2019**, *84*, 283-293.

[70]   Politeo, O.; Maravic, A.; Burčul, F.; Carev, I.; Kamenjarin, J. Phytochemical Composition and Antimicrobial Activity of Essential Oils of Wild Growing *Cistus* species in Croatia. *Nat. Prod. Commun.,* **2018**, *13*(6), 771-774.
       [http://dx.doi.org/10.1177/1934578X1801300631]

[71]   Maccioni, S.; Baldini, R.; Cioni, P.L.; Tebano, M.; Flamini, G. In vivo volatiles emission and essential oils from different organs and pollen of *Cistus albidus* from Caprione (Eastern Liguria, Italy). *Flavour Fragrance J.,* **2007**, *22*(1), 61-65.
       [http://dx.doi.org/10.1002/ffj.1759]

[72]   Llusià, J.; Peñuelas, J.; Ogaya, R.; Alessio, G. Annual and seasonal changes in foliar terpene content and emission rates in *Cistus albidus* L. submitted to soil drought in Prades forest (Catalonia, NE Spain). *Acta Physiol. Plant.,* **2010**, *32*(2), 387-394.
       [http://dx.doi.org/10.1007/s11738-009-0416-y]

[73]   Ormeño, E.; Fernandez, C.; Mévy, J.P. Plant coexistence alters terpene emission and content of Mediterranean species. *Phytochemistry,* **2007**, *68*(6), 840-852.
       [http://dx.doi.org/10.1016/j.phytochem.2006.11.033] [PMID: 17258247]

[74]   Palá-Paúl, J.; Velasco-Negueruela, A.; Pérez-Alonso, M.J.; Sanz, J. Seasonal variation in chemical composition of *Cistus albidus* L. from Spain. *J. Essent. Oil Res.,* **2005**, *17*(1), 19-22.
       [http://dx.doi.org/10.1080/10412905.2005.9698818]

[75]   Robles, C.; Garzino, S. Essential oil composition of *Cistus albidus* leaves. *Phytochemistry,* **1998**, *48*(8), 1341-1345.
       [http://dx.doi.org/10.1016/S0031-9422(97)01124-2]

[76]   Demetzos, C.; Katerinopoulos, H.; Kouvarakis, A.; Stratigakis, N.; Loukis, A.; Ekonomakis, C.; Spiliotis, V.; Tsaknis, J. Composition and antimicrobial activity of the essential oil of *Cistus creticus* subsp. *eriocephalus. Planta Med.,* **1997**, *63*(5), 477-479.
       [http://dx.doi.org/10.1055/s-2006-957742] [PMID: 9342956]

[77]   Demetzos, C.; Stahl, B.; Anastassaki, T.; Gazouli, M.; Tzouvelekis, L.S.; Rallis, M. Chemical analysis and antimicrobial activity of the resin Ladano, of its essential oil and of the isolated compounds. *Planta Med.,* **1999**, *65*(1), 76-78.
       [http://dx.doi.org/10.1055/s-2006-960444] [PMID: 10083849]

[78]   Falara, V.; Pichersky, E.; Kanellis, A.K. A copal-8-ol diphosphate synthase from the angiosperm *Cistus creticus* subsp. *creticus* is a putative key enzyme for the formation of pharmacologically active, oxygen-containing labdane-type diterpenes. *Plant Physiol.,* **2010**, *154*(1), 301-310.
       [http://dx.doi.org/10.1104/pp.110.159566] [PMID: 20595348]

[79]   Paolini, J.; Falchi, A.; Quilichini, Y.; Desjobert, J.M.; Cian, M.C.; Varesi, L.; Costa, J. Morphological, chemical and genetic differentiation of two subspecies of Cistus creticus L. (C. creticus subsp. eriocephalus and C. creticus subsp. corsicus). *Phytochemistry,* **2009**, *70*(9), 1146-1160.
       [http://dx.doi.org/10.1016/j.phytochem.2009.06.013] [PMID: 19660770]

[80]   Maggi, F.; Lucarini, D.; Papa, F.; Peron, G.; Dall'Acqua, S. Phytochemical Analysis of the Labdanum-poor *Cistus creticus* subsp. *eriocephalus* (Viv.) Greuter et Burdet Growing in Central Italy. *Biochem. Syst. Ecol.,* **2016**, *66*, 50-57.
       [http://dx.doi.org/10.1016/j.bse.2016.02.030]

[81]   Mastino, P.M.; Marchetti, M.; Costa, J.; Usai, M. Interpopulation Variability in the Essential Oil Composition of *Cistus creticus* subsp. *eriocephalus* from Sardinia. *Chem. Biodivers.,* **2018**, *15*(9), e1800151.
       [http://dx.doi.org/10.1002/cbdv.201800151] [PMID: 29959828]

[82]   Daglia, M. Polyphenols as antimicrobial agents. *Curr. Opin. Biotechnol.,* **2012**, *23*(2), 174-181.
        [http://dx.doi.org/10.1016/j.copbio.2011.08.007] [PMID: 21925860]

[83]   Küpeli, E.; Yesilada, E. Flavonoids with anti-inflammatory and antinociceptive activity from Cistus
        laurifolius L. leaves through bioassay-guided procedures. *J. Ethnopharmacol.,* **2007**, *112*(3), 524-530.
        [http://dx.doi.org/10.1016/j.jep.2007.04.011] [PMID: 17540523]

[84]   Mahmoudi, H.; Aouadhi, C.; Kaddour, R.; Gruber, M.; Zargouni, H.; Zaouali, W.; Ben Hamida, N.;
        Ben Nasri, M.; Ouerghi, Z.; Hosni, K. Comparison of antioxidant and antimicrobial activities of two
        cultivated Cistus species from Tunisia. *Biosci. J.,* **2016**, *32*(1), 226-237.
        [http://dx.doi.org/10.14393/BJ-v32n1a2016-30208]

[85]   Rebaya, A.; Belghith Igueld, S.; Hammrouni, S.; Amaaroufi, A.; Trabelsi Ayadi, M.; Cherif, J.K.
        Antibacterial and antifungal activities of *Halimium halimifolium, Cistus salviifolis* and *Cistus
        monspeliensis. International Journal of Pharmaceutical and Clinical Research,* **2016**, *8*, 243-247.

[86]   Mastino, P.M.; Marchetti, M.; Costa, J.; Juliano, C.; Usai, M. Analytical profiling of phenolic
        compounds in extracts of three *Cistus* species from Sardinia and their potential antimicrobial and
        antioxidant activity. Chem. Biodiversity, 2021. *Chem. Biodivers.,* **2021**, *18*(6), e2100053.
        [http://dx.doi.org/10.1002/cbdv.202100053] [PMID: 33932088]

[87]   Danne, A.; Petereit, F.; Nahrstedt, A. Flavan-3-ols, prodelphinidins and further polyphenols from
        Cistus salvifolius. Phytochemistry, **1994**, *37*(2), 533-538.
        [http://dx.doi.org/10.1016/0031-9422(94)85094-1] [PMID: 7765630]

[88]   Santagati, N.A.; Salerno, L.; Attaguile, G.; Savoca, F.; Ronsisvalle, G. Simultaneous determination of
        catechins, rutin, and gallic acid in *Cistus* species extracts by HPLC with diode array detection. *J.
        Chromatogr. Sci.,* **2008**, *46*(2), 150-156.
        [http://dx.doi.org/10.1093/chromsci/46.2.150] [PMID: 18366875]

[89]   Barrajón-Catalán, E.; Fernández-Arroyo, S.; Saura, D.; Guillén, E.; Fernández-Gutiérrez, A.; Segura-
        Carretero, A.; Micol, V. Cistaceae aqueous extracts containing ellagitannins show antioxidant and
        antimicrobial capacity, and cytotoxic activity against human cancer cells. *Food Chem. Toxicol.,* **2010**,
        48(8-9), 2273-2282.
        [http://dx.doi.org/10.1016/j.fct.2010.05.060] [PMID: 20510328]

[90]   Rodríguez Vaquero, M.J.; Aredes Fernández, P.A.; Manca de Nadra, M.C.; Strasser de Saad, A.M.
        Phenolic compound combinations on *Escherichia coli* viability in a meat system. *J. Agric. Food
        Chem.,* **2010**, *58*(10), 6048-6052.
        [http://dx.doi.org/10.1021/jf903966p] [PMID: 20438131]

[91]   Jayaraman, P.; Sakharkar, M.K.; Lim, C.S.; Tang, T.H.; Sakharkar, K.R. Activity and interactions of
        antibiotic and phytochemical combinations against *Pseudomonas aeruginosain vitro. Int. J. Biol. Sci.,*
        2010, *6*(6), 556-568.
        [http://dx.doi.org/10.7150/ijbs.6.556] [PMID: 20941374]

[92]   Talibi, I.; Askarne, L.; Boubaker, H.; Boudyach, E.H.; Saadi, B.; Ait Ben Aoumar, A. Antifungal
        activity of some Moroccan plants against *Geotrichum candidum*, the causal agent of postharvest citrus
        sour rot. *Crop Prot.,* **2012**, *35*, 41-46.
        [http://dx.doi.org/10.1016/j.cropro.2011.12.016]

[93]   Tomás-Menor, L.; Morales-Soto, A.; Barrajón-Catalán, E.; Roldán-Segura, C.; Segura-Carretero, A.;
        Micol, V. Correlation between the antibacterial activity and the composition of extracts derived from
        various Spanish *Cistus* species. *Food Chem. Toxicol.,* **2013**, *55*, 313-322.
        [http://dx.doi.org/10.1016/j.fct.2013.01.006] [PMID: 23333717]

[94]   Sassi, A.B.; Harzallah-Skhiri, F.; Aouni, M. Investigation of some medicinal plants from Tunisia for
        antimicrobial activities. *Pharm. Biol.,* **2007**, *45*(5), 421-428.
        [http://dx.doi.org/10.1080/13880200701215406]

[95]   Proestos, C.; Boziaris, I.S.; Nychas, G.J.E.; Komaitis, M. Analysis of flavonoids and phenolic acids in

Greek aromatic plants: investigation of their antioxidant capacity and antimicrobial activity. *Food Chem.,* **2006**, *95*(4), 664-671.
[http://dx.doi.org/10.1016/j.foodchem.2005.01.049]

[96] Boukhebti, H.; Chaker, A.N.; Belhadj, H.; Sahli, F.; Ramdhani, M.; Laouer, H.; Harzallah, D. Chemical composition and antibacterial activity of *Mentha pulegium* L. and *Mentha spicata* L. essential oils. *Pharm. Lett.,* **2011**, *3*, 267-275.

[97] Aligiannis, N.; Kalpoutzakis, E.; Mitaku, S.; Chinou, I.B. Composition and antimicrobial activity of the essential oils of two *Origanum* species. *J. Agric. Food Chem.,* **2001**, *49*(9), 4168-4170.
[http://dx.doi.org/10.1021/jf001494m] [PMID: 11559104]

[98] Srinivasan, D.; Nathan, S.; Suresh, T.; Lakshmana Perumalsamy, P. Antimicrobial activity of certain Indian medicinal plants used in folkloric medicine. *J. Ethnopharmacol.,* **2001**, *74*(3), 217-220.
[http://dx.doi.org/10.1016/S0378-8741(00)00345-7] [PMID: 11274820]

[99] Kähkönen, M.P.; Hopia, A.I.; Vuorela, H.J.; Rauha, J.P.; Pihlaja, K.; Kujala, T.S.; Heinonen, M. Antioxidant activity of plant extracts containing phenolic compounds. *J. Agric. Food Chem.,* **1999**, *47*(10), 3954-3962.
[http://dx.doi.org/10.1021/jf990146l] [PMID: 10552749]

[100] Pietta, P.G. Flavonoids as antioxidants. *J. Nat. Prod.,* **2000**, *63*(7), 1035-1042.
[http://dx.doi.org/10.1021/np9904509] [PMID: 10924197]

[101] Sadhu, S.K.; Okuyama, E.; Fujimoto, H.; Ishibashi, M.; Yesilada, E. Prostaglandin inhibitory and antioxidant components of Cistus laurifolius, a Turkish medicinal plant. *J. Ethnopharmacol.,* **2006**, *108*(3), 371-378.
[http://dx.doi.org/10.1016/j.jep.2006.05.024] [PMID: 16814498]

[102] Alsabri, S.G.; Zetrini, A.; Ermeli, N.; Mohamed, S.; Bensaber, S.; Hermann, A.; Gbaj, A. Study of eight medicinal plants for antioxidant activities. *J. Chem. Pharm. Res.,* **2012**, *4*, 4028-4031.

[103] Amensour, M.; Sendra, E.; Pérez-Alvarez, J.A.; Skali-Senhaji, N.; Abrini, J.; Fernández-López, J. Antioxidant activity and chemical content of methanol and ethanol extracts from leaves of rockrose (*Cistus ladaniferus*). *Plant Foods Hum. Nutr.,* **2010**, *65*(2), 170-178.
[http://dx.doi.org/10.1007/s11130-010-0168-2] [PMID: 20455024]

[104] Attaguile, G.; Russo, A.; Campisi, A.; Savoca, F.; Acquaviva, R.; Ragusa, N.; Vanella, A. Antioxidant activity and protective effect on DNA cleavage of extracts from *Cistus incanus* L. and *Cistus monspeliensis* L. *Cell Biol. Toxicol.,* **2000**, *16*(2), 83-90.
[http://dx.doi.org/10.1023/A:1007633824948] [PMID: 10917563]

[105] Christodoulakis, N.S.; Georgoudi, M.; Fasseas, C. Leaf Structure of *Cistus creticus* L. (Rock Rose), a Medicinal Plant Widely Used in Folk Remedies Since Ancient Times. *J. Herbs Spices Med. Plants,* **2014**, *20*(2), 103-114.
[http://dx.doi.org/10.1080/10496475.2013.839018]

[106] Vogt, T.; Proksch, P.; Gulz, P.G. Epicuticular Flavonoid aglycones in the Genus *Cistus* (*Cistaceae*). *J. Plant Physiol.,* **1987**, *131*(1-2), 25-36.
[http://dx.doi.org/10.1016/S0176-1617(87)80264-X]

Frontiers in Natural Product Chemistry, 2021, Vol. 10, 43-72 **43**

CHAPTER 2

Roles of Natural Abscisic Acids in Fruits during Fruit Development and under Environmental Stress

Bing Yuan[2], Qian Li[1], Yandan Xu[1] and Ping Leng[1,*]

[1] *College of Horticulture, China Agricultural University, Beijing 100193, P. R. China*

[2] *Environment, University of Melbourne, Melbourne, VIC 3010, Australia*

Abstract: Phytohormone abscisic acid (ABA) regulates the growth and development of plants as well as their response to environmental changes. Recently, the regulations of ABA during fruit ripening and stress resistance were discovered in two types of fruits (climacteric and non-climacteric fruits). However, it is challenging to understand the physiological, biochemical, and molecular biological mechanisms in fruit ripening and stress response controlled by ABA. ABA is involved in fruit development processes, including young fruit growth, fruit ripening onset, ripening process and quality formation. Meanwhile, ABA plays an important role in fruit adapting to environmental stresses. ABA works through the adjustment of its concentration and signal transduction. This review summarizes the current knowledge regarding ABA in the regulation of fruit development and ripening as well as in responses to environmental stresses.

Keywords: ABA, ABA receptor, ABA signalling, Abiotic stress, Drought, Fruit ripening, Fruit quality, Strawberry, Tomato.

INTRODUCTION

Fleshy fruits play an important role in the evolution of angiosperms; meanwhile, they provide indispensable sources of nutrients to the human body and are a vital pillar in the world economy [1, 2]. The ripening process of fleshy fruit shows a remarkable evolutionary advantage as it can protect the seeds during fruit development and seed dispersion [3 - 5]. Fleshy fruits can be broadly classified as climacteric (tomato, apple, peach, apricot) and non-climacteric (strawberry, grape, sweet cherry, citrus) fruits based on their respiration pattern during ripening [6, 7]. The climacteric fruit ripening is considered to be associated with an ethylene burst

---

* **Corresponding author Ping Leng:** College of Horticulture, China Agricultural University, Beijing 100193, P. R. China; Tel: 086-010-62731638; E-mails: pleng@cau.edu.cn

during ripening, while the ripening mechanism of non-climact eric fruit is still unclear [8]. Both types of fruits share the same regulatory pathways during ripening activation, and their main difference is whether to release ethylene during fruit ripening. Among fleshy fruits, tomato and strawberry are the most popular fruit crops which represent the climacteric and non-climacteric fruits, respectively, and are used as model fruits to study fruit biological characteristics and their important commercial traits [9, 10]. Fruit ripening is a genetically programmed and highly coordinated process which leads to structural and biochemical changes, such as fruit colouring, softening, and the increased contents of sugar, volatile compounds, and vitamins [9]. Large-scale analysis of various omics, such as transcriptome and proteome, has indicated that phytohormone abscisic acid (ABA) involves in the regulation of the development and ripening of both fruit types [11 - 13].

On the other hand, global warming and population soaring force us to increase grain yield, including the economic fruit crops. The new strategy to enhance the stress resistance of crops, especially improving their water efficiency, is crucial in food productions in near future [14 - 16]. Plants cannot run away as humans and animals do from encountered dangers, such as the abiotic stress of drought, high in salt and alkali, as well as the biotic stress of plant diseases and insect pests. They can only tolerate the stresses because their roots penetrate deep into the soil.

Therefore, plants have evolved for a long time to avoid damage. It has been found that ABA plays a key role in the regulation of crops responding to biotic and abiotic stresses to improve their growth and development [17, 18]. For example, during photosynthesis, plants lose most of their water through transpiration which is controlled by the movements of stomata. And the opening and closing of stomata in plants is adjusted by ABA [19 - 21].

ABA acts by adjusting its concentration and signalling. The core components in ABA biosynthetic and degradation pathways and ABA glycosylation have been identified through molecular, physiological and multi-omics approaches for decades [22, 23]. ABA signalling pathway consists of the ABA receptors PYR1/PYL/RCAR (afterwards PYL), group A protein phosphatase 2Cs (PP2Cs) and sucrose non-fermenting-1 (SNF1)-related protein kinases 2 (SnRK2) [24, 25]. How does the ABA signal transduction pathway work? For example, during fruit ripening or under drought stress, the ABA level raises, which is perceived by the PYL proteins binding to ABA to promote the formation of a PYL-ABA-PP2C ternary complex to suppress the activity of PP2Cs [24, 26]. The inhibition of PP2Cs activates (1) SnRK2s, which regulates the activity of downstream genes related to fruit development and ripening, and/or (2) a stress-activated kinase nalling network controls the osmotic pressure and stomatal closure of guard cells [17, 27, 28].

In the review, we summarize the roles of ABA in fleshy fruit development and ripening, as well as in response to environmental stress. We discuss the related mechanisms of ABA regulation in these processes under the genetic, molecular, and physiological levels. The study of ABA can be applied in optimizing the yield and quality of fruits and the postharvest storage condition of fruits.

Metabolism, (de) Conjugation, and Signalling of ABA

The biosynthesis of ABA in plants starts with the cleavage of C_{40} carotenoid molecules, which is catalysed by Zeaxanthin (C_{40}) epoxidase (ZEP). 9-*cis*-epoxycarotenoid dioxygenase (NCED) is the rate-limiting enzyme that catalyses the conversion of 9'-*cis*-neoxanthin and 9'-*cis*-violaxanthin to xanthoxin in plastids. In cytoplasm, the C_{15} xanthoxin is converted by alcohol dehydrogenase to abscisic aldehyde which is oxidized into ABA *via* AAO3. ABA can be degraded to phasic acid (PA) catalyzed by CYP707As. PA is then transferred to dihydrophaseic acid (DPA) or DPA-4-O-β-D-glucoside (DPAG) by PA reductase (PAR). In ABA conjugation pathway, ABA can be glycosylated into ABA-glucose ester (ABA-GE) by UDP-glucosyltransferase (ABA UGT), and ABA β-glucosidases (BGs) can transform ABA-GE to active ABA.

As shown in Fig. (**1**), ABA is a sesquiterpene derived from carotenoid to form all-*trans*-violaxanthin, which can either transfer to 9'-*cis*-neoxanthin or form 9'-*cis*-violaxanthin [29 - 31]. Both 9'-*cis*-neoxanthin and 9'-*cis*-violaxanthin are cleaved to create C_{15} xanthoxin catalysed by NCED [32, 33]. Finally, in cytoplasm, xanthoxin is converted into abscisic aldehyde *via* a short-chain alcohol dehydrogenase, which is eventually oxidized to ABA [34, 35]. The reduction of ABA content can be achieved in two ways, namely, the hydroxylation of ABA and the glycosylation of ABA. In the reaction of ABA hydroxylation, ABA is hydroxylated into phasic acid (PA) catalysed by CYP707As [36]. PA is then degraded to dihydrophasic acid (DPA), which binds to sugar to further form DPA-glucoside (DPAG) [37, 38]. To date, a large number of mutants of the synthetic and degradation genes have been discovered in each step of the ABA metabolic process in different plant species [39, 40].

In addition, the ABA accumulation in cell can be affected by the glycosylation of ABA. In plants, most hormones can be inactivated through glycosylation, such as ABA, auxin, gibberellin, salicylic acid, brassinosteroid, and cytokinin [41]. ABA can be glycosylated by UDP-glucosyltransferase (UGT) to ABA-glucose ester (ABA-GE), which can exit the cytosol and enter a membrane compartment for storage through the recognition by transporters [42]. By contrast, ABA level can be enhanced through β-glucosidases (BGs), which hydrolyses ABA-GE to release free ABA [43, 44]. The glycosylation of ABA is a reversible, one-step reaction, which is extremely important in quickly adjusting ABA levels to meet the requirements of different development and responses to stresses. This part is discussed in more detail in the back part.

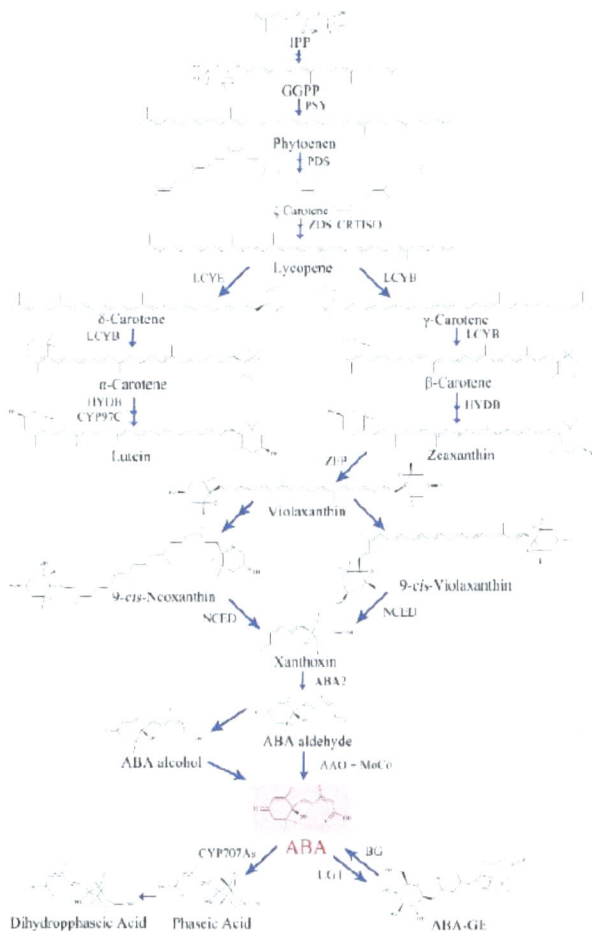

Fig. (1). ABA metabolism and (de) conjugation in plants.

On the other hand, great progress has been made recently in the identification and characterization of core ABA signalling components, especially in the ABA receptor protein family [45]. ABA signal transduction is initiated by the ABA receptor PYLs, and in the absence of ABA, PP2Cs can repress the activity of SnRK2. In the presence of ABA, ABA-bound PYL proteins interact and inhibit the activity of PP2Cs, thus, activates SnRK2 [26, 46, 47] and phosphorylates the AREB/ABFs proteins [48, 49]. AREB/ABFs are ABA-response element binding factors, containing a basic leucine zipper family (zip)-type DNA-binding domain, which bind the ABA-responsive element motifs and plays a crucial role in activating the ABA-response gene [50, 51].

The PP2C is considered to be a co-receptor of ABA and acts as a relay station in ABA signalling system. ABA receptor PYLs are generally divided into three subfamilies: subfamilies I and II have monomeric structures with high basal activity, while subfamily III has a dimeric structure in solution with low basal activity [52, 53]. The activity and conformation of ABA receptor PYLs are impacted by phosphorylation, nitration and ubiquitination, which influence the responses of ABA to demand fruit development and abiotic stress during ABA signalling [54, 55]. The (de) phosphorylation of PYL is essential to maintain the stability of ABA signal during the fruit development and response to environmental stresses [56].

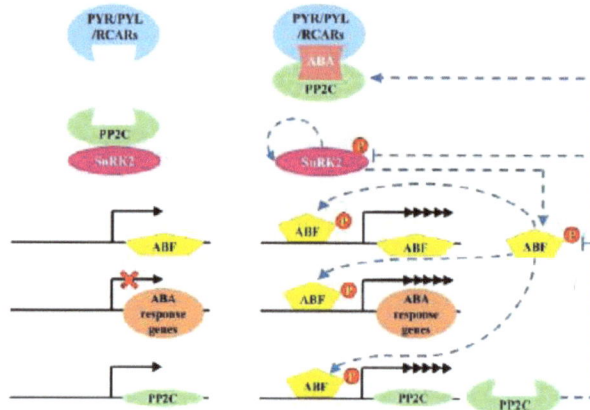

Fig. (2). ABA signalling core components and their transduction pathways. The ABA signalling pathway consists of receptors RCAR/PYL/PYR (PYLs), PP2C (protein phosphatases of type 2C), SnRK2s (sucrose non-fermenting-1 (SNF1)-related protein kinase 2), and ABFs (ABA-responsive element-binding factors).

PP2Cs are negative regulators of ABA signalling, which can be reduced by ABA receptor PYLs and several other regulators. On the contrary, SnRK2s are the positive regulators in ABA signalling, which can be activated by several kinases, such as Raff-like MAKKKs, RAF10 and ARK. In addition, SnRK2s are repressed by the positive signals from fruit growth and development, such as brassinosteroid (BR) [57] and nitric oxide (NO) signalling [58, 59]. Furthermore, it can be stimulated by environmental stresses.

Transcriptional Regulation of the Core Components in ABA Metabolism and Signalling Pathway

A large number of studies for the two types of fruits have suggested a close relationship between the ABA concentration and fruit maturation [7, 60]. The ABA level in fruit depends mainly on balance between the de novo biosynthesis of ABA and the ABA catabolism by ABA 8'- hydroxylase, which regulated by *NCED* gene family and *CYP707A* family, respectively [61, 62]. Meanwhile, the ABA accumulation is adjusted by the glycosylation of ABA under a reversible reaction of β-glucosidases and UDP-glucosyltransferase. To date, the genes in ABA metabolism and in ABA glycosylation pathway have been identified and characterized in various climacteric fruits (tomato, apple, peach, melon, *etc.*) and non-climacteric fruits (orange, sweet cherry, strawberry, *etc.*). In climacteric fruits, the complete sequencing of genome [63] shows that numerous genes are involved in ABA metabolism and ABA glycosylation, participating in the regulation of fruit development and ripening. For example, in tomato, *SlNCED1* and *CYP707A2* are the most important genes among *NCEDs* and *CYP707As* during ABA metabolism [64]. In ABA-deficient mutant and fruits silencing *SlNCED1* gene, the ethylene release is delayed due to the reduction of endogenous ABA during mature green stage and breaker stage, and thereby, the fruit ripening onset is delayed compared to the wild type (WT) [65, 66]. By contrast, if *SlNCED1* is overexpressed in tomato, the ABA accumulation is enhanced, which inducts the ethylene release and accelerates fruit ripening. Both the overexpression and suppression of the *SlNCED1* gene affect the pollen development and germination [67], and cause deterioration in various aspects during flower organ development in tomato [68]. Besides, the expression of *CYP707A* can alter the dynamic balance of ABA in plant tissue because the region of *CYP707A* gene promoter contains the ABA-responsive elements (ABREs) [69]. The suppression of *SlCYP707A2* can accelerate fruit ripening, while the overexpression of *SlCYP707A2* delays fruits ripening in tomato [64]. In addition, the regulation of genes related to ABA conjugation also affects the cellular ABA levels. β-glucosidases (BGs) can catalyse the hydrolysis of glucose esters (GE) of hormone, such as ABA, auxin, and cytokinin, to release free ABA or IAA [44, 70]. Several BG genes are identified in fruits can hydrolyte the ABA glucose ester (ABA-GE) to release free ABA both *in vitro* and *vivo*. For example, in tomato plants with overexpressed persimmon *DkBG1*, fruit ripening is accelerative and fruit quality is impacted compared to WT fruits [71]. These ABA BG genes participate in the regulation of ABA accumulation in several fleshy fruits, such as grape [72], strawberry [73] and persimmon [71]. On the contrary, UDP-glucosyltransferase (UGT) can glycosylate ABA to form ABA-glucose ester (ABA-GE) [74], which reduces the ABA accumulation [75]. If a tomato *SlUGT75C1* is suppressed, the plants become more sensitive to ABA under strong drought stress with delayed seed germination and post-germination growth and advanced fruit ripening compared to WT fruits [76]. Both BG and UGT protein families are encoded by multi-genes, and they play roles in the regulation of ABA level during fruit development and in response to abiotic stress. In addition, ABA accumulation is also impacted by the crosstalk of other hormones, such as ethylene. For example, PpERF2, an ethylene response factor of peach, suppresses the expressions of *PpNCED2* and *PpeNCED3* in ABA biosynthetic pathway, thereby affects the ABA level during fruit ripening [77]. All these results suggest that ABA plays an important role in the regulation of fruit development and ripening.

• In contrast to climacteric fruits, the key regulatory genes to control the ripening of non-climacteric fruits are still unclear. Strawberry (*Fragaria* × *ananassa* Duch.) is a typical non-climacteric fruit with unique flavour and aroma. The strawberry flesh is enlarged from the flower receptacle, and on the flesh surface, actual fruits (achenes) are embedded. Although the ethylene treatment can impact strawberry ripening [78 - 80], ethylene is not generally considered to be necessary to initiate and/or maintain fruit ripening [81]. ABA is thought to be the main phytohormone to control strawberry ripening [18]. In addition, the application of exogenous ABA can induce the grape colouring *via* the enhanced expression of synthetic enzyme genes in anthocyanin metabolic pathway [72]. ABA overproduction through the over-expression of ABA synthetic gene during fruit ripening can induce more production of the phenylpropanoid pathway (PPP), thereby increases the productions of flavonoids, monolignols, phenolic acids, stilbenes, coumarins and other related molecules [82]. In recent research, ABA can induce calcium (Ca^{2+}), Ca^{2+}-dependent protein kinases (CDPKs) and reactive oxygen species (ROS) to affect PPP [83]. In sweet cherry, the application of exogenous ABA can accelerate the accumulation of anthocyanin and fruit ripening through the up-regulated of the key genes in the anthocyanin synthetic pathway [73, 84]. The suppression of *PavNCED1* expression leads to lower ABA content, reduced anthocyanin accumulation and delayed fruit ripening in sweet cherry fruits [85]. RNA-seq analysis showed that in ABA- and NDGA (nordihydroguaiaretic acid)-treated strawberry [86], ABA regulates the expressions of genes in multiple metabolism pathways simultaneously, such as hormone signalling, anthocyanin synthesis, and flavonoids synthesis. These results show that ABA plays a crucial role in the regulation of fruit colouring and ripening onset in non-climacteric fruits.

Generally, ABA acts in the coordinating physiological processes mainly through the interactions with proteins for signalling. It is worth noting that all ABA signalling proteins identified in recent years are encoded by multi-gene families, and it is difficult to distinguish the role of each member in the family. How do multiple ABA receptor PYLs coordinate in response to developmental signals and environmental changes? Many points remain unknown, lacking thorough and systematic research. The over-expression of PYL strategy to enhance plant drought resistance has been extensively validated in many food crops, such as rice, maize, wheat, *etc* [87, 88]. However, in fleshy fruits, their biological effects are still evaluated and have not been applied to practical production yet. Although the ABA signalling pathway is universal in land plants [89], ABA receptors are differentially expressed at different times and spaces in plants [90]. Here, we summarize the recently published studies on the core components in the ABA signaling pathway.

ABA receptor PYLs can influence fruit physiological characteristics and ripening. These PYL proteins are different in binding with ABA, and show different effects on the inhibition of the type 2C phosphatase (PP2C) [91]. In tomato, ABA signalling genes of PYL, PP2C and SnRK2 are expressed in all the tissues and organs during fruit development. For example, the overexpression or suppression of the ABA receptor *SlPYL9* gene causes an advanced or delayed fruit ripening and an increased or decreased drought resistance in transgenic tomato [68]. ABA receptors can be used in different plants beyond the limitation of species. For example, *Arabidopsis* thaliana has enhanced drought resistance after the introduction of tomato PYL [92, 93].

In addition, the PP2C family mediates the second step in ABA signalling, which negatively regulates the PYL ABA receptor family on the downstream during ABA signalling. In tomato fruits, if the expression of *SlPP2C1* gene is suppressed, the release of ethylene is advanced, and fruit ripens earlier than WT fruits [94]. Suppression of *SlPP2C1* can increase the plants sensitive to ABA, leading to delayed seed germination and primary root growth, as well as increased drought resistance. At the same time, *SlPP2C1*-RNAi causes abnormal pollens and ovaries during floral organ development [94]. These results suggest that SlPP2C1 is a negative regulator in the ABA signalling pathway, which is involved in the regulation of flower and fruit development. PP2C, a relay station for ABA signal transmission, selectively interacts with upstream ABA receptors and downstream SnRK2 kinases. In tomato plants, *SlPP2C3*-RNAi can enhance the plant sensitivity to ABA and accelerates fruit ripening. Suppressing the expression of *SlPP2C3* dulls the fruit glossiness through altering the expressions of cuticle-related genes, which affect the outer epidermis structure of pericarp. These results suggest that PP2C affects fruit glossiness *via* transcriptional control in tomato [67].

At present, ABA receptor PYLs have become the ideal targets in the manipulation of ABA sensitivity to enhance the stress resistance in plants [95]. In *Arabidopsis*, the overexpression of PYLs as an effective mean is extensively used to improve water efficiency *via* increased ABA sensitivity [92, 96] and similar technical methods is attempted in many food crops [16]. Compared to dimeric PYLs, monomeric PYLs with high activity is widely used to improve the drought resistance of food crops. In addition, a few manipulations are tried on the dimer PYLs in crops as well.

ABA Regulates Fruit Ripening Onset

Fruit ripening is a very complex biochemical process [8]. Beginning with the fruit maturation accompanied by the degradation of chlorophyll and the accumulation of carotenoids or anthocyanin, colour changes from green to yellow or red with fruit softening [4, 97]. A number of hormones are involved in the regulation of fruit ripening onset (Fig. **3**), and among them, ABA seems to play an important role triggered the start of fruit maturity. Moreover, ABA treatment influences the ripening-related parameters, such as the sugar and anthocyanin content [85].

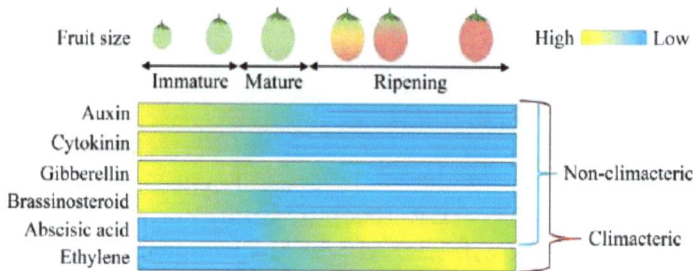

Fig. (3). The variations of key hormones in a fruit life. A description of key hormones in different fruit developmental stages, their relationship and changes in the content of auxin, gibberellin, cytokinin, ethylene, and ABA in both climacteric and non-climacteric fruits.

During ABA signalling, ABA-response element binding factors (AREB/ABFs) located below SnRK2 activate the downstream ABA-response genes through binding to ABREs (ABA-responsive elements), which exist in the promoter region of target genes [98, 99]. Recent research shows that the transcription of AREB/ABFs can be fully activated by ABA signalling, suggesting that ABA-dependent phosphorylation of AREB/ABFs may be necessary to activate the downstream genes [99]. In tomato, two AREB transcription factor genes are identified (*SlAREB1* and *SlAREB2*) and can be detected in all tissues of tomato plants [100] which can be significantly induced by the exogenous ABA [101]. In tomato, SlAREB1 plays a crucial role in the regulation of genes related to stress responses, while the role of SlAREB2 is limited [98]. Besides, SlAREB1 is involved in the regulation of basic metabolic substances in fruits during development [99, 102]. In fruits, the over-expressions of SlAREB1, organic acids, sugars and amino acids are due to the enhanced transcription levels of related genes, which impact the fruit quality [102]. During fruit ripening, ABA and ethylene interact to each other through complex signalling networks [103].

The synthesis, accumulation and peak value of ABA are earlier than those of ethylene during ripening onset, which is necessary to trigger maturation initiation [104]. In addition, *SlAREB1*-OE can increase the expressions of ethylene biosynthetic genes (*SlACS2/4* and *SlACO1*), while *SlAREB1*-RNAi decreases these expressions [99], suggesting that SlAREB1 can induce the ethylene release through mediating ABA signalling. Moreover, SlAREB1 can specifically activate NOR transcription *via* the binding of the ABRE motif to its promoter region. All these results suggest that SlAREB1 positively regulates ethylene release.

After decades of hard work, a number of crucial proteins regulating the climacteric fruit ripening have been found through ripening-impaired mutants in tomato, such as MADS-box TFs, RIN, TAGL1, CNR, NOR, AP2/ERF and AP2a [105 - 110]. These transcription factors are involved in the regulation of fruit development, ripening and quality [111]. In *nor* mutant, fruit cannot reach maturation due to lack of ethylene, and the application of exogenous ethylene does not work, suggesting that ripening regulator NOR may be located on the upstream of ethylene [112, 113]. NOR plays an important role in various physiological processes during fruit ripening [7, 114], and the expression of the NOR gene is positively regulated by ABA [115]. It is found that the transcription level of *NOR* influences fruit softening, colouring and quality during ripening [12, 116]. The expression of the NOR gene can be modulated by SlNAP2, and the suppression of SlNAP2 can impact sugar content, carotenoids accumulation, and ethylene release during fruit ripening [117, 118].

On the other hand, several transcription factors, such as ABF and MYB regulate ripening in non-climacteric fruits. For example, grape VvABF2 belongs to group A of the zip family, and the over-expression of *VvABF2* can enhance the sensitivity of transgenic plants to ABA, which affects the accumulation of phenolic compounds related to fruit quality [119, 120]. FaMYB10 affects the anthocyanin accumulation in fruits by regulating the genes expressions in flavonoid pathway, and the expression of FaMYB10 can be up/down-regulated by ABA or auxins in strawberry fruits [121]. FvCDPK1, a member of calcium-dependent protein kinases (CDPKs), is involved in the regulation of the development and ripening of strawberries fruits which can be activated by ABA treatment [122]. These results suggest the crucial regulatory roles of these transcription factors in non-climacteric fruit ripening. To date, there is mounting evidence that transcription factors play an important role to integrate multiple signals in a complex network of ripening control.

ABA Regulates The Fruit Ripening Process And Fruit Quality

Both climacteric and non-climacteric fruits exhibit similar fluctuations, such as fruit softening, colouring, and the accumulation of sugar, organic acid, and aroma when fruits enter the ripening stage. The only difference is that non-climacteric fruits do not exhibit ethylene burst during ripening process.

Fruit Colouring

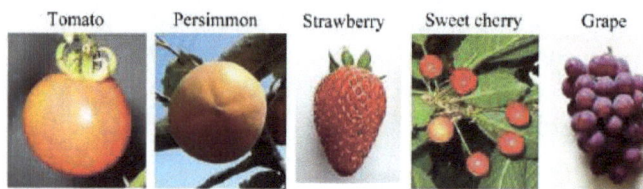

Fig. (4). Different kinds of fresh fruits during ripening stage.

In tomato, mango, persimmon and citrus fruits, fruit colour is mediated by carotenoids, lycopene and lutein. In other fruits, like strawberry, sweet cherry, and grape, anthocyanins are the most important colouring molecules [123]. During ripening, the fruit colour changes from green to red, which is accompanied by the transition from chloroplasts to chromoplasts and the accumulation of carotenoids or anthocyanin in fruits [6]. ABA acts in different ways in the above process for climacteric and non-climacteric fruits. In the synthesis pathway of carotenoid (Fig. **1**), phytoene synthase (PSY) is a key rate-limiting enzyme [123]. Under PSY, GGPP is transformed to 15-*cis*-phytoene which is induced by PDS, ZISO, ZDS, and CRTISO transcriptionally to *all trans*-lycopene. The concentrations of lycopene and β-carotene are increased by the up-regulated *SlPSY1* and endogenous ABA in tomato fruits [124]. In tomato, increased ABA accumulation during pre-breaker stage can trigger fruit ripening onset by inducing the ethylene release regulated by ethylene synthetic genes (SlACS2/4 and SlACO1). For example, SlPYL9 is an ABA receptor, and DkBG1 is an enzyme which can catalyse the hydrolyzation of ABA-GE. The over-expressed *SlPYL9* or *DkBG1* can accelerate fruit colouring during tomato fruit ripening [68, 71]. Conversely, the suppression of *SlPYL9* or *DkBG1* delays fruit ripening [68]. LCY-B catalyses the conversion of lycopene to β-carotene. Therefore, an increased activity of LCY-B can decrease the lycopene accumulation but increase the β-carotene and ABA levels [66, 72, 76]. The over-expression of LCY-B gene enhances the β-carotene content and delays the colouring due to the increased ABA content and decreased ethylene release causing by *LCY-B*-OE [125]. On the contrary, lycopene is highly synthesized in the tomato mutant of high-pigment 3 (hp3), which is caused by an altered gene for zeaxanthin epoxidase (Zep) [126]. In addition, *SlSGR1* is widely known as a stay-green protein inhibiting the degradation of chlorophyll in fruits [127].

ABA adjusts the biosynthesis of anthocyanin and flavonoid in fruits as well. In grapes, the application of ABA increases the accumulation of anthocyanin and antioxidants *via* the promotion of phenols metabolism [128]. In bilberry (*Vaccinium myrtillus* L.), several key genes in the anthocyanin biosynthetic pathway rapidly increase with the increased ABA [129]. Besides, ABA affects the expressions of significant genes related to the synthesis of phenylpropanoid, flavonoid and anthocyanin in grape berries [72, 130].

Fruit Softening

As fruit ripens, the flesh becomes soft and juicy with a large change of physical properties, such as solubilization of pectin, depolymerization of cellulose and hemicellulose, loosening of xyloglucan-cellulose network and the increase of wall porosity [131]. Cell wall degradation depends on a large number of hydrolases, such as poly-galacturonate (PG), pectin methylesterase (PME), pectate lyase (PL) and β-galactosidase (TBG), xyloglucan endotransglucosylase (XTH), endo-glucans (CEL) and expansions (EXP) [132, 133]. Ethylene can induce the enzymatic activities of these hydrolases in fruits during ripening [134], involving the regulation of fruit softening. Mounting evidence shows ABA's involvement in fruit softening recently [66, 72]. ABA also affects the fruit texture, for example, the over-expression or suppression of the key genes in the ABA metabolic pathway can alter the expression levels of hydrolytic enzyme genes, like PG, PL, PME, TBG, XTH, CEL and EXP, which are responsible for the disintegration of cell wall structures, thereby affecting the fruit texture in transgenic tomato [66, 71].

Fruit Size And Fruit Shape

ABA regulates fruit development in many aspects through ABA signalling, affecting fruit ripening and quality. There are many factors related to fruit quality, such as fruit shape index, fruit size, colour, volatile compounds. In tomato fruits, two or more fused carpels form locules, which are separated by fleshy septa, and the number of carpels in a flower determines the final number of locules (or compartments) in mature fruit. In the ABA deficient mutants of tomato, the fruit size is small, and the number of locules (or compartments) is less than that of WT fruits [65]. Several genes are found in tomato [77], such as quantitative trait loci *fasciated* (*fas*) [135] and *locule number* (*lc*) [136], regulating the locule number and the fruit size. To date, *fw2.2* is the only locus which affects the fruit weight, although the mature fruit weight is varied by fruit shape as well [137]. Two loci, *fas* (chromosome 11) and *lc* (chromosome 2), are thought to be associated with fruit size with the influence of the number of carpels in a flower. The multi-locular tomato fruits are found carrying one or both fruit size-related genes [138]. In tomato fruits, the overexpression or suppression of *SlNCED1, SlPYL9* and *SlBG*, significantly alters the shape and size of the transgenic fruits. These reports indicate that ABA may involve in the regulation of fruit size and fruit shape *via* ABA signalling, although the exact mechanism remains unclear.

ABA Regulates Sugar And Acid Metabolism

During fruit ripening, the sugar accumulation increases while the acid content decreases. The balance of the two contents is critical to fruit quality. The application of ABA promotes the uptake of sugar in apple pulp [139] and in citrus fruits [140]. In *Arabidopsis*, ABA signalling impacts the sugar signal in sugar-sensitive mutants. Many sugar mutants are hype-sensitive or insensitive to ABA, and ABA and sugar often exert similar or antagonistic effects on plant development [141, 142]. For example, sugar treatment can promote seed germination *via* relieving the inhibition of ABA on it [143]. In addition, the suppression of a sucrose *FaSUT1* can delay the fruit ripening by decreasing the sucrose content as well as the ABA accumulation [18]. These results suggest that the presence of multiple signalling pathways in fruits, such as all kinds of hormones and sugar signalling, influence the fruit ripening and quality. In addition, the suppression of tomato *SlORE1S02* can enhance carbon assimilation and fruit yield with a longer fruits shelf life and higher quality [144].

ABA Influences Fruit Glossiness

It is found that *SlPP2Cs* can affect fruit glossiness. For example, the suppression of *SlPP2C3* leads to a dull fruit surface in transgenic tomato fruits [145]. Scanning electron microscopy analysis reveals that the change of glossiness in *SlPP2C3*-RNAi fruits is caused by the alteration of cuticle/wax metabolism. RNA-seq analysis indicates that abundant genes are involved in the metabolism of cuticle and wax in transgenic pericarps. For instance, the expression of transcription factor *SlMYB96* is down-regulated, while *SlMYB106* is upregulated in *SlPP2C3*-RNAi fruits, and both promoter regions contain ABA response elements [145]. Orthologs in *Arabidopsis* are found to be involved in the regulation of cuticle metabolism [146, 147]. In addition, there are numerous genes associated with fruit glossiness, such as genes related to cuticle transporter, cutin synthase [148], cutin biosynthesis [149], *CYP450s* [150], *SlHTH* (formation of dicarboxylic fatty acids) [151], and glycerol-3-phosphate acyltransferase (involve in the final step of cutin monomer biosynthesis) [152]. These results suggest that dull fruit glossiness in *SlPP2C3*-RNAi fruits is caused by changing the cuticle metabolism related to ABA signalling.

ABA Regulates Seed Dormancy

Fruits can protect seeds during development and help seed dispersion in angiosperms. Seed dormancy is important during the long-term evolution of plants, which prevents seed precocious germination such as seed vivipary [153]. Seed dormancy is partly influenced by the organizational structure surrounding a seed. However, the mechanism is not fully understood yet [154]. The dormancy of seeds also depends on a balance between ABA and gibberellins in cell: ABA can induce, regulate and maintain seed dormancy, while gibberellins rouse seeds from dormancy and promote seed germination [154]. Transgenic tomato fruits with the overexpressed/suppressed ABA synthetic enzyme *SlNCED1* help us to extend our biochemical knowledge on the seed precocious germination process. The transcriptomes data shows that when ABA receptor SlPYL9 is over-expressed, seeds exhibit a higher sensibility to ABA, and seeds from *SlPYL9*-RNAi lines behave oppositely [68]. The accumulation of ABA in seeds is earlier than that in pulp [89]. Some genes related to gibberellins synthesis and catabolism are expressed in fruits at different stages, which may be involved in the regulation of seed dormancy and germination. In addition, several genes associated with embryo development and seed dormancy are found in fruits/seeds, such as IPK2β, an inositol polyphosphate kinase induced by ABA [51]. Shortly, ABA plays an essential role in the regulation of seed dormancy and germination. Besides, ABA finely tunes the physiological traits of fruits to avoid seed vivipary in fruits.

ABA Regulates The Adapting Of Fruit/Plant To Environmental Changes

So far, numerous studies proved that plants have developed a complete defense system to avoid danger. ABA is a major regulator in plants under various environmental stresses, such as the regulation of plant response to heat, drought, salinity and osmotic stress [155]. Most of the transcription factors and genes have dual attributes, which means these transcription factors and genes related to fruit development and ripening are originally classified as stress-responsive genes [156]. For example, NOR-like1 is a ripening regulator in the upstream of RIN (RIPENING-INHIBITOR) and NOR (NON-RIPENING), which affects the fruit ripening and quality through directly binding to the promoter of genes involved in ethylene synthesis, cell wall modification, pigmentation, and flavor substances [157, 158]. However, NOR-like1 gains considerable attention as *SlNAC3* negatively regulates the ABA-mediated response to drought stress [159]. Later, *SlNAC3* is found to play an essential role in the regulation of embryo and endosperm during seed development [160]. NOR-like SNAC4 (SlNAC48) is verified as a regulator under high salt and drought stress [158]. The suppression of *SNAC4* leads to a decreased carotenoid synthesis, delayed chlorophyll breakdown and ethylene release during fruit ripening [157]. In addition, *SlNAC1* involves in the regulation of defensive response to heat or chilling stress and to Pseudomonas syringe [161, 162]. *SlNAC1* regulates fruit ripening and quality formation through binding to genes in the regulatory regions related to ethylene release, cell wall modification and lycopene biosynthesis. The manipulation of the expression of *SlNAC1* can alter flesh texture, flavor substance, and fruit appearance quality [163, 164]. These studies indicate that most of the transcription factors and genes regulate the fruit development and ripening and stress responses concurrently in plants.

When plant is subjected to abiotic stresses, ABA accumulation rises to trigger the ABA signalling networks for stress response [30]. ABA adjusts the response to drought stress, and the water efficiency is improved in plants through ABA accumulation and signalling [165]. For example, in tomato *SlNCED1*-OE plants, the ABA content increases which leads to more closed stomas closed stoma to reduce the water loss in leaves [166]. Generally, ABA metabolic *CYP707A* genes in fruits can be up regulated under exogenous ABA treatment and down regulated under drought stress [84, 167]. In tomato plants with the over-expressed *SlPYL9,* an ABA receptor gene, the drought resistance is enhanced due to the increased plant sensitivity to ABA. By contrast, the drought resistance is decreased in the *SlPYL9*-RNAi plants [68]. Besides, the suppression of *SlPP2C1* or *SlPP2C3* in tomato leads to various ABA-hypersensitization phenotypes, including slower seed germination and enhanced drought resistance compared to WT plants. This result indicates that *SlPP2C1* and *SlPP2C3* of ABA signalling core components negatively regulate ABA signalling in tomato plants during fruit development as well as under environmental stresses.

On the other hand, ABA signalling affects the stress resistance of fruit during fruit growth and after fruit harvest. During fruit expansion, the thickness of cuticle and the expansion of fruit epidermis must be coordinated to maintain the normal development of fruit pericarp [168, 169]. The outer epidermis of fruit is a crucial barrier which protects plants against abiotic stresses, plant diseases and insect pests. The changes in cuticle architecture and composition are proved to be the integral elements in the formation of fruit texture [168, 170]. The outer pericarp of fruit contains a large polymer cutin and cuticular wax, and reducing them causes a thinner cuticle, which leads to reduced fruit resistance and a postharvest shelf life [171, 172]. ABA influences cuticle formation through adjusting the expressions of genes related to cuticle metabolism under water deficit conditions in *Arabidopsis* and tomato [144, 173]. According to the reports, core components in ABA signalling (PYL, PP2C and SnRK2) affect cuticle formation and thickness during *Arabidopsis* development. In ABA-deficient tomato mutants, the cutin and wax compositions are reduced, and the expressions of cuticle biosynthesis genes are downregulated in leaves [174]. To date, the intricate mechanisms on the formation of cuticle and its influencing factors remain unknown. The transcription factors belonging to zinc finger superfamily regulate plant growth and development in many aspects, especially in the regulation of plant response to abiotic stresses. SlZF2 is a cysteine-2/histidine-2-type zinc finger protein which can be induced by exogenous ABA and drought stress. *35S::SlZF2* can promote ABA accumulation and it is speculated to be involved in the ABA biosynthesis and signalling in tomato [175]. It's not hard to see that most studies on the abiotic stress caused by environmental changes have been implemented for the whole plants, and seldom of them focus on fruits. Research on the ability and mechanism of fruit resistance to abiotic stresses is far from enough compared to other fruit properties. Abiotic and biotic stresses due to environmental anomaly on fruit need further study, especially on the mechanism of fruit resistance.

CONCLUDING REMARKS

ABA can induce fruit ripening and response to abiotic stress in both climacteric and non-climacteric fleshy fruits through the adjustment of concentration and signal transduction. ABA-PP2C-SnRK2-mediated ABA signalling pathway is a control centre to assist the linkage and synergy of plant hormones, transcription factors and downstream genes during fruit development and under abiotic stresses. It is a crucial regulator in fruit development, ripening, quality traits and stress response. All the core components in ABA signalling are encoded by multiple gene families, suggesting the functional redundancy in their signal transduction pathways. Moreover, ABA accumulation and ABA signalling activity vary in different tissues and developmental stages and are affected by many internal and external factors. This complexity shows that it is challenging to reveal the mechanism and the regulatory networks of ABA signalling in fruits.

FUNDING

This work is financially supported by the Israel Science Foundation (ISF)–National Natural Science Foundation of China (NSFC) Joint Scientific Research Program [grant No. 31661143046] and the NSFC (Nos. 31572095 and 31772270].

CONSENT FOR PUBLICATION

Not applicable.

CONFLICT OF INTEREST

The author declares no conflict of interest, financial or otherwise.

ACKNOWLEDGEMENTS

Declared none.

REFERENCES

[1]   Wallace, T.C.; Bailey, R.L.; Blumberg, J.B.; Burton-Freeman, B.; Chen, C.O.; Crowe-White, K.M.; Drewnowski, A.; Hooshmand, S.; Johnson, E.; Lewis, R.; Murray, R.; Shapses, S.A.; Wang, D.D. Fruits, vegetables, and health: A comprehensive narrative, umbrella review of the science and recommendations for enhanced public policy to improve intake. *Crit. Rev. Food Sci. Nutr.,* **2020**, *60*(13), 2174-2211.
        [http://dx.doi.org/10.1080/10408398.2019.1632258] [PMID: 31267783]

[2]   Mason-D'Croz, D.; Bogard, J.R.; Sulser, T.B.; Cenacchi, N.; Dunston, S.; Herrero, M.; Wiebe, K. Gaps between fruit and vegetable production, demand, and recommended consumption at global and national levels: an integrated modelling study. *Lancet Planet. Health,* **2019**, *3*(7), e318-e329.
        [http://dx.doi.org/10.1016/S2542-5196(19)30095-6] [PMID: 31326072]

[3]   Knapp, S. Tobacco to tomatoes: a phylogenetic perspective on fruit diversity in the Solanaceae. *J. Exp. Bot.,* **2002**, *53*(377), 2001-2022.
        [http://dx.doi.org/10.1093/jxb/erf068] [PMID: 12324525]

[4]   McAtee, P.; Karim, S.; Schaffer, R.; David, K. A dynamic interplay between phytohormones is required for fruit development, maturation, and ripening. *Front. Plant Sci.,* **2013**, *4*(4), 79.
        [http://dx.doi.org/10.3389/fpls.2013.00079] [PMID: 23616786]

[5]   Zhong, W.; Gao, Z.; Zhuang, W.; Shi, T.; Zhang, Z.; Ni, Z. Genome-wide expression profiles of seasonal bud dormancy at four critical stages in Japanese apricot. *Plant Mol. Biol.,* **2013**, *83*(3), 247-264.
        [http://dx.doi.org/10.1007/s11103-013-0086-4] [PMID: 23756818]

[6]   Klee, H.J.; Giovannoni, J.J. Genetics and control of tomato fruit ripening and quality attributes. *Annu. Rev. Genet.,* **2011**, *45*, 41-59.
        [http://dx.doi.org/10.1146/annurev-genet-110410-132507] [PMID: 22060040]

[7]   Osorio, S.; Alba, R.; Nikoloski, Z.; Kochevenko, A.; Fernie, A.R.; Giovannoni, J.J. Integrative comparative analyses of transcript and metabolite profiles from pepper and tomato ripening and development stages uncovers species-specific patterns of network regulatory behavior. *Plant Physiol.,* **2012**, *159*(4), 1713-1729.
        [http://dx.doi.org/10.1104/pp.112.199711] [PMID: 22685169]

[8]   Alexander, L.; Grierson, D. Ethylene biosynthesis and action in tomato: a model for climacteric fruit ripening. *J. Exp. Bot.,* **2002**, *53*(377), 2039-2055.
        [http://dx.doi.org/10.1093/jxb/erf072] [PMID: 12324528]

[9]   Giovannoni, J. Ripening activator turned repressor. *Nat. Plants,* **2017**, *3*(12), 920-921.
        [http://dx.doi.org/10.1038/s41477-017-0062-0] [PMID: 29133904]

[10]   Osorio, S.; Vallarino, J.G.; Szecowka, M.; Ufaz, S.; Tzin, V.; Angelovici, R.; Galili, G.; Fernie, A.R. Alteration of the interconversion of pyruvate and malate in the plastid or cytosol of ripening tomato fruit invokes diverse consequences on sugar but similar effects on cellular organic acid, metabolism, and transitory starch accumulation. *Plant Physiol.,* **2013**, *161*(2), 628-643.
        [http://dx.doi.org/10.1104/pp.112.211094] [PMID: 23250627]

[11]   Zhang, M.; Yuan, B.; Leng, P. The role of ABA in triggering ethylene biosynthesis and ripening of

tomato fruit. *J. Exp. Bot.,* **2009**, *60*(6), 1579-1588.
[http://dx.doi.org/10.1093/jxb/erp026] [PMID: 19246595]

[12]   Gapper, N.E.; Giovannoni, J.J.; Watkins, C.B. Understanding development and ripening of fruit crops in an 'omics' era. *Hortic. Res.,* **2014**, *1*, 14034.
[http://dx.doi.org/10.1038/hortres.2014.34] [PMID: 26504543]

[13]   Guo, J.; Wang, S.; Yu, X.; Dong, R.; Li, Y.; Mei, X.; Shen, Y. Polyamines Regulate Strawberry Fruit Ripening by Abscisic Acid, Auxin, and Ethylene. *Plant Physiol.,* **2018**, *177*(1), 339-351.
[http://dx.doi.org/10.1104/pp.18.00245] [PMID: 29523717]

[14]   Pennisi, E. Plant genetics. The blue revolution, drop by drop, gene by gene. *Science,* **2008**, *320*(5873), 171-173.
[http://dx.doi.org/10.1126/science.320.5873.171] [PMID: 18403686]

[15]   Morison, J.I.L.; Baker, N.R.; Mullineaux, P.M.; Davies, W.J. Improving water use in crop production. *Philos. Trans. R. Soc. Lond. B Biol. Sci.,* **2008**, *363*(1491), 639-658.
[http://dx.doi.org/10.1098/rstb.2007.2175] [PMID: 17652070]

[16]   Mega, R.; Abe, F.; Kim, J.S.; Tsuboi, Y.; Tanaka, K.; Kobayashi, H.; Sakata, Y.; Hanada, K.; Tsujimoto, H.; Kikuchi, J.; Cutler, S.R.; Okamoto, M. Tuning water-use efficiency and drought tolerance in wheat using abscisic acid receptors. *Nat. Plants,* **2019**, *5*(2), 153-159.
[http://dx.doi.org/10.1038/s41477-019-0361-8] [PMID: 30737511]

[17]   Deluc, L.G.; Grimplet, J.; Wheatley, M.D.; Tillett, R.L.; Quilici, D.R.; Osborne, C.; Schooley, D.A.; Schlauch, K.A.; Cushman, J.C.; Cramer, G.R. Transcriptomic and metabolite analyses of Cabernet Sauvignon grape berry development. *BMC Genomics,* **2007**, *8*, 429.
[http://dx.doi.org/10.1186/1471-2164-8-429] [PMID: 18034876]

[18]   Jia, H.F.; Chai, Y.M.; Li, C.L.; Lu, D.; Luo, J.J.; Qin, L.; Shen, Y.Y. Abscisic acid plays an important role in the regulation of strawberry fruit ripening. *Plant Physiol.,* **2011**, *157*(1), 188-199.
[http://dx.doi.org/10.1104/pp.111.177311] [PMID: 21734113]

[19]   Finkelstein, R.R.; Gampala, S.S.; Rock, C.D. Abscisic acid signaling in seeds and seedlings. *Plant Cell,* **2002**, *14* Suppl., S15-S45.
[http://dx.doi.org/10.1105/tpc.010441] [PMID: 12045268]

[20]   Yamaguchi-Shinozaki, K.; Shinozaki, K. Transcriptional regulatory networks in cellular responses and tolerance to dehydration and cold stresses. *Annu. Rev. Plant Biol.,* **2006**, *57*, 781-803.
[http://dx.doi.org/10.1146/annurev.arplant.57.032905.105444] [PMID: 16669782]

[21]   Cutler, S.R.; Rodriguez, P.L.; Finkelstein, R.R.; Abrams, S.R. Abscisic acid: emergence of a core signaling network. *Annu. Rev. Plant Biol.,* **2010**, *61*, 651-679.
[http://dx.doi.org/10.1146/annurev-arplant-042809-112122] [PMID: 20192755]

[22]   Cornforth, J.W.; Milborrow, B.V.; Ryback, G. Synthesis of (±)–abscisin II. *Nature,* **1965**, *206*, 715.
[http://dx.doi.org/10.1038/206715a0]

[23]   Addicott, F.T.; Lyon, J.L.; Ohkuma, K.; Thiessen, W.E.; Carns, H.R.; Smith, O.E.; Cornforth, J.W.; Milborrow, B.V.; Ryback, G.; Wareing, P.F. Abscisic acid: a new name for abscisin II (dormin). *Science,* **1968**, *159*(3822), 1493.
[http://dx.doi.org/10.1126/science.159.3822.1493.b] [PMID: 5732498]

[24]   Ma, Y.; Szostkiewicz, I.; Korte, A.; Moes, D.; Yang, Y.; Christmann, A.; Grill, E. Regulators of PP2C phosphatase activity function as abscisic acid sensors. *Science,* **2009**, *324*(5930), 1064-1068.
[http://dx.doi.org/10.1126/science.1172408] [PMID: 19407143]

[25]   Park, S.Y.; Fung, P.; Nishimura, N.; Jensen, D.R.; Fujii, H.; Zhao, Y.; Lumba, S.; Santiago, J.; Rodrigues, A.; Chow, T.F.; Alfred, S.E.; Bonetta, D.; Finkelstein, R.; Provart, N.J.; Desveaux, D.; Rodriguez, P.L.; McCourt, P.; Zhu, J.K.; Schroeder, J.I.; Volkman, B.F.; Cutler, S.R. Abscisic acid inhibits type 2C protein phosphatases *via* the PYR/PYL family of START proteins. *Science,* **2009**, *324*(5930), 1068-1071.

[http://dx.doi.org/10.1126/science.1173041] [PMID: 19407142]

[26]   Fujii, H.; Chinnusamy, V.; Rodrigues, A.; Rubio, S.; Antoni, R.; Park, S.Y.; Cutler, S.R.; Sheen, J.; Rodriguez, P.L.; Zhu, J.K. *In vitro* reconstitution of an abscisic acid signalling pathway. *Nature,* **2009**, *462*(7273), 660-664.
       [http://dx.doi.org/10.1038/nature08599] [PMID: 19924127]

[27]   Çakir, B.; Agasse, A.; Gaillard, C.; Saumonneau, A.; Delrot, S.; Atanassova, R. A grape ASR protein involved in sugar and abscisic acid signaling. *Plant Cell,* **2003**, *15*(9), 2165-2180.
       [http://dx.doi.org/10.1105/tpc.013854] [PMID: 12953118]

[28]   Zhao, C.; Liu, B.; Piao, S.; Wang, X.; Lobell, D.B.; Huang, Y.; Huang, M.; Yao, Y.; Bassu, S.; Ciais, P.; Durand, J.L.; Elliott, J.; Ewert, F.; Janssens, I.A.; Li, T.; Lin, E.; Liu, Q.; Martre, P.; Müller, C.; Peng, S.; Peñuelas, J.; Ruane, A.C.; Wallach, D.; Wang, T.; Wu, D.; Liu, Z.; Zhu, Y.; Zhu, Z.; Asseng, S. Temperature increase reduces global yields of major crops in four independent estimates. *Proc. Natl. Acad. Sci. USA,* **2017**, *114*(35), 9326-9331.
       [http://dx.doi.org/10.1073/pnas.1701762114] [PMID: 28811375]

[29]   Audran, C.; Liotenberg, S.; Gonneau, M. Localisation and expression of zeaxanthin epoxidase mRNA in Arabidopsis in response to drought stress and during seed development. *Aust. J. Plant Physiol.,* **2001**, *28*, 1161-1173.

[30]   Nambara, E.; Marion-Poll, A. Abscisic acid biosynthesis and catabolism. *Annu. Rev. Plant Biol.,* **2005**, *56*, 165-185.
       [http://dx.doi.org/10.1146/annurev.arplant.56.032604.144046] [PMID: 15862093]

[31]   North, H.M.; De Almeida, A.; Boutin, J.P.; Frey, A.; To, A.; Botran, L.; Sotta, B.; Marion-Poll, A. The Arabidopsis ABA-deficient mutant aba4 demonstrates that the major route for stress-induced ABA accumulation is *via* neoxanthin isomers. *Plant J.,* **2007**, *50*(5), 810-824.
       [http://dx.doi.org/10.1111/j.1365-313X.2007.03094.x] [PMID: 17470058]

[32]   Anstis, P.J.P.; Friend, J.; Gardner, D.C.J. Role of xanthoxin in inhibition of pea seedling growth by red–light. *Phytochemistry,* **1975**, *14*, 31-35.
       [http://dx.doi.org/10.1016/0031-9422(75)85002-3]

[33]   Schwartz, S.H.; Léon-Kloosterziel, K.M.; Koornneef, M.; Zeevaart, J.A. Biochemical characterization of the aba2 and aba3 mutants in Arabidopsis thaliana. *Plant Physiol.,* **1997**, *114*(1), 161-166.
       [http://dx.doi.org/10.1104/pp.114.1.161] [PMID: 9159947]

[34]   Bittner, F.; Oreb, M.; Mendel, R.R. ABA3 is a molybdenum cofactor sulfurase required for activation of aldehyde oxidase and xanthine dehydrogenase in Arabidopsis thaliana. *J. Biol. Chem.,* **2001**, *276*(44), 40381-40384.
       [http://dx.doi.org/10.1074/jbc.C100472200] [PMID: 11553608]

[35]   Schwartz, S.H.; Qin, X.; Zeevaart, J.A.D. Elucidation of the indirect pathway of abscisic acid biosynthesis by mutants, genes, and enzymes. *Plant Physiol.,* **2003**, *131*(4), 1591-1601.
       [http://dx.doi.org/10.1104/pp.102.017921] [PMID: 12692318]

[36]   Kushiro, T.; Okamoto, M.; Nakabayashi, K.; Yamagishi, K.; Kitamura, S.; Asami, T.; Hirai, N.; Koshiba, T.; Kamiya, Y.; Nambara, E. The Arabidopsis cytochrome P450 CYP707A encodes ABA 8′-hydroxylases: key enzymes in ABA catabolism. *EMBO J.,* **2004**, *23*(7), 1647-1656.
       [http://dx.doi.org/10.1038/sj.emboj.7600121] [PMID: 15044947]

[37]   Setha, S.; Kondo, S.; Hirai, N.; Ohigashi, H. Quantification of ABA and its metabolites in sweet cherries using deuterium–labeled internal standards. *Plant Growth Regul.,* **2005**, *45*, 183-188.
       [http://dx.doi.org/10.1007/s10725-005-3088-7]

[38]   Weng, J.K.; Ye, M.; Li, B.; Noel, J.P. Co–evolution of hormone metabolism and signaling networks expands plant adaptive plasticity. *Cell,* **2016**, *166*(4), 881-893.
       [http://dx.doi.org/10.1016/j.cell.2016.06.027] [PMID: 27518563]

[39]   Huo, H.; Dahal, P.; Kunusoth, K.; McCallum, C.M.; Bradford, K.J. Expression of 9-ci-

-EPOXYCAROTENOID DIOXYGENASE4 is essential for thermoinhibition of lettuce seed germination but not for seed development or stress tolerance. *Plant Cell,* **2013**, *25*(3), 884-900.
[http://dx.doi.org/10.1105/tpc.112.108902] [PMID: 23503626]

[40] Nitsch, L.M.C.; Oplaat, C.; Feron, R.; Ma, Q.; Wolters-Arts, M.; Hedden, P.; Mariani, C.; Vriezen, W.H. Abscisic acid levels in tomato ovaries are regulated by LeNCED1 and SlCYP707A1. *Planta,* **2009**, *229*(6), 1335-1346.
[http://dx.doi.org/10.1007/s00425-009-0913-7] [PMID: 19322584]

[41] Jenkins, J.; Lo Leggio, L.; Harris, G.; Pickersgill, R. Beta-glucosidase, beta-galactosidase, family A cellulases, family F xylanases and two barley glycanases form a superfamily of enzymes with 8-fold beta/alpha architecture and with two conserved glutamates near the carboxy-terminal ends of beta-strands four and seven. *FEBS Lett.,* **1995**, *362*(3), 281-285.
[http://dx.doi.org/10.1016/0014-5793(95)00252-5] [PMID: 7729513]

[42] Liu, Z.; Yan, J.P.; Li, D.K.; Luo, Q.; Yan, Q.; Liu, Z.B.; Ye, L.M.; Wang, J.M.; Li, X.F.; Yang, Y. UDP-glucosyltransferase71c5, a major glucosyltransferase, mediates abscisic acid homeostasis in Arabidopsis. *Plant Physiol.,* **2015**, *167*(4), 1659-1670.
[http://dx.doi.org/10.1104/pp.15.00053] [PMID: 25713337]

[43] Lee, K.H.; Piao, H.L.; Kim, H.Y.; Choi, S.M.; Jiang, F.; Hartung, W.; Hwang, I.; Kwak, J.M.; Lee, I.J.; Hwang, I. Activation of glucosidase via stress-induced polymerization rapidly increases active pools of abscisic acid. *Cell,* **2006**, *126*(6), 1109-1120.
[http://dx.doi.org/10.1016/j.cell.2006.07.034] [PMID: 16990135]

[44] Xu, Z.Y.; Lee, K.H.; Dong, T.; Jeong, J.C.; Jin, J.B.; Kanno, Y.; Kim, D.H.; Kim, S.Y.; Seo, M.; Bressan, R.A.; Yun, D.J.; Hwang, I. A vacuolar β-glucosidase homolog that possesses glucose-conjugated abscisic acid hydrolyzing activity plays an important role in osmotic stress responses in Arabidopsis. *Plant Cell,* **2012**, *24*(5), 2184-2199.
[http://dx.doi.org/10.1105/tpc.112.095935] [PMID: 22582100]

[45] Antoni, R.; Gonzalez-Guzman, M.; Rodriguez, L.; Peirats-Llobet, M.; Pizzio, G.A.; Fernandez, M.A.; De Winne, N.; De Jaeger, G.; Dietrich, D.; Bennett, M.J.; Rodriguez, P.L. PYRABACTIN RESISTANCE1-LIKE8 plays an important role for the regulation of abscisic acid signaling in root. *Plant Physiol.,* **2013**, *161*(2), 931-941.
[http://dx.doi.org/10.1104/pp.112.208678] [PMID: 23370718]

[46] Li, J.; Assmann, S.M. An abscisic acid–activated and calcium–independent protein kinase from guard cells of fava bean. *Plant Cell,* **1996**, *8*(12), 2359-2368.
[http://dx.doi.org/10.2307/3870474] [PMID: 12239380]

[47] Umezawa, T.; Sugiyama, N.; Mizoguchi, M.; Hayashi, S.; Myouga, F.; Yamaguchi-Shinozaki, K.; Ishihama, Y.; Hirayama, T.; Shinozaki, K. Type 2C protein phosphatases directly regulate abscisic acid-activated protein kinases in Arabidopsis. *Proc. Natl. Acad. Sci. USA,* **2009**, *106*(41), 17588-17593.
[http://dx.doi.org/10.1073/pnas.0907095106] [PMID: 19805022]

[48] Hubbard, K.E.; Nishimura, N.; Hitomi, K.; Getzoff, E.D.; Schroeder, J.I. Early abscisic acid signal transduction mechanisms: newly discovered components and newly emerging questions. *Genes Dev.,* **2010**, *24*(16), 1695-1708.
[http://dx.doi.org/10.1101/gad.1953910] [PMID: 20713515]

[49] Weiner, J.J.; Peterson, F.C.; Volkman, B.F.; Cutler, S.R. Structural and functional insights into core ABA signaling. *Curr. Opin. Plant Biol.,* **2010**, *13*(5), 495-502.
[http://dx.doi.org/10.1016/j.pbi.2010.09.007] [PMID: 20934900]

[50] Choi, H.; Hong, J.; Ha, J.; Kang, J.; Kim, S.Y. ABFs, a family of ABA-responsive element binding factors. *J. Biol. Chem.,* **2000**, *275*(3), 1723-1730.
[http://dx.doi.org/10.1074/jbc.275.3.1723] [PMID: 10636868]

[51] Yoshida, T.; Fujita, Y.; Maruyama, K.; Mogami, J.; Todaka, D.; Shinozaki, K.; Yamaguchi-Shinozaki,

K. Four Arabidopsis AREB/ABF transcription factors function predominantly in gene expression downstream of SnRK2 kinases in abscisic acid signalling in response to osmotic stress. *Plant Cell Environ.,* **2015**, *38*(1), 35-49.
[http://dx.doi.org/10.1111/pce.12351] [PMID: 24738645]

[52]   Yin, P.; Fan, H.; Hao, Q.; Yuan, X.; Wu, D.; Pang, Y.; Yan, C.; Li, W.; Wang, J.; Yan, N. Structural insights into the mechanism of abscisic acid signaling by PYL proteins. *Nat. Struct. Mol. Biol.,* **2009**, *16*(12), 1230-1236.
[http://dx.doi.org/10.1038/nsmb.1730] [PMID: 19893533]

[53]   Santiago, J.; Dupeux, F.; Round, A.; Antoni, R.; Park, S.Y.; Jamin, M.; Cutler, S.R.; Rodriguez, P.L.; Márquez, J.A. The abscisic acid receptor PYR1 in complex with abscisic acid. *Nature,* **2009**, *462*(7273), 665-668.
[http://dx.doi.org/10.1038/nature08591] [PMID: 19898494]

[54]   Wang, B.; Li, C.; Kong, X.; Li, Y.; Liu, Z.; Wang, J.; Li, X.; Yang, Y. AtARRE, an E3 ubiquitin ligase, negatively regulates ABA signaling in Arabidopsis thaliana. *Plant Cell Rep.,* **2018**, *37*(9), 1269-1278.
[http://dx.doi.org/10.1007/s00299-018-2311-8] [PMID: 29947951]

[55]   Li, D.; Mou, W.; Xia, R.; Li, L.; Zawora, C.; Ying, T.; Mao, L.; Liu, Z.; Luo, Z. Integrated analysis of high-throughput sequencing data shows abscisic acid-responsive genes and miRNAs in strawberry receptacle fruit ripening. *Hortic. Res.,* **2019**, *6*, 26.
[http://dx.doi.org/10.1038/s41438-018-0100-8] [PMID: 30729016]

[56]   Zhu, J.K. Abiotic Stress Signaling and Responses in Plants. *Cell,* **2016**, *167*(2), 313-324.
[http://dx.doi.org/10.1016/j.cell.2016.08.029] [PMID: 27716505]

[57]   Cai, Z.; Liu, J.; Wang, H.; Yang, C.; Chen, Y.; Li, Y.; Pan, S.; Dong, R.; Tang, G.; Barajas-Lopez, Jde.D.; Fujii, H.; Wang, X. GSK3-like kinases positively modulate abscisic acid signaling through phosphorylating subgroup III SnRK2s in Arabidopsis. *Proc. Natl. Acad. Sci. USA,* **2014**, *111*(26), 9651-9656.
[http://dx.doi.org/10.1073/pnas.1316717111] [PMID: 24928519]

[58]   Wang, P.; Du, Y.; Hou, Y.J.; Zhao, Y.; Hsu, C.C.; Yuan, F.; Zhu, X.; Tao, W.A.; Song, C.P.; Zhu, J.K. Nitric oxide negatively regulates abscisic acid signaling in guard cells by S-nitrosylation of OST1. *Proc. Natl. Acad. Sci. USA,* **2015**, *112*(2), 613-618.
[http://dx.doi.org/10.1073/pnas.1423481112] [PMID: 25550508]

[59]   Zhao, M.; Li, Q.; Chen, Z.; Lv, Q.; Bao, F.; Wang, X.; He, Y. Regulatory Mechanism of ABA and ABI3 on Vegetative Development in the Moss *Physcomitrella patens. Int. J. Mol. Sci.,* **2018**, *19*(9), E2728.
[http://dx.doi.org/10.3390/ijms19092728] [PMID: 30213069]

[60]   Han, Y.; Dang, R.; Li, J.; Jiang, J.; Zhang, N.; Jia, M.; Wei, L.; Li, Z.; Li, B.; Jia, W. SUCROSE NONFERMENTING1-RELATED PROTEIN KINASE2.6, an ortholog of OPEN STOMATA1, is a negative regulator of strawberry fruit development and ripening. *Plant Physiol.,* **2015**, *167*(3), 915-930.
[http://dx.doi.org/10.1104/pp.114.251314] [PMID: 25609556]

[61]   Burbidge, A.; Grieve, T.M.; Jackson, A.; Thompson, A.; McCarty, D.R.; Taylor, I.B. Characterization of the ABA-deficient tomato mutant notabilis and its relationship with maize Vp14. *Plant J.,* **1999**, *17*(4), 427-431.
[http://dx.doi.org/10.1046/j.1365-313X.1999.00386.x] [PMID: 10205899]

[62]   Saito, S.; Hirai, N.; Matsumoto, C.; Ohigashi, H.; Ohta, D.; Sakata, K.; Mizutani, M. Arabidopsis CYP707As encode (+)-abscisic acid 8′-hydroxylase, a key enzyme in the oxidative catabolism of abscisic acid. *Plant Physiol.,* **2004**, *134*(4), 1439-1449.
[http://dx.doi.org/10.1104/pp.103.037614] [PMID: 15064374]

[63]   Sato, S.; Tabata, S.; Hirakawa, H. The tomato genome sequence provides insights into fleshy fruit

evolution. *Nature,* **2012**, *485*(7400), 635-641.
[http://dx.doi.org/10.1038/nature11119] [PMID: 22660326]

[64] Ji, K.; Kai, W.; Zhao, B.; Sun, Y.; Yuan, B.; Dai, S.; Li, Q.; Chen, P.; Wang, Y.; Pei, Y.; Wang, H.; Guo, Y.; Leng, P. SlNCED1 and SlCYP707A2: key genes involved in ABA metabolism during tomato fruit ripening. *J. Exp. Bot.,* **2014**, *65*(18), 5243-5255.
[http://dx.doi.org/10.1093/jxb/eru288] [PMID: 25039074]

[65] Galpaz, N.; Wang, Q.; Menda, N.; Zamir, D.; Hirschberg, J. Abscisic acid deficiency in the tomato mutant high-pigment 3 leading to increased plastid number and higher fruit lycopene content. *Plant J.,* **2008**, *53*(5), 717-730.
[http://dx.doi.org/10.1111/j.1365-313X.2007.03362.x] [PMID: 17988221]

[66] Sun, L.; Sun, Y.; Zhang, M.; Wang, L.; Ren, J.; Cui, M.; Wang, Y.; Ji, K.; Li, P.; Li, Q.; Chen, P.; Dai, S.; Duan, C.; Wu, Y.; Leng, P. Suppression of 9-cis-epoxycarotenoid dioxygenase, which encodes a key enzyme in abscisic acid biosynthesis, alters fruit texture in transgenic tomato. *Plant Physiol.,* **2012**, *158*(1), 283-298.
[http://dx.doi.org/10.1104/pp.111.186866] [PMID: 22108525]

[67] Dai, S.; Kai, W.; Liang, B.; Wang, J.; Jiang, L.; Du, Y.; Sun, Y.; Leng, P. The functional analysis of SlNCED1 in tomato pollen development. *Cell. Mol. Life Sci.,* **2018**, *75*(18), 3457-3472.
[http://dx.doi.org/10.1007/s00018-018-2809-9] [PMID: 29632966]

[68] Kai, W.B.; Wang, J.; Liang, B. Role of an ABA receptor SlPYL9 in tomato fruit ripening. *J. Exp. Bot.,* **2019**, *70*, 6305-6319.
[http://dx.doi.org/10.1093/jxb/erz396] [PMID: 31504753]

[69] Umezawa, T.; Okamoto, M.; Kushiro, T.; Nambara, E.; Oono, Y.; Seki, M.; Kobayashi, M.; Koshiba, T.; Kamiya, Y.; Shinozaki, K. CYP707A3, a major ABA 8'-hydroxylase involved in dehydration and rehydration response in Arabidopsis thaliana. *Plant J.,* **2006**, *46*(2), 171-182.
[http://dx.doi.org/10.1111/j.1365-313X.2006.02683.x] [PMID: 16623881]

[70] Brzobohatý, B.; Moore, I.; Kristoffersen, P.; Bako, L.; Campos, N.; Schell, J.; Palme, K. Release of active cytokinin by a beta-glucosidase localized to the maize root meristem. *Science,* **1993**, *262*(5136), 1051-1054.
[http://dx.doi.org/10.1126/science.8235622] [PMID: 8235622]

[71] Liang, B.; Zheng, Y.; Wang, J.; Zhang, W.; Fu, Y.; Kai, W.; Xu, Y.; Yuan, B.; Li, Q.; Leng, P. Overexpression of the persimmon abscisic acid β-glucosidase gene (DkBG1) alters fruit ripening in transgenic tomato. *Plant J.,* **2020**, *102*(6), 1220-1233.
[http://dx.doi.org/10.1111/tpj.14695] [PMID: 31960511]

[72] Sun, L.; Zhang, M.; Ren, J.; Qi, J.; Zhang, G.; Leng, P. Reciprocity between abscisic acid and ethylene at the onset of berry ripening and after harvest. *BMC Plant Biol.,* **2010**, *10*, 257.
[http://dx.doi.org/10.1186/1471-2229-10-257] [PMID: 21092180]

[73] Li, Q.; Ji, K.; Sun, Y.; Luo, H.; Wang, H.; Leng, P. The role of FaBG3 in fruit ripening and B. cinerea fungal infection of strawberry. *Plant J.,* **2013**, *76*(1), 24-35.
[PMID: 23802911]

[74] Liu, Z.; Yan, J.P.; Li, D.K.; Luo, Q.; Yan, Q.; Liu, Z.B.; Ye, L.M.; Wang, J.M.; Li, X.F.; Yang, Y. UDP-glucosyltransferase71c5, a major glucosyltransferase, mediates abscisic acid homeostasis in Arabidopsis. *Plant Physiol.,* **2015**, *167*(4), 1659-1670.
[http://dx.doi.org/10.1104/pp.15.00053] [PMID: 25713337]

[75] Tikunov, Y.M.; Molthoff, J.; de Vos, R.C.; Beekwilder, J.; van Houwelingen, A.; van der Hooft, J.J.; Nijenhuis-de Vries, M.; Labrie, C.W.; Verkerke, W.; van de Geest, H.; Viquez Zamora, M.; Presa, S.; Rambla, J.L.; Granell, A.; Hall, R.D.; Bovy, A.G. Non-smoky glycosyltransferase1 prevents the release of smoky aroma from tomato fruit. *Plant Cell,* **2013**, *25*(8), 3067-3078.
[http://dx.doi.org/10.1105/tpc.113.114231] [PMID: 23956261]

[76] Sun, Y.; Ji, K.; Liang, B.; Du, Y.; Jiang, L.; Wang, J.; Kai, W.; Zhang, Y.; Zhai, X.; Chen, P.; Wang,

H.; Leng, P. Suppressing ABA uridine diphosphate glucosyltransferase (SlUGT75C1) alters fruit ripening and the stress response in tomato. *Plant J.,* **2017**, *91*(4), 574-589.
[http://dx.doi.org/10.1111/tpj.13588] [PMID: 28482127]

[77]   Wang, Y.T.; Chen, Z.Y.; Jiang, Y. Involvement of ABA and antioxidant system in brassinosteroid–induced water stress tolerance of grapevine (Vitis vinifera L.). *Sci. Hortic. (Amsterdam),* **2019**, 256.
[http://dx.doi.org/10.1016/j.scienta.2019.108596]

[78]   Trainotti, L.; Pavanello, A.; Casadoro, G. Different ethylene receptors show an increased expression during the ripening of strawberries: does such an increment imply a role for ethylene in the ripening of these non-climacteric fruits? *J. Exp. Bot.,* **2005**, *56*(418), 2037-2046.
[http://dx.doi.org/10.1093/jxb/eri202] [PMID: 15955790]

[79]   Villarreal, N.M.; Rosli, H.G.; Martínez, G.A. Polygalacturonase activity and expression of related genes during ripening of strawberry cultivars with con– trasting fruit firmness. *Postharvest Biol. Technol.,* **2008**, *47*, 141-150.
[http://dx.doi.org/10.1016/j.postharvbio.2007.06.011]

[80]   Sun, Y.F.; Chen, P.; Duan, C.R. Transcriptional regulation of genes encoding key enzymes of abscisic acid metabolism during melon (Cucumis melo L.) fruit development and ripening. *J. Plant Growth Regul.,* **2013**, *32*, 233-244.
[http://dx.doi.org/10.1007/s00344-012-9293-5]

[81]   Seymour, G.B.; Østergaard, L.; Chapman, N.H.; Knapp, S.; Martin, C. Fruit development and ripening. *Annu. Rev. Plant Biol.,* **2013**, *64*, 219-241.
[http://dx.doi.org/10.1146/annurev-arplant-050312-120057] [PMID: 23394500]

[82]   Deng, Y.; Lu, S. Biosynthesis and regulation of phenylpropanoids in plants. *Crit. Rev. Plant Sci.,* **2017**, *36*, 257-290.
[http://dx.doi.org/10.1080/07352689.2017.1402852]

[83]   Vighi, I.L.; Crizel, R.L.; Perin, E.C. Crosstalk during fruit ripening and stress response among abscisic acid, calcium–dependent protein kinase and phenylpropanoid. *Crit. Rev. Plant Sci.,* **2019**, *38*, 99-116.
[http://dx.doi.org/10.1080/07352689.2019.1602959]

[84]   Ren, J.; Chen, P.; Dai, S.J. Role of abscisic acid and ethylene in. sweet cherry fruit maturation: molecular aspects. *N. Z. J. Crop Hortic. Sci.,* **2011**, *39*, 1-14.
[http://dx.doi.org/10.1080/01140671.2011.563424]

[85]   Shen, X.; Zhao, K.; Liu, L.; Zhang, K.; Yuan, H.; Liao, X.; Wang, Q.; Guo, X.; Li, F.; Li, T. A role for PacMYBA in ABA-regulated anthocyanin biosynthesis in red-colored sweet cherry cv. Hong Deng (Prunus avium L.). *Plant Cell Physiol.,* **2014**, *55*(5), 862-880.
[http://dx.doi.org/10.1093/pcp/pcu013] [PMID: 24443499]

[86]   Li, X.; Kong, X.; Huang, Q.; Zhang, Q.; Ge, H.; Zhang, L.; Li, G.; Peng, L.; Liu, Z.; Wang, J.; Li, X.; Yang, Y. CARK1 phosphorylates subfamily III members of ABA receptors. *J. Exp. Bot.,* **2019**, *70*(2), 519-528.
[http://dx.doi.org/10.1093/jxb/ery374] [PMID: 30380101]

[87]   Saez, A.; Robert, N.; Maktabi, M.H.; Schroeder, J.I.; Serrano, R.; Rodriguez, P.L. Enhancement of abscisic acid sensitivity and reduction of water consumption in Arabidopsis by combined inactivation of the protein phosphatases type 2C ABI1 and HAB1. *Plant Physiol.,* **2006**, *141*(4), 1389-1399.
[http://dx.doi.org/10.1104/pp.106.081018] [PMID: 16798945]

[88]   Santiago, J.; Rodrigues, A.; Saez, A.; Rubio, S.; Antoni, R.; Dupeux, F.; Park, S.Y.; Márquez, J.A.; Cutler, S.R.; Rodriguez, P.L. Modulation of drought resistance by the abscisic acid receptor PYL5 through inhibition of clade A PP2Cs. *Plant J.,* **2009**, *60*(4), 575-588.
[http://dx.doi.org/10.1111/j.1365-313X.2009.03981.x] [PMID: 19624469]

[89]   Hauser, F.; Waadt, R.; Schroeder, J.I. Evolution of abscisic acid synthesis and signaling mechanisms. *Curr. Biol.,* **2011**, *21*(9), R346-R355.

[http://dx.doi.org/10.1016/j.cub.2011.03.015] [PMID: 21549957]

[90] Gonzalez-Guzman, M.; Pizzio, G.A.; Antoni, R.; Vera-Sirera, F.; Merilo, E.; Bassel, G.W.; Fernández, M.A.; Holdsworth, M.J.; Perez-Amador, M.A.; Kollist, H.; Rodriguez, P.L. Arabidopsis PYR/PYL/RCAR receptors play a major role in quantitative regulation of stomatal aperture and transcriptional response to abscisic acid. *Plant Cell,* **2012**, *24*(6), 2483-2496.
[http://dx.doi.org/10.1105/tpc.112.098574] [PMID: 22739828]

[91] Chen, P.; Pei, Y.L.; Liang, B. Role of abscisic acid in regulating fruit set and ripening in squash (Cucurbita pepo L.). *N. Z. J. Crop Hortic. Sci.,* **2016**, *44*, 274-290.
[http://dx.doi.org/10.1080/01140671.2016.1212907]

[92] Mosquna, A.; Peterson, F.C.; Park, S.Y.; Lozano-Juste, J.; Volkman, B.F.; Cutler, S.R. Potent and selective activation of abscisic acid receptors *in vivo* by mutational stabilization of their agonist-bound conformation. *Proc. Natl. Acad. Sci. USA,* **2011**, *108*(51), 20838-20843.
[http://dx.doi.org/10.1073/pnas.1112838108] [PMID: 22139369]

[93] Pizzio, G.A.; Rodriguez, L.; Antoni, R.; Gonzalez-Guzman, M.; Yunta, C.; Merilo, E.; Kollist, H.; Albert, A.; Rodriguez, P.L. The PYL4 A194T mutant uncovers a key role of PYR1-LIKE4/PROTEIN PHOSPHATASE 2CA interaction for abscisic acid signaling and plant drought resistance. *Plant Physiol.,* **2013**, *163*(1), 441-455.
[http://dx.doi.org/10.1104/pp.113.224162] [PMID: 23864556]

[94] Zhang, Y.; Li, Q.; Jiang, L.; Kai, W.; Liang, B.; Wang, J.; Du, Y.; Zhai, X.; Wang, J.; Zhang, Y.; Sun, Y.; Zhang, L.; Leng, P. Suppressing type 2C protein phosphatases alters fruit ripening and the stress response in tomato. *Plant Cell Physiol.,* **2018**, *59*(1), 142-154.
[http://dx.doi.org/10.1093/pcp/pcx169] [PMID: 29121241]

[95] Tischer, S.V.; Wunschel, C.; Papacek, M.; Kleigrewe, K.; Hofmann, T.; Christmann, A.; Grill, E. Combinatorial interaction network of abscisic acid receptors and coreceptors from *Arabidopsis thaliana. Proc. Natl. Acad. Sci. USA,* **2017**, *114*(38), 10280-10285.
[http://dx.doi.org/10.1073/pnas.1706593114] [PMID: 28874521]

[96] Yang, Z.; Liu, J.; Tischer, S.V.; Christmann, A.; Windisch, W.; Schnyder, H.; Grill, E. Leveraging abscisic acid receptors for efficient water use in Arabidopsis. *Proc. Natl. Acad. Sci. USA,* **2016**, *113*(24), 6791-6796.
[http://dx.doi.org/10.1073/pnas.1601954113] [PMID: 27247417]

[97] Giovannoni, J.J. Genetic regulation of fruit development and ripening. *Plant Cell,* **2004**, *16* Suppl., S170-S180.
[http://dx.doi.org/10.1105/tpc.019158] [PMID: 15010516]

[98] Orellana, S.; Yañez, M.; Espinoza, A.; Verdugo, I.; González, E.; Ruiz-Lara, S.; Casaretto, J.A. The transcription factor SlAREB1 confers drought, salt stress tolerance and regulates biotic and abiotic stress-related genes in tomato. *Plant Cell Environ.,* **2010**, *33*(12), 2191-2208.
[http://dx.doi.org/10.1111/j.1365-3040.2010.02220.x] [PMID: 20807374]

[99] Fujita, Y.; Yoshida, T.; Yamaguchi-Shinozaki, K. Pivotal role of the AREB/ABF-SnRK2 pathway in ABRE-mediated transcription in response to osmotic stress in plants. *Physiol. Plant.,* **2013**, *147*(1), 15-27.
[http://dx.doi.org/10.1111/j.1399-3054.2012.01635.x] [PMID: 22519646]

[100] Bastías, A.; López-Climent, M.; Valcárcel, M.; Rosello, S.; Gómez-Cadenas, A.; Casaretto, J.A. Modulation of organic acids and sugar content in tomato fruits by an abscisic acid-regulated transcription factor. *Physiol. Plant.,* **2011**, *141*(3), 215-226.
[http://dx.doi.org/10.1111/j.1399-3054.2010.01435.x] [PMID: 21128945]

[101] Yáñez, M.; Cáceres, S.; Orellana, S.; Bastías, A.; Verdugo, I.; Ruiz-Lara, S.; Casaretto, J.A. An abiotic stress-responsive bZIP transcription factor from wild and cultivated tomatoes regulates stress-related genes. *Plant Cell Rep.,* **2009**, *28*(10), 1497-1507.
[http://dx.doi.org/10.1007/s00299-009-0749-4] [PMID: 19652975]

[102] Bastías, A.; Yañez, M.; Osorio, S.; Arbona, V.; Gómez-Cadenas, A.; Fernie, A.R.; Casaretto, J.A. The transcription factor AREB1 regulates primary metabolic pathways in tomato fruits. *J. Exp. Bot.,* **2014**, *65*(9), 2351-2363.
[http://dx.doi.org/10.1093/jxb/eru114] [PMID: 24659489]

[103] Chervin, C.; Tira-Umphon, A.; Terrier, N.; Zouine, M.; Severac, D.; Roustan, J.P. Stimulation of the grape berry expansion by ethylene and effects on related gene transcripts, over the ripening phase. *Physiol. Plant.,* **2008**, *134*(3), 534-546.
[http://dx.doi.org/10.1111/j.1399-3054.2008.01158.x] [PMID: 18785902]

[104] Gapper, N.E.; McQuinn, R.P.; Giovannoni, J.J. Molecular and genetic regulation of fruit ripening. *Plant Mol. Biol.,* **2013**, *82*(6), 575-591.
[http://dx.doi.org/10.1007/s11103-013-0050-3] [PMID: 23585213]

[105] Vrebalov, J.; Ruezinsky, D.; Padmanabhan, V.; White, R.; Medrano, D.; Drake, R.; Schuch, W.; Giovannoni, J. A MADS-box gene necessary for fruit ripening at the tomato ripening-inhibitor (rin) locus. *Science,* **2002**, *296*(5566), 343-346.
[http://dx.doi.org/10.1126/science.1068181] [PMID: 11951045]

[106] Vrebalov, J.; Pan, I.L.; Arroyo, A.J.M.; McQuinn, R.; Chung, M.; Poole, M.; Rose, J.; Seymour, G.; Grandillo, S.; Giovannoni, J.; Irish, V.F. Fleshy fruit expansion and ripening are regulated by the Tomato SHATTERPROOF gene TAGL1. *Plant Cell,* **2009**, *21*(10), 3041-3062.
[http://dx.doi.org/10.1105/tpc.109.066936] [PMID: 19880793]

[107] Manning, K.; Tör, M.; Poole, M.; Hong, Y.; Thompson, A.J.; King, G.J.; Giovannoni, J.J.; Seymour, G.B. A naturally occurring epigenetic mutation in a gene encoding an SBP-box transcription factor inhibits tomato fruit ripening. *Nat. Genet.,* **2006**, *38*(8), 948-952.
[http://dx.doi.org/10.1038/ng1841] [PMID: 16832354]

[108] Lin, Z.; Hong, Y.; Yin, M.; Li, C.; Zhang, K.; Grierson, D. A tomato HD-Zip homeobox protein, LeHB-1, plays an important role in floral organogenesis and ripening. *Plant J.,* **2008**, *55*(2), 301-310.
[http://dx.doi.org/10.1111/j.1365-313X.2008.03505.x] [PMID: 18397374]

[109] Itkin, M.; Seybold, H.; Breitel, D.; Rogachev, I.; Meir, S.; Aharoni, A. TOMATO AGAMOUS-LIKE 1 is a component of the fruit ripening regulatory network. *Plant J.,* **2009**, *60*(6), 1081-1095.
[http://dx.doi.org/10.1111/j.1365-313X.2009.04064.x] [PMID: 19891701]

[110] Chung, M.Y.; Vrebalov, J.; Alba, R.; Lee, J.; McQuinn, R.; Chung, J.D.; Klein, P.; Giovannoni, J. A tomato (Solanum lycopersicum) APETALA2/ERF gene, SlAP2a, is a negative regulator of fruit ripening. *Plant J.,* **2010**, *64*(6), 936-947.
[http://dx.doi.org/10.1111/j.1365-313X.2010.04384.x] [PMID: 21143675]

[111] Bemer, M.; Karlova, R.; Ballester, A.R.; Tikunov, Y.M.; Bovy, A.G.; Wolters-Arts, M.; Rossetto, Pde.B.; Angenent, G.C.; de Maagd, R.A. The tomato FRUITFULL homologs TDR4/FUL1 and MBP7/FUL2 regulate ethylene-independent aspects of fruit ripening. *Plant Cell,* **2012**, *24*(11), 4437-4451.
[http://dx.doi.org/10.1105/tpc.112.103283] [PMID: 23136376]

[112] Su, L.; Diretto, G.; Purgatto, E.; Danoun, S.; Zouine, M.; Li, Z.; Roustan, J.P.; Bouzayen, M.; Giuliano, G.; Chervin, C. Carotenoid accumulation during tomato fruit ripening is modulated by the auxin-ethylene balance. *BMC Plant Biol.,* **2015**, *15*, 114.
[http://dx.doi.org/10.1186/s12870-015-0495-4] [PMID: 25953041]

[113] Yokotani, N.; Tamura, S.; Nakano, R. Comparison of ethylene– and wound–induced responses in fruit of wild–type, rin and nor tomatoes. *Postharvest Biol. Technol.,* **2004**, *32*, 247-252.
[http://dx.doi.org/10.1016/j.postharvbio.2004.01.001]

[114] Martel, C.; Vrebalov, J.; Tafelmeyer, P.; Giovannoni, J.J. The tomato MADS-box transcription factor RIPENING INHIBITOR interacts with promoters involved in numerous ripening processes in a COLORLESS NONRIPENING-dependent manner. *Plant Physiol.,* **2011**, *157*(3), 1568-1579.
[http://dx.doi.org/10.1104/pp.111.181107] [PMID: 21941001]

[115] Breitel, D.A.; Chappell-Maor, L.; Meir, S.; Panizel, I.; Puig, C.P.; Hao, Y.; Yifhar, T.; Yasuor, H.; Zouine, M.; Bouzayen, M.; Granell Richart, A.; Rogachev, I.; Aharoni, A. AUXIN RESPONSE FACTOR 2 Intersects Hormonal Signals in the Regulation of Tomato Fruit Ripening. *PLoS Genet.,* **2016,** *12*(3), e1005903.
[http://dx.doi.org/10.1371/journal.pgen.1005903] [PMID: 26959229]

[116] Ríos, P.; Argyris, J.; Vegas, J.; Leida, C.; Kenigswald, M.; Tzuri, G.; Troadec, C.; Bendahmane, A.; Katzir, N.; Picó, B.; Monforte, A.J.; Garcia-Mas, J. ETHQV6.3 is involved in melon climacteric fruit ripening and is encoded by a NAC domain transcription factor. *Plant J.,* **2017,** *91*(4), 671-683.
[http://dx.doi.org/10.1111/tpj.13596] [PMID: 28493311]

[117] Ma, X.; Zhang, Y.; Turečková, V.; Xue, G.P.; Fernie, A.R.; Mueller-Roeber, B.; Balazadeh, S. The NAC transcription factor SLNAP2 regulates leaf senescence and fruit yield in tomato. *Plant Physiol.,* **2018,** *177*(3), 1286-1302.
[http://dx.doi.org/10.1104/pp.18.00292] [PMID: 29760199]

[118] Kou, X.; Zhao, Y.; Wu, C. SNAC4 and SNAC9 transcription factors show contrasting effects on tomato carotenoids biosynthesis and softening. *Postharvest Biol. Technol.,* **2018,** *144*, 9-19.
[http://dx.doi.org/10.1016/j.postharvbio.2018.05.008]

[119] Nicolas, P.; Lecourieux, D.; Kappel, C.; Cluzet, S.; Cramer, G.; Delrot, S.; Lecourieux, F. The basic leucine zipper transcription factor ABSCISIC ACID RESPONSE ELEMENT-BINDING FACTOR2 is an important transcriptional regulator of abscisic acid-dependent grape berry ripening processes. *Plant Physiol.,* **2014,** *164*(1), 365-383.
[http://dx.doi.org/10.1104/pp.113.231977] [PMID: 24276949]

[120] Nijhawan, A.; Jain, M.; Tyagi, A.K.; Khurana, J.P. Genomic survey and gene expression analysis of the basic leucine zipper transcription factor family in rice. *Plant Physiol.,* **2008,** *146*(2), 333-350.
[http://dx.doi.org/10.1104/pp.107.112821] [PMID: 18065552]

[121] Medina-Puche, L.; Cumplido-Laso, G.; Amil-Ruiz, F.; Hoffmann, T.; Ring, L.; Rodríguez-Franco, A.; Caballero, J.L.; Schwab, W.; Muñoz-Blanco, J.; Blanco-Portales, R. MYB10 plays a major role in the regulation of flavonoid/phenylpropanoid metabolism during ripening of Fragaria x ananassa fruits. *J. Exp. Bot.,* **2014,** *65*(2), 401-417.
[http://dx.doi.org/10.1093/jxb/ert377] [PMID: 24277278]

[122] Feng, Y.M.; We, X.K.; Liao, W.X. Molecular analysis of the. annexin gene family in soybean. *Biol. Plant.,* **2013,** *57*, 655-662.
[http://dx.doi.org/10.1007/s10535-013-0334-0]

[123] Fraser, P.D.; Enfissi, E.M.; Halket, J.M.; Truesdale, M.R.; Yu, D.; Gerrish, C.; Bramley, P.M. Manipulation of phytoene levels in tomato fruit: effects on isoprenoids, plastids, and intermediary metabolism. *Plant Cell,* **2007,** *19*(10), 3194-3211.
[http://dx.doi.org/10.1105/tpc.106.049817] [PMID: 17933904]

[124] Kachanovsky, D.E.; Filler, S.; Isaacson, T.; Hirschberg, J. Epistasis in tomato color mutations involves regulation of phytoene synthase 1 expression by cis-carotenoids. *Proc. Natl. Acad. Sci. USA,* **2012,** *109*(46), 19021-19026.
[http://dx.doi.org/10.1073/pnas.1214808109] [PMID: 23112190]

[125] Diretto, G; Frusciante, S Manipulation of b–carotene levels in tomato fruits results in increased ABA content and extended shelf life. *Plant Biotechnol. J.,* **2019,** 1-15.
[PMID: 31646753]

[126] Kolotilin, I.; Koltai, H.; Tadmor, Y.; Bar-Or, C.; Reuveni, M.; Meir, A.; Nahon, S.; Shlomo, H.; Chen, L.; Levin, I. Transcriptional profiling of high pigment-2dg tomato mutant links early fruit plastid biogenesis with its overproduction of phytonutrients. *Plant Physiol.,* **2007,** *145*(2), 389-401.
[http://dx.doi.org/10.1104/pp.107.102962] [PMID: 17704236]

[127] Hörtensteiner, S. Stay-green regulates chlorophyll and chlorophyll-binding protein degradation during senescence. *Trends Plant Sci.,* **2009,** *14*(3), 155-162.

[http://dx.doi.org/10.1016/j.tplants.2009.01.002] [PMID: 19237309]

[128] Lacampagne, S.; Gagne, S.; Geny, L. Involvement of abscisic acid in controlling the proanthocyanidin biosynthesis pathway in grape skin. *J. Plant Growth Regul.,* **2009**, *29*, 81-90.
[http://dx.doi.org/10.1007/s00344-009-9115-6]

[129] Karppinen, K.; Hirvelä, E.; Nevala, T.; Sipari, N.; Suokas, M.; Jaakola, L. Changes in the abscisic acid levels and related gene expression during fruit development and ripening in bilberry (Vaccinium myrtillus L.). *Phytochemistry,* **2013**, *95*, 127-134.
[http://dx.doi.org/10.1016/j.phytochem.2013.06.023] [PMID: 23850079]

[130] Koyama, K.; Sadamatsu, K.; Goto-Yamamoto, N. Abscisic acid stimulated ripening and gene expression in berry skins of the Cabernet Sauvignon grape. *Funct. Integr. Genomics,* **2010**, *10*(3), 367-381.
[http://dx.doi.org/10.1007/s10142-009-0145-8] [PMID: 19841954]

[131] Carpita, N.C.; Gibeaut, D.M. Structural models of primary cell walls in flowering plants: consistency of molecular structure with the physical properties of the walls during growth. *Plant J.,* **1993**, *3*(1), 1-30.
[http://dx.doi.org/10.1111/j.1365-313X.1993.tb00007.x] [PMID: 8401598]

[132] Uluisik, S.; Chapman, N.H.; Smith, R.; Poole, M.; Adams, G.; Gillis, R.B.; Besong, T.M.; Sheldon, J.; Stiegelmeyer, S.; Perez, L.; Samsulrizal, N.; Wang, D.; Fisk, I.D.; Yang, N.; Baxter, C.; Rickett, D.; Fray, R.; Blanco-Ulate, B.; Powell, A.L.; Harding, S.E.; Craigon, J.; Rose, J.K.; Fich, E.A.; Sun, L.; Domozych, D.S.; Fraser, P.D.; Tucker, G.A.; Grierson, D.; Seymour, G.B. Genetic improvement of tomato by targeted control of fruit softening. *Nat. Biotechnol.,* **2016**, *34*(9), 950-952.
[http://dx.doi.org/10.1038/nbt.3602] [PMID: 27454737]

[133] Cosgrove, D.J. Expansive growth of plant cell walls. *Plant Physiol. Biochem.,* **2000**, *38*(1-2), 109-124.
[http://dx.doi.org/10.1016/S0981-9428(00)00164-9] [PMID: 11543185]

[134] Nishiyama, K.; Guis, M.; Rose, J.K.C.; Kubo, Y.; Bennett, K.A.; Wangjin, L.; Kato, K.; Ushijima, K.; Nakano, R.; Inaba, A.; Bouzayen, M.; Latche, A.; Pech, J.C.; Bennett, A.B. Ethylene regulation of fruit softening and cell wall disassembly in Charentais melon. *J. Exp. Bot.,* **2007**, *58*(6), 1281-1290.
[http://dx.doi.org/10.1093/jxb/erl283] [PMID: 17308329]

[135] van der Knaap, E.; Chakrabarti, M.; Chu, Y.H.; Clevenger, J.P.; Illa-Berenguer, E.; Huang, Z.; Keyhaninejad, N.; Mu, Q.; Sun, L.; Wang, Y.; Wu, S. What lies beyond the eye: the molecular mechanisms regulating tomato fruit weight and shape. *Front. Plant Sci.,* **2014**, *5*, 227.
[http://dx.doi.org/10.3389/fpls.2014.00227] [PMID: 24904622]

[136] Xu, K.K.; Yang, W.J.; Tian, Y.; Wu, Y.B.; Wang, J.J. Insulin signaling pathway in the oriental fruit fly: The role of insulin receptor substrate in ovarian development. *Gen. Comp. Endocrinol.,* **2015**, *216*, 125-133.
[http://dx.doi.org/10.1016/j.ygcen.2014.11.022] [PMID: 25499646]

[137] Tanksley, S.D. The genetic, developmental, and molecular bases of fruit size and shape variation in tomato. *Plant Cell,* **2004**, *16* Suppl., S181-S189.
[http://dx.doi.org/10.1105/tpc.018119] [PMID: 15131251]

[138] Lippman, Z.; Tanksley, S.D. Dissecting the genetic pathway to extreme fruit size in tomato using a cross between the small-fruited wild species Lycopersicon pimpinellifolium and L. esculentum var. Giant Heirloom. *Genetics,* **2001**, *158*(1), 413-422.
[http://dx.doi.org/10.1093/genetics/158.1.413] [PMID: 11333249]

[139] Yamaki, S.; Asakura, T. Stimulation of the uptake of sorbitol into vacuoles from apple fruit flesh by abscisic acid and into protoplasts by indoleacetic acid. *Plant Cell Physiol.,* **1991**, *32*, 315-318.
[http://dx.doi.org/10.1093/oxfordjournals.pcp.a078082]

[140] Kojima, K.; Yamada, Y.; Yamamoto, M. Effects of abscisic acid injection on sugar and organic acid contents of citrus fruit. *Japanese Society for Horticultural Science.,* **1995**, *64*, 17-21.
[http://dx.doi.org/10.2503/jjshs.64.17]

[141]   Finkelstein, R.R.; Gibson, S.I. ABA and sugar interactions regulating development: cross-talk or voices in a crowd? *Curr. Opin. Plant Biol.,* **2002**, *5*(1), 26-32.
[http://dx.doi.org/10.1016/S1369-5266(01)00225-4] [PMID: 11788304]

[142]   Gambetta, G.A.; Matthews, M.A.; Shaghasi, T.H.; McElrone, A.J.; Castellarin, S.D. Sugar and abscisic acid signaling orthologs are activated at the onset of ripening in grape. *Planta,* **2010**, *232*(1), 219-234.
[http://dx.doi.org/10.1007/s00425-010-1165-2] [PMID: 20407788]

[143]   Price, J.; Li, T.C.; Kang, S.G.; Na, J.K.; Jang, J.C. Mechanisms of glucose signaling during germination of Arabidopsis. *Plant Physiol.,* **2003**, *132*(3), 1424-1438.
[http://dx.doi.org/10.1104/pp.103.020347] [PMID: 12857824]

[144]   Kosma, D.K.; Bourdenx, B.; Bernard, A.; Parsons, E.P.; Lü, S.; Joubès, J.; Jenks, M.A. The impact of water deficiency on leaf cuticle lipids of Arabidopsis. *Plant Physiol.,* **2009**, *151*(4), 1918-1929.
[http://dx.doi.org/10.1104/pp.109.141911] [PMID: 19819982]

[145]   Liang, B.; Sun, Y.F.; Wang, J. Tomato Protein Phosphatase 2C (SlPP2C3). influences fruit ripening onset and fruit glossiness. *J. Exp. Bot.,* **2021**.
[http://dx.doi.org/10.1093/jxb/eraa593]

[146]   Seo, P.J.; Lee, S.B.; Suh, M.C.; Park, M.J.; Go, Y.S.; Park, C.M. The MYB96 transcription factor regulates cuticular wax biosynthesis under drought conditions in Arabidopsis. *Plant Cell,* **2011**, *23*(3), 1138-1152.
[http://dx.doi.org/10.1105/tpc.111.083485] [PMID: 21398568]

[147]   Oshima, Y.; Shikata, M.; Koyama, T.; Ohtsubo, N.; Mitsuda, N.; Ohme-Takagi, M. MIXTA-like transcription factors and WAX INDUCER1/SHINE1 coordinately regulate cuticle development in Arabidopsis and Torenia fournieri. *Plant Cell,* **2013**, *25*(5), 1609-1624.
[http://dx.doi.org/10.1105/tpc.113.110783] [PMID: 23709630]

[148]   Bessire, M.; Borel, S.; Fabre, G.; Carraça, L.; Efremova, N.; Yephremov, A.; Cao, Y.; Jetter, R.; Jacquat, A.C.; Métraux, J.P.; Nawrath, C. A member of the PLEIOTROPIC DRUG RESISTANCE family of ATP binding cassette transporters is required for the formation of a functional cuticle in Arabidopsis. *Plant Cell,* **2011**, *23*(5), 1958-1970.
[http://dx.doi.org/10.1105/tpc.111.083121] [PMID: 21628525]

[149]   Schnurr, J.; Shockey, J.; Browse, J. The acyl-CoA synthetase encoded by LACS2 is essential for normal cuticle development in Arabidopsis. *Plant Cell,* **2004**, *16*(3), 629-642.
[http://dx.doi.org/10.1105/tpc.017608] [PMID: 14973169]

[150]   Shi, J.X.; Adato, A.; Alkan, N.; He, Y.; Lashbrooke, J.; Matas, A.J.; Meir, S.; Malitsky, S.; Isaacson, T.; Prusky, D.; Leshkowitz, D.; Schreiber, L.; Granell, A.R.; Widemann, E.; Grausem, B.; Pinot, F.; Rose, J.K.C.; Rogachev, I.; Rothan, C.; Aharoni, A. The tomato SlSHINE3 transcription factor regulates fruit cuticle formation and epidermal patterning. *New Phytol.,* **2013**, *197*(2), 468-480.
[http://dx.doi.org/10.1111/nph.12032] [PMID: 23205954]

[151]   Kurdyukov, S.; Faust, A.; Trenkamp, S.; Bär, S.; Franke, R.; Efremova, N.; Tietjen, K.; Schreiber, L.; Saedler, H.; Yephremov, A. Genetic and biochemical evidence for involvement of HOTHEAD in the biosynthesis of long-chain alpha-,omega-dicarboxylic fatty acids and formation of extracellular matrix. *Planta,* **2006**, *224*(2), 315-329.
[http://dx.doi.org/10.1007/s00425-005-0215-7] [PMID: 16404574]

[152]   Li, Y.; Beisson, F.; Koo, A.J.; Molina, I.; Pollard, M.; Ohlrogge, J. Identification of acyltransferases required for cutin biosynthesis and production of cutin with suberin-like monomers. *Proc. Natl. Acad. Sci. USA,* **2007**, *104*(46), 18339-18344.
[http://dx.doi.org/10.1073/pnas.0706984104] [PMID: 17991776]

[153]   Cota–Sánchez, J.H. Precocious germination (vivipary) in tomato: a link to economic loss? *Proc. Natl. Acad. Sci., India, Sect. B Biol. Sci.,* **2018**, *88*, 1443-1451.
[http://dx.doi.org/10.1007/s40011-017-0878-4]

[154] Matilla, A.J. Seed dormancy: Molecular control of its induction and alleviation. *Plants,* **2020**, *9*(10), 1402.
[http://dx.doi.org/10.3390/plants9101402] [PMID: 33096840]

[155] Vishwakarma, K.; Upadhyay, N.; Kumar, N.; Yadav, G.; Singh, J.; Mishra, R.K.; Kumar, V.; Verma, R.; Upadhyay, R.G.; Pandey, M.; Sharma, S. Abscisic Acid Signaling and Abiotic Stress Tolerance in Plants: A Review on Current Knowledge and Future Prospects. *Front. Plant Sci.,* **2017**, *8*, 161.
[http://dx.doi.org/10.3389/fpls.2017.00161] [PMID: 28265276]

[156] Jin, J.F.; Wang, Z.Q.; He, Q.Y.; Wang, J.Y.; Li, P.F.; Xu, J.M.; Zheng, S.J.; Fan, W.; Yang, J.L. Genome-wide identification and expression analysis of the NAC transcription factor family in tomato (Solanum lycopersicum) during aluminum stress. *BMC Genomics,* **2020**, *21*(1), 288.
[http://dx.doi.org/10.1186/s12864-020-6689-7] [PMID: 32264854]

[157] Kou, X.; Liu, C.; Han, L.; Wang, S.; Xue, Z. NAC transcription factors play an important role in ethylene biosynthesis, reception and signaling of tomato fruit ripening. *Mol. Genet. Genomics,* **2016**, *291*(3), 1205-1217.
[http://dx.doi.org/10.1007/s00438-016-1177-0] [PMID: 26852223]

[158] Gao, Y.; Wei, W.; Zhao, X.; Tan, X.; Fan, Z.; Zhang, Y.; Jing, Y.; Meng, L.; Zhu, B.; Zhu, H.; Chen, J.; Jiang, C.Z.; Grierson, D.; Luo, Y.; Fu, D.Q. A NAC transcription factor, NOR-like1, is a new positive regulator of tomato fruit ripening. *Hortic. Res.,* **2018**, *5*(1), 75.
[http://dx.doi.org/10.1038/s41438-018-0111-5] [PMID: 30588320]

[159] Han, Q.; Zhang, J.; Li, H.; Luo, Z.; Ziaf, K.; Ouyang, B.; Wang, T.; Ye, Z. Identification and expression pattern of one stress-responsive NAC gene from Solanum lycopersicum. *Mol. Biol. Rep.,* **2012**, *39*(2), 1713-1720.
[http://dx.doi.org/10.1007/s11033-011-0911-2] [PMID: 21637957]

[160] Han, Q.Q.; Song, Y.Z.; Zhang, J.Y.; Liu, L.F. Studies on the role of the SlNAC3 gene in regulating seed development in tomato (Solanum lycopersicum). *J. Hortic. Sci. Biotechnol.,* **2014**, *89*, 423-429.
[http://dx.doi.org/10.1080/14620316.2014.11513101]

[161] Liang, X.Q.; Ma, N.N.; Wang, G.D. Suppression of. SlNAC1 reduces heat resistance in tomato plants. *Biol. Plant.,* **2014**, *59*, 92-98.
[http://dx.doi.org/10.1007/s10535-014-0477-7]

[162] Huang, W.; Miao, M.; Kud, J.; Niu, X.; Ouyang, B.; Zhang, J.; Ye, Z.; Kuhl, J.C.; Liu, Y.; Xiao, F. SlNAC1, a stress-related transcription factor, is fine-tuned on both the transcriptional and the post-translational level. *New Phytol.,* **2013**, *197*(4), 1214-1224.
[http://dx.doi.org/10.1111/nph.12096] [PMID: 23278405]

[163] Ma, N.; Feng, H.; Meng, X.; Li, D.; Yang, D.; Wu, C.; Meng, Q. Overexpression of tomato SlNAC1 transcription factor alters fruit pigmentation and softening. *BMC Plant Biol.,* **2014**, *14*, 351.
[http://dx.doi.org/10.1186/s12870-014-0351-y] [PMID: 25491370]

[164] Meng, C.; Yang, D.; Ma, X.; Zhao, W.; Liang, X.; Ma, N.; Meng, Q. Suppression of tomato SlNAC1 transcription factor delays fruit ripening. *J. Plant Physiol.,* **2016**, *193*, 88-96.
[http://dx.doi.org/10.1016/j.jplph.2016.01.014] [PMID: 26962710]

[165] Deluc, L.G.; Quilici, D.R.; Decendit, A.; Grimplet, J.; Wheatley, M.D.; Schlauch, K.A.; Mérillon, J.M.; Cushman, J.C.; Cramer, G.R. Water deficit alters differentially metabolic pathways affecting important flavor and quality traits in grape berries of Cabernet Sauvignon and Chardonnay. *BMC Genomics,* **2009**, *10*(1), 212.
[http://dx.doi.org/10.1186/1471-2164-10-212] [PMID: 19426499]

[166] Thompson, A.J.; Jackson, A.C.; Symonds, R.C.; Mulholland, B.J.; Dadswell, A.R.; Blake, P.S.; Burbidge, A.; Taylor, I.B. Ectopic expression of a tomato 9-cis-epoxycarotenoid dioxygenase gene causes over-production of abscisic acid. *Plant J.,* **2000**, *23*(3), 363-374.
[http://dx.doi.org/10.1046/j.1365-313x.2000.00789.x] [PMID: 10929129]

[167] Li, Q; Ji, K; Sun, YF The role of FaBG3in fruit ripening and B. cinerea fungal infection of strawberry. *The Plant Journa,* **2013**, *176*, 24-35.

[168] Saladié, M.; Matas, A.J.; Isaacson, T.; Jenks, M.A.; Goodwin, S.M.; Niklas, K.J.; Xiaolin, R.; Labavitch, J.M.; Shackel, K.A.; Fernie, A.R.; Lytovchenko, A.; O'Neill, M.A.; Watkins, C.B.; Rose, J.K. A reevaluation of the key factors that influence tomato fruit softening and integrity. *Plant Physiol.,* **2007**, *144*(2), 1012-1028.
[http://dx.doi.org/10.1104/pp.107.097477] [PMID: 17449643]

[169] Leide, J.; Hildebrandt, U.; Reussing, K.; Riederer, M.; Vogg, G. The developmental pattern of tomato fruit wax accumulation and its impact on cuticular transpiration barrier properties: effects of a deficiency in a beta-ketoacyl-coenzyme A synthase (LeCER6). *Plant Physiol.,* **2007**, *144*(3), 1667-1679.
[http://dx.doi.org/10.1104/pp.107.099481] [PMID: 17468214]

[170] Romero, P.; Rose, J.K.C. A relationship between tomato fruit softening, cuticle properties and water availability. *Food Chem.,* **2019**, *295*, 300-310.
[http://dx.doi.org/10.1016/j.foodchem.2019.05.118] [PMID: 31174762]

[171] Yeats, T.H.; Rose, J.K. The formation and function of plant cuticles. *Plant Physiol.,* **2013**, *163*(1), 5-20.
[http://dx.doi.org/10.1104/pp.113.222737] [PMID: 23893170]

[172] Isaacson, T.; Kosma, D.K.; Matas, A.J.; Buda, G.J.; He, Y.; Yu, B.; Pravitasari, A.; Batteas, J.D.; Stark, R.E.; Jenks, M.A.; Rose, J.K. Cutin deficiency in the tomato fruit cuticle consistently affects resistance to microbial infection and biomechanical properties, but not transpirational water loss. *Plant J.,* **2009**, *60*(2), 363-377.
[http://dx.doi.org/10.1111/j.1365-313X.2009.03969.x] [PMID: 19594708]

[173] Curvers, K.; Seifi, H.; Mouille, G.; de Rycke, R.; Asselbergh, B.; Van Hecke, A.; Vanderschaeghe, D.; Höfte, H.; Callewaert, N.; Van Breusegem, F.; Höfte, M. Abscisic acid deficiency causes changes in cuticle permeability and pectin composition that influence tomato resistance to Botrytis cinerea. *Plant Physiol.,* **2010**, *154*(2), 847-860.
[http://dx.doi.org/10.1104/pp.110.158972] [PMID: 20709830]

[174] Martin, L.B.B.; Romero, P.; Fich, E.A.; Domozych, D.S.; Rose, J.K.C. Cuticle biosynthesis is developmentally regulated by abscisic acid. *Plant Physiol.,* **2017**, *174*(3), 1384-1398.
[http://dx.doi.org/10.1104/pp.17.00387] [PMID: 28483881]

[175] Hichri, I.; Muhovski, Y.; Žižkova, E.; Dobrev, P.I.; Franco-Zorrilla, J.M.; Solano, R.; Lopez-Vidriero, I.; Motyka, V.; Lutts, S. The Solanum lycopersicum Zinc Finger2 cysteine-2/histidine-2 repressor-like transcription factor regulates development and tolerance to salinity in tomato and Arabidopsis. *Plant Physiol.,* **2014**, *164*(4), 1967-1990.
[http://dx.doi.org/10.1104/pp.113.225920] [PMID: 24567191]

CHAPTER 3

Progress in the Research of Naturally Occurring Biflavonoids: A Look Through

Dilip Gorai[1], Shyamal K. Jash[2] and Debasish Kundu[3,*]

[1] *Department of Chemistry, Bolpur College, Bolpur, Birbhum - 731204, West Bengal, India*

[2] *Department of Chemistry, Krishna Chandra College, Hetampur, Birbhum - 731124, West Bengal, India*

[3] *Department of Chemistry, Govt. Degree College, Mangalkote, Burdwan - 713132, West Bengal, India*

Abstract: Biflavonoids are dimers of monomeric flavonoids and have reported to exhibit several pharmacological activities, like anti-microbial, anti-inflammatory, anti-enzymatic, antioxidant, anticancer, anti-Perkinson, anti-ulcer, anti-hypertensive, anti-diabetic, anti-depressant and anti-protozoan. Extensive research work on this important segment of natural compounds is in progress. In this chapter, we report the progress of research on natural biflavonoids from the period of 2005 to early 2020; it includes enlisting newly isolated bioflavonoids from plant sources, biological activities exhibited by the known as well as new compounds and synthetic strategies developed for synthesizing such compounds. In this time period, a total of 247 biflavonoids have been reported either in terms of their first-time appearance or evaluation of their biological activities or both. Out of the reported 247 biflavonoids, 176 have been reported as new compounds from natural plant sources. They have been reported to exhibit a wide range of biological and pharmacological properties, including anti-microbial and antiviral, cytotoxic and anti-cancer, anti-diabetic, anti-anoxic, antioxidant, NO-inhibitory activity, anti-enzymatic, anti-HIV, anti thrombin, anti-allergic, cytoprotective, neuroprotective and anti-inflammatory, which have been discussed in a comprehensive manner. Different synthetic strategies that have been reported for the synthesis of structurally different biflavonoids are also included. This chapter cites 177 references.

Keywords: Anti-cancer, Anti-diabetic, Anti-enzymatic, Anti-microbial, Antioxidant, Antiviral, Biflavonoids, Biological activities, Cytotoxic, Natural distribution, Nomenclature, Occurrence, Structural aspects, Synthesis.

---

* **Corresponding author Debasish Kundu:** Department of Chemistry, Govt. Degree College, Mangalkote, Burdwan - 713132, West Bengal, India; E-mail:chem.debasishkundu@mangalkotegovtcollege.org

Atta-ur-Rahman (Ed.)

INTRODUCTION

The term '*Flavonoid*' may be regarded as a broad assemblage of naturally available compounds that contain a C6-C3-C6 carbon framework, *i.e.* phenylbenzopyran functionality [1]. On the basis of the position at which the aromatic ring links with the benzopyrano functionality, this group of natural compounds can be divided into three classes: the flavonoids (2-phenylbenzopyrans) (Fig. **1A**), isoflavonoids (3-phenylbenzopyrans) (Fig. **1B**) and the neoflavonoids (4-phenylbenzopyrans) (Fig. **1C**). Keeping in mind the biogenesis pathway, these groups generally share a common precursor, chalcone (Fig. **1D**), and as expected, they are structurally and biogenetically related [2 - 6].

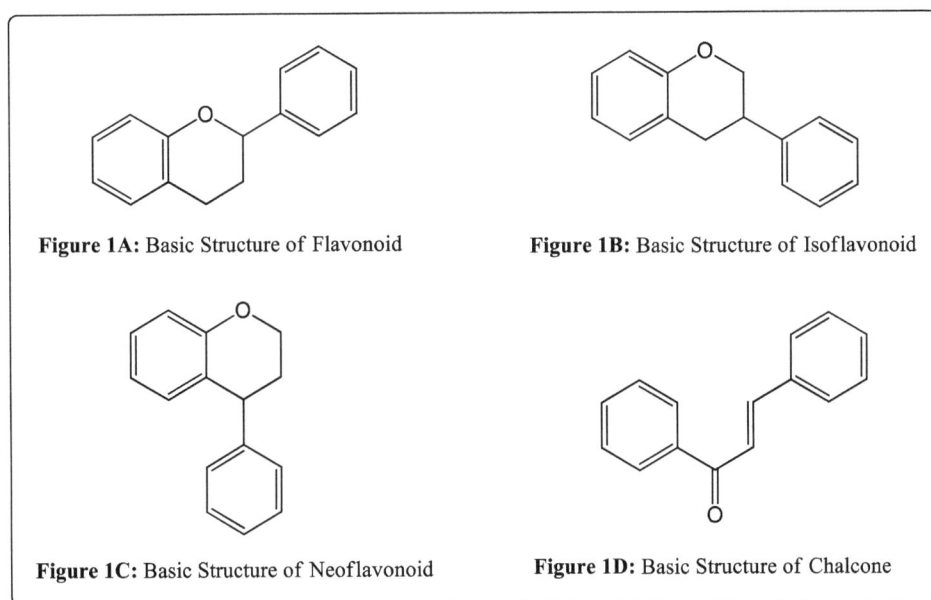

Figure 1A: Basic Structure of Flavonoid

Figure 1B: Basic Structure of Isoflavonoid

Figure 1C: Basic Structure of Neoflavonoid

Figure 1D: Basic Structure of Chalcone

Fig. (1). (1A) Basic Structure of Flavonoid; **(1B)** Basic Structure of Isoflavonoid **(1C)** Basic Structure of NeoFlavonoid **(1D)** Basic Structure of Chalcone.

Biflavonoids are dimers of monomeric flavonoid, namely flavone, chalcone, flavonol, flavanone or flavanol (Fig. **2**), and due to their dimeric nature, biflavones are phenolic compounds, constituted by the same or different flavonoid units linked with each other either in symmetric or asymmetric fashion involving variable length of alkyl or ether spacer chains [7].

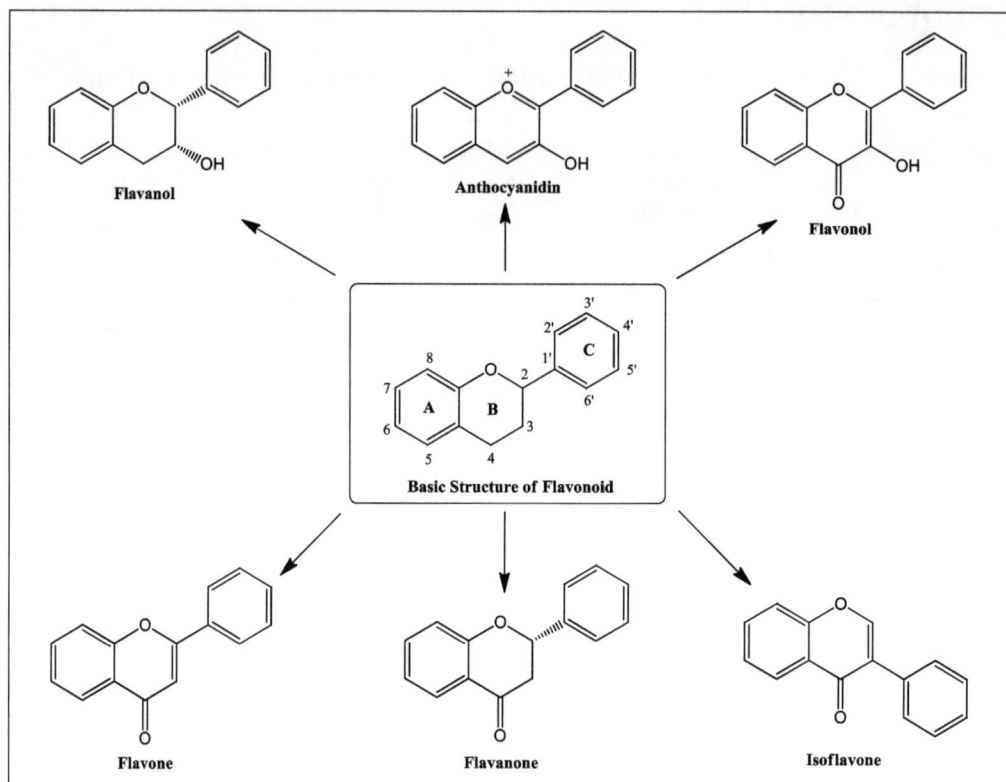

Fig. (2). Basic structures of flavonoid subclasses.

Therefore, a large structural diversity of biflavonoids is expected owing to variations in flavonflavonoidic units, as well as a large number of substitution possibilities in different positions and the nature of inter-flavonoidic linkage [7, 8]. Biflavonoids are thus regarded as a subclass of the family of natural flavonoids and are distributed to several species in the plant kingdom. These natural constituents have been found to be very abundant in nature, and are available in many vegetal tissues such as leaves, roots, fruits, seeds, charcoal and pollen [9]. Structurally, they are characterized as dimeric flavonoids, differing from other oligomers, such as proanthocyanidins, by the biogenetic origin of their constitutional units [9].

Till now, more than 250 biflavonoids have been isolated from different plant sources, and this number is gradually improving day by day as a consequence of continuous research in this direction [10]. These natural products are extensively reported in the literature for their several pharmacological properties, like anti-microbial, anti-inflammatory, anti-enzymatic, antioxidant, anticancer, anti-Parkinson, anti-ulcer, anti-hypertensive, anti-diabetic, anti-depressant and anti-protozoan [8, 11 - 14]. Research on this important class of natural constituents is in progress. Besides original research works, a few review works have been published in different reputed journals [8, 11, 12].

In this chapter, we report the development of research on natural biflavonoids from the period of 2005 to early 2020; it includes enlisting newly isolated bioflavonoids from plant sources, biological activities exhibited by the known as well as new compounds and synthetic strategies developed for synthesizing such compounds. In this period, a total of 247 biflavonoids have been reported either in terms of their first-time appearance or evaluation of their biological activities or both. Out of the reported 247 biflavonoids, 176 have been reported as new compounds from natural plant sources. They have been reported to exhibit a wide range of biological and pharmacological properties, including anti-microbial and antiviral, cytotoxic and anti-cancer, anti-diabetic, anti-anoxic, antioxidant, NO-inhibitory activity, anti-enzymatic, anti-HIV, anti thrombin, anti-allergic, cytoprotective, neuroprotective and anti-inflammatory activities, and have been discussed here in a comprehensive manner. Synthesis of biflavonoids always remains a challenging task for organic chemists as large numbers of variations are possible in the parent flavonoid units coupled with a large number of permutations in the position and nature of the inter-flavonoid linkage, which introduce significant structural diversity. Different synthetic strategies that have been reported for the synthesis of structurally different biflavonoids are also discussed in detail.

NOMENCLATURE AND STRUCTURAL ASPECTS

Biflavonoids are formed due to the inter-flavonoidic linkage between two flavonoids. The majority of such compounds are formed by flavone-flavone, flavone-flavonone, flavonone-flavonone linkages, as well as dimers of chalcones and isoflavones in a few cases [15]. When both structural subunits are the same, the flavonoids belong to the *bis*-flavonoids class, and when there are different subunits, biflavonoids are formed. Flavonoidic subunits could be interconnected either by C-C or C-O-C bonds, involving rings A, B or C of the monomer (Fig. **3**) [15]. However, bonding could be done in different positions (*e.g.* 3-4"' or 4'-4"). Changes in the oxidation level of precursors are rarely observed, except for 5, 7 and 4' positions, and eventually on position 3' [9, 16]. Numbering on biflavonoid structure is done by attributing ordinary numbers for the carbon atoms on rings A and C and primed (') numbers for ring B of one of the monomers. For the second unit, a double primed (") ordinary numbering to the nuclei A and C and ordinary triple primed ("') numbers to the core B are employed [15]. According to the carbon atoms involved in the linkage between the structural units, dimers are classified into groups of biflavonoids, as chalcones dimers with C-3→O-C-4''' (luxenchalcones) [17] and C-3'→C-3'' (brackenines) [18] and isoflavones dimers with C-2→C-2'' (hexaspermones) [19]. In some cases, methylated hydroxyl groups can occur, leading to the correspondent methyl ethers, which are required to be named especially [20].

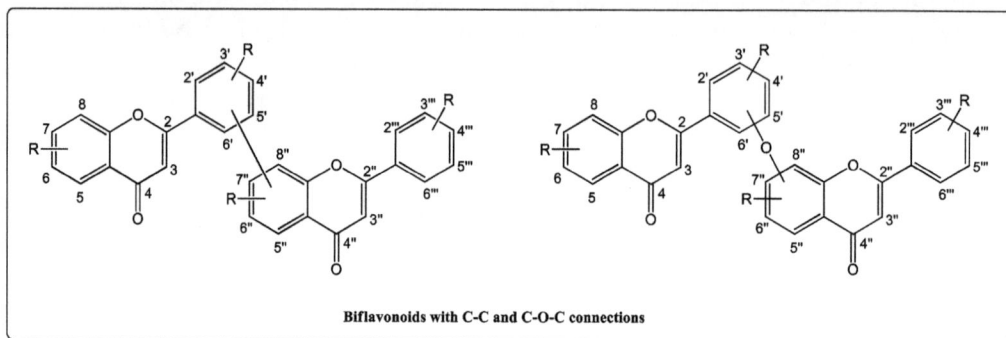

Biflavonoids with C-C and C-O-C connections

Fig. (3). Examples of chemical structures of biflavonoids with C-C and C-*O*-Cbonds.

OCCURRENCE AND DISTRIBUTION

In the literature survey, natural biflavonoids have been reported to occur in many families, including Anacardiaceae, Berberidaceae, Burseraceae, Caprifoliaceae, Casuarinaceae, Euphorbiaceae, Guttiferae (especially *Garcinia*), Haemcdoraceae, Iridaceae, Labiatae, Lamiaceae, Leguminosae, Loganiaceae, Ochnaceae, Papilionaceae, Piperaceae, Rhamnaceae, Rubiaceae, Rutaceae, Salicaceae, Solanaceae, Thymelaeaceae and Velloziaceae [10]. Among all genera, biflavonoids are especially abundant in species of *Daphne* (Thymelaeaceae), *Calycopteris* (Combretaceae), *Selaginella* (Selaginellaceae), *Lophira* as well as *Ochna* (Ochnaceae) [11]. We have extensively compiled these natural constituents in a multi-informational table (Table **1**), mentioning their family, genus, species, plant parts used for isolation as well as biological activities reported so far, if any. Moreover, the connectivity patterns have also been included in this table for an easy understanding of the readers. Some polyflavonoids are also enlisted in the last part of the table, owing to their structural similarity with the biflavonoids. Structures of the reported biflavonoids have been shown in Figs. (**4** - **5**), and in Fig. (**6**), chemical structures of polyflavonoids are shown.

Table 1. Biflavonoids reported in the literature, classified by type of connection and the corresponding plant and other sources.

Sl. No.	Compounds (Str. No.)	Connectivity	Source [Plant Spp. (Family) /Purchased/Other]	Plant Parts	Bioactivity	Ref.
1.	(I-2S)-I-5,II-5,I-7,II-7,I-2',II-2',I-5',II-5'-octahydroxy-[I-6,II-6']-flavanonylflavone (1)	(6→ 6')	*Scutellaria amabilis* (Lamiaceae)	Roots	—	[21]
2.	(I-2S)-I-5,II-5,I-7,II-7,I-2',II-2',II-5'-heptahydroxy-[I-6,II-6']-flavanonyl-flavone (2)	(6→ 6')	*Scutellaria amabilis* (Lamiaceae)	Roots	—	[21]
3.	(I-3,II-3)-biliquiritigenin (3)	(3→ 3")	*Ochna integerrima* (Ochnaceae)	Inner barks	Antimalarial activity	[22]
			Ormocarpum kirkii (Papilionaceae)	Roots	Antiplasmodial activity	[23]
4.	2',8"-biapigenin (4)*	(2'→ 8")	*Selaginella tamariscina* (Selaginellaceae)	Whole plants	Matrix metalloproteinase in human skin fibroblasts	[24]
				Aerial parts	Antidiabetic activity	[25]
5.	2",3"-dihydroamentoflavone-4'-methyl ether (5)	(3'→ 8")	*Selaginella uncinata* (Selaginellaceae)	Whole herbs	Protective effect against anoxia	[26]
6.	2", 3"-dihydro-3', 3'"-biapigenin (6)*	(3'→ 3'")	*Selaginella doederleinii* (Selaginellaceae)	Whole plants	Anti-tumor activity	[27, 28]
7.	2", 3"-dihydroochnaflavone (7)	(3'- O-4'")	*Lexembugia nobilis* (Ochnaceae)	Leaves	Cytotoxic activity	[29]
8.	2,2",3,3"-tetrahydro robustaflavone-7,4',7"-trimethylether (8)	(3'→ 6")	*Selaginella doederleinii* (Selaginellaceae)	Whole plant	Cytotoxic activity	[30]
9.	2,2"-bisteppogenin (9)	(3→ 3")	*Daphne aurantiaca* (Thymelaeaceae)	Stem barks	—	[31]
10.	2,2"-bisteppogenin 7-O-β-glucopyranoside (10)	(3→ 3")	*Daphne aurantiaca* (Thymelaeaceae)	Stem barks	—	[31]
11.	2,3-dihidro-6-methylginkgetin (11)*	(3'→ 8")	*Cephalotaxus harringtonia* (Cephalotaxaceae)	—	β-Secretase (BACE-1) inhibitory effect: Alzheimer	[117]
12.	2,3-dihydro-4',4'"-di-O-methyl-amentoflavone (12)	(3'→ 8")	*Podocarpus macrophyllus* (Popocarpaceae)	Leaves	Anti-tyrosinase effect	[32]
13.	2,3-dihydro-4'"-O-methyl amentoflavone (13)	(3'→ 8")	*Cycas beddomei* (Cycadacea)	Cones	—	[33]
14.	2,3-dihydro-4'-O-methylamentoflavone (14)	(3'→ 8")	*Selaginella uncinata* (Selaginellaceae)	Whole plants	Anti-oxidant activities	[34]
15.	2,3-dihydro-5,5",7,7",4'-pentahydroxi-6,6"-dimethyl-[3'-O-4'"]-biflavone (15)	(3'- O-4'")	*Selaginella labordei* (Selaginellacea)	Herbs	—	[35]
16.	2,3-dihydroamentoflavone (16)*	(3'→ 8")	*Cycas circinalis* (Cycadaceae)	Leaflets	Antibacterial activity	[36]
			Selaginella bryopteris (Selaginellaceae)	Whole plants	Antiplasmodial and leishmanicidal activity	[37]
			Selaginella uncinata (Selaginellaceae)	Whole herbs	Protective effect against anoxia	[26]
17.	2",3"-dihydroamentoflavone (17)*	(3'→ 8")	*Selaginella bryopteris* (Selaginellaceae)	Whole plants	Antiplasmodial and leishmanicidal activity	[37]
			Selaginella uncinata (Selaginellaceae)	Whole herbs	Protective effect against anoxia	[26]

(Table 1) cont.....

No.	Name	Linkage	Source	Part	Activity	Ref.
18.	2,3-dihydroamentoflavone-4'-methyl ether (**18**)	(3'→ 8")	*Selaginella uncinata* (Selaginellaceae)	Whole herbs	Protective effect against anoxia	[26]
				Whole plants	Antibacterial activity	[34]
19.	2,3,2",3"-tetrahydro-4'-O-methyl-amentoflavone (**19**)	(3'→ 8")	*Selaginella uncinata* (Selaginellaceae)	Whole plants	Antibacterial activity	[34]
				Whole herbs	Protective effect against anoxia	[26]
			Cycas circinalis (Cycadaceae)	Leaflets	Antibacterial activity	[36]
20.	(2S, 2"S)-tetrahydrorobustaflavone (**20**)*	(3'→ 6")	*Selaginella uncinata* (Selaginellaceae)	Whole herbs	Anti-anoxic effect	[159]
21.	2,3-dihydrohinokiflavone (**21**)*	(4'- O-6")	*Selaginella bryopteris* (Selaginellaceae)	Whole plants	Antiplasmodial and leishmanicidal activity	[37]
22.	2",3"-dihydrohinokiflavone (**22**)	(4'-O-6")	*Cycas beddomei* (Cycadaceae)	Cones	—	[38]
			Selaginella bryopteris (Selaginellaceae)	Whole plant	Antiplasmodial and leishmanicidal activity	[37]
23.	2,3-dihydroochnaflavone 7"-O-methyl ether (**23**)	(3'-O-4''')	*Ochna lanceolata* (Ochnaceae)	Stem bark	—	[39]
24.	2,3-dihydrorobustaflavone 7,7"-dimethyl ether (**24**)	(3'→ 6")	*Selaginella doederleinii* (Selaginellaceae)	Whole plant	—	[40]
25.	2,3-dihydrosciadopitysin (**25**)*	(3'→ 8")	*Podocarpus macrophyllus* (Popocarpaceae)	Leaves	Anti-tyrosinase effect	[32]
26.	2'''-dehydroxy-2,2"-bisteppogenin (**26**)	(3→ 3")	*Daphne aurantiaca* (Thymelaeaceae)	Stem bark	—	[31]
27.	2'''-dehydroxy-2,2"-bisteppogenin 7-O-β-glucopyranoside (**27**)	(3→ 3")	*Daphne aurantiaca* (Thymelaeaceae)	Stem bark	—	[31]
28.	2'-hydroxy-6,4',6",4'''-tetramethoxy-{7-O-7"}-bisisoflavone (**28**)	(7-O-7")	*Platymiscium floribundum* (Leguminosae)	Heartwood	—	[41]
29.	2"-hydroxygenkwanol A (**29**)	(8 → 3")	*Daphne linearifolia* (Thymelaeaceae)	Aerial parts	Anti-cancer activity	[42]
30.	2"-methoxy daphnodorin C (**30**)	(8 → 3")	*Daphne feddei* (Thymelaeaceae)	Stem bark	Activities against Nitric Oxide Production	[43]
31.	2"-methoxy-2-epi-daphnodorin C (**31**)	(8 → 3")	*Daphne feddei* (Thymelaeaceae)	Stem bark	Activities against Nitric Oxide Production	[43]
32.	3"-hydroxyamentoflavone (**32**)	(3' → 8")	*Aristolochia contorta* (Aristolochiaceae)	Fruits	—	[44]
33.	3"-hydroxyamentoflavone-7-O-methyl ether (**33**)	(3' → 8")	*Aristolochia contorta* (Aristolochiaceae)	Fruits	—	[44]
34.	3,5,7,3',4',3",5",7",3''',4'''-decahydroxyl-[8-CH₂-8'']-biflavone (**34**)	(8-CH₂-8'')	*Galium verum* (Rubiaceae)	Whole herbs	—	[46]
35.	3',8"-biisokaempferide (**35**)	(3' → 8")	*Namuza plicata* (Velloziaceae)	Whole plant	Cytotoxicity	[47]
36.	3', 3'''-binaringenin (**36**)*	(3'→ 3''')	*Selaginella doederleinii* (Selaginellaceae)	Whole plants	Anti-tumour activity	[27, 28]
37.	3',4',7,8-tetrahydroxyflavone-(3,4)-ent-epimesquitol (**37**)	(3 → 4")	*Acacia nigrescens* (Leguminosae)	Heartwood	—	[48]
38.	3"-epidiphysin (**38**)	(3 → 3")	*Ormocarpum trichocarpum* (Papilionaceae)	Aerial part	Antiplasmodial activity and antibacterial activity	[49]
39.	3'-hydroxydaphnodorin A (**39**)	(8 → 3")	*Wikstroemia indica* (Thymelaeaceae)	Rhizome	Anticancer /cytotoxic activity	[50]
40.	3'-O-methylloniflavone [5,5",7,7"-tetrahydroxy 3'-methoxy 4',4"-biflavonyl ether] (**40**)	(4'-O-4'')	*Lonicera japonica* (Caprifoliaceae)	Leaves	—	[51]
41.	3-hydroxy 2,3-dihydroapegenyl-{1-4',O, II-3'}dihydrokaempferol [Sulcatone A] (**41**)	(3'- O-4''')	*Ouratea sulcata* (Ochnaceae)	Aerial parts	Antimicrobial activities	[52]

(Table 1) cont.....

42.	3-O-α-L-rhamnopyranosylmyricetinyl-(I-2″,II-2″)-3-O-α-L-rhamnopyrano-yl-myricetin (42)	(2′ → 2‴)	*Baeckea frutescens* (Myrtaceae)	Leaves	Inhibition of copper-induced LDL oxidation	[53]
43.	4,4″-dimethoxylophirone A (43)	(3 → 3′)	*Allexis cauliflora* (Violaceae)	Root	Antibacterial activities, good antiplasmodial activity	[54]
44.	4′,5-dihydroxy-2′,3′-dimethoxy-7-(5-hydroxychromen-7yl)-isoflavanone (44)	(7′-O-7″)	*Uraria picta* (Papilionaceae)	Roots	Antimicrobial activity	[55]
45.	4′,7″-di-O-methyl-amentoflavone (45)	(3 → 8″)	*Cephalotaxus koreana* (Cephalotaxaceae)	Leaves and twigs	Osteoblast differentiation	[56]
46.	4‴-methoxyamentoflavone (46)*	(3 → 8″)	*Garcinia prainiana* (Guttiferae)	Stem barks	Antibacterial, antioxidant, Anti-tyrosinase	[57]
47.	4′-methoxydaphnodorin E (47)	(8 → 3″)	*Wikstroemia indica* (Thymelaeaceae)	Root	Antiviral activity	[58]
48.	4′-methylgenkwanol A (48)	(8 → 3″)	*Daphne linearifolia* (Thymelaeaceae)	Aerial parts	Anti-cancer activity	[42]
49.	4‴-O-methylagatisflavone (49)	(6 → 8″)	*Campylospermum flavum* (Ochnaceae)	Stem bark	—	[59]
50.	4‴-O-methyl-I3,II8-biapigenin (50)	(3 → 8″)	*Garcinia bakeriana* (Clusiaceae)	Leaves	—	[60]
51.	5,5″-di-O-methyldiphysin (51)	(3 → 3″)	*Ormocarpum kirkii* (Papilionaceae)	Roots	Antiplasmodial activity	[23]
52.	5-hydroxy-4′,7-dimethoxyflavone-(6-C-6″)-5″-hydroxy-3‴,4‴,7″-trimethoxyflavone (52)	(6 → 6″)	*Miconia cabucu* (Melastomataceae)	Aerial parts	—	[61]
53.	7,4′,7″,4″-tetramethylisochamaejasmin (53)	(3 → 3″)	*Ochna lanceolata* (Ochnaceae)	Stem bark	—	[39]
			Cephalotaxus harringtonia (Cephalotaxaceae)	—	β-Secretase (BACE-1) inhibitory effect: Alzheimer	[117]
54.	7,4′,7″,4‴-tetra-O-methylamentoflavone (54)*	(3′ → 8″)	*Araucaria angustifolia* (Araucariacea)	Needles	Protective agents against DNA damage and lipoperoxidation	[62]
			Cephalotaxus koreana (Cephalotaxaceae)	Leaves and twigs	Osteoblast differentiation	[56]
			Selaginella doederleinii (Selaginellaceae)	Whole plants	Anti-tumour activity	[27]
55.	7,7″-di-O-methylchamaejasmin (55)	(3 → 3″)	*Ormocarpum trichocarpum* (Papilionaceae)	Aerial part	Antiplasmodial activity and antibacterial activity	[49]
56.	7,7″-di-O-methylisochamaejasmin (56)	(3 → 3″)	*Ormocarpum trichocarpum* (Papilionaceae)	Aerial part	Antiplasmodial activity and antibacterial activity	[49]
57.	7-hydroxy-5,8-dimethoxyflavan-(4β→3′)-2′,6′-dihydroxy-4′-methoxy-chalcone (57)	(4 → 3′)	*Sarcandra hainanensis* (Chloranthaceae)	Whole plants	Anti-HIV activity	[63]
58.	7-hydroxy-6,6′-dimethoxy-3,7′-O-bis-coumarin (58)	(3- O-7′)	*Erycibe hainanesis* (Convolvulaceae)	Roots and stems	Hepatoprotective activities	[64]
59.	7-methoxy chamaejasmin (59)	(3 → 3″)	*Stellera chamaejasme* (Thymelaeaceae)	Roots	Aldose reductase inhibitors	[65]
60.	7-methoxy neochamaejasmin (60)*	(3 → 3″)	*Stellera chamaejasme* (Thymelaeaceae)	Roots	Aldose reductase inhibitors	[65]
61.	7-methoxyneochamaejasmin B (61)	(3 → 3″)	*Daphne aurantiaca* (Thymelaeaceae)	Stem bark	—	[31]
62.	7″-O-methylamentoflavone (62)*	(3′ → 8″)	*Campylospermum excavatum* (Ochnaceae)	Leaves	Antiparasitic activities	[66]
63.	7-O-methylhinokiflavone (63)*	(4′- O-6″)	*Selaginella bryopteris* (Selaginellaceae)	Whole plant	Antiplasmodial and leishmanicidal activity	[37]

(Table 1) cont.....

64.	7-*O*-methyl-isoginkgetin (**64**)*	(3' → 8")	*Cephalotaxus koreana* (Cephalotaxaceae)	Leaves and twigs	Osteoblast differentiation	[56]
65.	7-*O*-methylochnaflavone (**65**)	(3'- O-4"')	*Campylospermum excavatum* (Ochnaceae)	Leaves	Antiparasitic activities	[66]
66.	7-*O*-β-D-glucopyranosyldiphysin (**66**)	(3 → 3")	*Ormocarpum kirkii* (Papilionaceae)	Roots	Antiplasmodial activity	[23]
67.	7-*O*-β-D-glucopyranosylchamaejasmin (**67**)	(3 → 3")	*Ormocarpum kirkii* (Papilionaceae)	Roots	Antiplasmodial activity	[23]
68.	8,8"-biapigeninyl (**68**)*	(8 → 8")	*Cupressus sempervirens* (Cupressaceae)	Fruits	Inhibits osteoclast And adipocyte functions	[67]
69.	8,8"-bisbaicalein (**69**)	(8 → 8")	*Oroxylum indicum* (Bignoniaceae)	Stem barks	—	[68]
70.	8-methylsocotrin-3-methoxy-4-ol (**70**)	(γ → 6)	*Dracaena cambodiana* (Agavaceae)	Stem	—	[69]
71.	8-methylsocotrin-4-methoxy-3-ol (**71**)	(γ → 6)	*Dracaena cambodiana* (Agavaceae)	Stem	—	[69]
72.	8-methylsocotrin-4'-ol (**72**)	(γ → 6)	*Dracaena cochinchinensis* (Agavaceae)	Stems	Anti-Helicobacter pylori and Thrombin Inhibitory activity	[69, 70]
73.	9'-methoxyl rutarensin (**73**)	(3-O-7')	*Boenninghausenia sessilicarpa* (Rutaceae)	Whole plant	—	[71]
74.	Absienol A (**74**)	(2'→ 8")	*Abies sachalinensis* (Pinaceae)	Bark	Anti-tumor-initiating activity	[72, 72a]
75.	Absienol B (**75**)	(2'→ 8")	*Abies sachalinensis* (Pinaceae)	Bark	Anti-tumor-initiating activity	[72, 72a]
76.	Absienol C (**76**)	(2'→ 8")	*Abies sachalinensis* (Pinaceae)	Bark	Anti-tumor-initiating activity	[72, 72a]
77.	Absienol D (**77**)	(2'→ 8")	*Abies sachalinensis* (Pinaceae)	Bark	Anti-tumor-initiating activity	[72, 72a]
78.	Absienol E (**78**)	(2'→ 8")	*Abies sachalinensis* (Pinaceae)	Bark	Anti-tumor-initiating activity	[72, 72a]
79.	Absienol F (**79**)	(2'→ 8")	*Abies sachalinensis* (Pinaceae)	Bark	Anti-tumor-initiating activity	[72, 72a]
80.	Absienol G (**80**)	(2'→ 8")	*Abies sachalinensis* (Pinaceae)	Bark	—	[72a]
81.	Absienol H (**81**)	(2'→ 8")	*Abies sachalinensis* (Pinaceae)	Bark	—	[72a]
82.	Agathisflavone (**82**)*	(6 → 8")	*Ochna schweinfurthiana* (Ochnaceae)	Barks	Anti-Inflammatory activity	[73]
			Rhus pyroides (Anacardiaceae)	Leaves	3H-Ro 15-1788 (flumazenil) binding assay	[74]

(Table 1) cont.....

No.	Name		Plant (Family)	Part	Activity	Ref.
83.	Amentoflavone (**83**)*	(3 → 8″)	*Campylospermum excavatum* (Ochnaceae)	Leaves	Antiparasitic activities	[66]
			Dietes bicolor (Iridaceae)	Leaves	Anti-inflammatory activity	[75]
			Garcinia prainiana (Guttiferae)	Stem barks	Antibacterial, antioxidant, Anti-tyrosinase	[57]
			Garcinia subelliptica (Clusiaceae)	Leaves	Strongly inhibited hypoxia-inducible factor-1 in human embryonic kidney 293 cells Under hypoxic conditions.	[76]
			Hypericum connatum (Guttiferae)	Aerial parts	Antiviral activity	[77]
			Ochna schweinfurthiana (Ochnaceae)	Barks	Anti-Inflammatory activity	[73]
			Rhus pyroides (Anacardiaceae)	Leaves	3H-Ro 15-1788 (flumazenil) binding assay	[74]
			Selaginella doederleinii (Selaginellaceae)	Whole plants	Anti-tumour activity	[27, 28]
			Selaginella moellendorffii (Selaginellacea)	Herbs	Anti HBV activity	[78]
			Selaginella tamariscina (Selaginellaceae)	Whole plants	Matrix metalloproteinase in human skin fibroblasts	[24]
					Antifungal activity	[79]
					Antidiabetic activity	[25]
				Aerial parts	CYP2C8 and CYP2C9 enzyme inhibitory activity	[80]
			Selaginella uncinata (Selaginellaceae)	Whole herbs	Protective effect against anoxia	[26]
			Torreya nucifera (Taxaceae)	Leaves	SARS-cov 3clpro inhibition	[89]
			Purchased from Shanghai Yuan Ye Biotechnology Co., Ltd. (Shanghai, China)	—	Potential hepatic and renal toxicity	[81]
			Chemical structure was retrieved from NCBI PubChem database	—	α-Glucosidase, tyrosinase, 15-lipoxygenase inhibitory activity	[82]
84.	Apigeninyl-(I-3,II-3)-naringenin (**84**)	(3 → 3″)	*Ormocarpum kirkii* (Papilionaceae)	Roots	Antiplasmodial activity	[23]
85.	Asteryomenin (**85**)	(3 → 3″)	*Aster yomena* (Asteraceae)	Aerial parts	IL-6 inhibitory activity	[83]
86.	Baeckein C (**86**)	(3-O-4″)	*Baeckea frutescens* (Myrtaceae)	Roots	—	[84]
					Cytoprotective activity	[85]
87.	Baeckein D (**87**)	(3-O-4″)	*Baeckea frutescens* (Myrtaceae)	Roots	—	[84]
					Cytoprotective activity	[85]
88.	Baeckein E (**88**)	(3-O-4″)	*Baeckea frutescens* (Myrtaceae)	Roots	Cytoprotective activity	[85]
89.	Beilschmieflavonoid A (**89**)	(4-O-4″)	*Beilschmiedia zenkeri* (Lauraceae)	Stem bark	Antibacterial activity	[86]

(Table 1) cont.....

90.	Beilschmieflavonoid B (**90**)	(4-O-4″)	*Beilschmiedia zenkeri* (Lauraceae)	Stem bark	Antibacterial activity	[86]
91.	Bilobetin (**91**)*	(3′→ 8″)	*Araucaria angustifolia* (Araucariaceae)	Leaves	Antiviral activity	[87]
			Cephalotaxus koreana (Cephalotaxaceae)	Leaves and twigs	Osteoblast differentiation	[56]
			Gingko biloba (Ginkgoaceae)	—	Neuroprotective effects	[88]
			Selaginella bryopteris (Selaginellaceae)	Whole plant	Antiplasmodial and leishmanicidal activity	[37]
			Selaginella moellendorffii (Selaginellaceae)	—	β-Secretase (BACE-1) inhibitory effect: Alzheimer	[117]
			Torreya nucifera (Taxaceae)	Leaves	SARS-cov 3clpro inhibition	[89]
			Purchased from Shanghai Yuan Ye Biotechnology Co., Ltd. (Shanghai, China)	—	Potential hepatic and renal toxicity	[81]
92.	Bioflavonoid (**92**)	(3 → 3″)	*Butea monosperma* (Fabaceae)	Flowers	Influenza A neuraminidase inhibitory activity and DPPH Free-radical scavenging activity.	[90]
93.	Bioflavonoid (**93**)	(3 → 6″)	*Butea monosperma* (Fabaceae)	Flowers	Influenza A neuraminidase inhibitory activity and DPPH Free-radical scavenging activity.	[90]
94.	Bioflavonoid (**94**)	—	*Butea monosperma* (Fabaceae)	Flowers	Influenza A neuraminidase inhibitory activity and DPPH Free-radical scavenging activity.	[90]
95.	Binaringenin-7″-*O*-β-glucoside (**95**)	(3 → 8″)	*Clusia paralicola* (Clusiaceae)	Green fruits	Antioxidant activity	[91]
96.	Bismurrangain (**96**)	(9-O-9′)	*Murraya exotica* (Rutaceae)	Vegetative Branches	—	[92]
97.	Buchananiflavonol (**97**)	(3 → 8″)	*Garcinia buchananii* (Guttiferae)	Stem barks	Anti-oxidant activities	[93]
98.	Buchananiflavanone (**98**)	(3 → 8″)	*Garcinia buchananii* (Guttiferae)	Stem barks	Anti-oxidant activities	[94]
99.	Caesalflavone (**99**)	(3′→ 6″)	*Caesalpinia pyramidalis* (Fabaceae)	Leaves	—	[95]
100.	Campylospermone A (**100**)	(3′→ 3″)	*Campylospermum mannii* (Ochnaceae)	Leaves and stem bark	—	[96]
101.	Campylospermone B (**101**)	(3′→ 3″)	*Campylospermum mannii* (Ochnaceae)	Leaves and stem bark	—	[96]
102.	CGY-1 (**102**)	(3′→ 8″)	*Cardiocrinum giganteum* (Liliaceae)	Seeds	Neuroprotective effect	[97]
103.	Chamaechromone (**103**)*	(3 → 3″)	*Stellera chamaejasme* (Thymelaeaceae)	Roots	Aldose reductase inhibitors	[65]
					Antiviral effect	[120]
104.	Chamaeflavone A (**104**)	(3 → 3″)	*Stellera chamaejasme* (Thymelaeaceae)	Roots	Anti-HIV, cytotoxicity	[98]

(Table 1) cont.....

					Anti-cancer activity	[99]
105.	Chamaejasmenin B (**105**)*	(3 → 3")	*Stellera chamaejasme* (Thymelaeaceae)	Roots	Cytotoxic activity	[100]
					Aldose reductase inhibitors	[65]
106.	Chamaejasmenin E (**106**)	(3 → 3")	*Stellera chamaejasme* (Thymelaeaceae)	Roots	Cytotoxic activity	[100]
107.	Chamaejasmin (**107**)*	(3 → 3")	*Ormocarpum kirkii* (Papilionaceae)	Roots	Antiplasmodial activity	[23]
			Ormocarpum trichocarpum (Papilionaceae)	Aerial parts	Antiplasmodial activity and antibacterial activity	[49]
			Stellera chamaejasme (Thymelaeaceae)	Roots	Aldose reductase inhibitors	[65]
				Whole plants	Cytotoxic activity	[101]
108.	Chamaejasmin D (**108**)	(3 → 3")	*Stellera chamaejasme* (Thymelaeaceae)	Roots	Cytotoxic activity	[100]
109.	Cochinchinenene A (**109**)	(γ → 4)	*Dracaena cochinchinensis* (Agavaceae)	Stems	Anti-Helicobacter pylori and Thrombin Inhibitory activity	[70]
110.	Cochinchinenene B (**110**)	(γ → 2)	*Dracaena cochinchinensis* (Agavaceae)	Stems	Anti-Helicobacter pylori and Thrombin Inhibitory activity	[70]
111.	Cochinchinenene C (**111**)	(γ → 2)	*Dracaena cochinchinensis* (Agavaceae)	Stems	Anti-Helicobacter pylori and Thrombin Inhibitory activity	[70]
112.	Cochinchinenene D (**112**)	(γ → 2)	*Dracaena cochinchinensis* (Agavaceae)	Stems	Anti-Helicobacter pylori and Thrombin Inhibitory activity	[70]
113.	Cochinchinenin B (**113**)	(γ → 5)	*Dracaena cochinchinensis* (Agavaceae)	Stems	Anti-Helicobacter pylori and Thrombin Inhibitory activity	[70]
114.	Cochinchinenin C (**114**)	(γ → 5)	*Dracaena cochinchinensis* (Agavaceae)	Stems	Anti-Helicobacter pylori and Thrombin Inhibitory activity	[70]
115.	Cupressuflavone (**115**)*	(8 → 8")	*Selaginella tamariscina* (Selaginellaceae)	Aerial parts	Antidiabetic activity	[25]
					CYP2C8 and CYP2C9 enzyme inhibitory activity	[80]
116.	Daphnodorin B (**116**)*	—	*Wikstroemia indica* (Thymelaeaceae)	Rhizome	Anticancer / cytotoxic activity	[50]
117.	Daphnodorin G (**117**)*	—	*Wikstroemia indica* (Thymelaeaceae)	Rhizome	Anticancer / cytotoxic activity	[50]
118.	Daphnodorin H (**118**)*	—	*Wikstroemia indica* (Thymelaeaceae)	Rhizome	Anticancer / cytotoxic activity	[50]
119.	Daphnodorin J (**119**)*	—	*Wikstroemia indica* (Thymelaeaceae)	Rhizome	Anticancer / cytotoxic activity	[50]
120.	Daphnodorin M (**120**)*	—	*Daphne feddei* (Thymelaeaceae)	Stem bark	Activities against Nitric Oxide Production	[43]
121.	Daphnodorin N (**121**)*	—	*Daphne feddei* (Thymelaeaceae)	Stem bark	Activities against Nitric Oxide Production	[43]
122.	Daphnogirins A (**122**)	(8 → 3")	*Daphne giraldii* (Thymelaeaceae)	Roots	Antioxidative activity	[102]
123.	Daphnogirins B (**123**)	(8 → 3")	*Daphne giraldii* (Thymelaeaceae)	Roots	Antioxidative activity	[102]
124.	Dehydrolophirone C (**124**)	—	*Ochna holtzii* (Ochnaceae)	Root and Stem barks	Antimicrobial activity	[103]
125.	Delicaflavone (**125**)*	(3-O-4''')	*Selaginella doederleinii* (Selaginellaceae)	Whole plants	Anti-tumor activity	[28]
126.	De-O-methyl rotundaflavanochalcone (**126**)	(β → 6)	*Boesenbergia rotunda* (Zingiberaceae)	Roots	α-Glucosidase and pancreatic lipase inhibitory activity	[104]

(Table 1) cont.....

127.	Diphysin (**127**)*	(3 → 3")	*Ormocarpum kirkii* (Papilionaceae)	Roots	Antiplasmodial activity	[23]
			Ormocarpum trichocarpum (Papilionaceae)	Aerial parts	Antiplasmodial activity and antibacterial activity	[49]
128.	*ent*-naringeninyl-(I-3α,II-8)-4'-*O*-methylnaringenin (**128**)	(3 → 8")	*Garcinia livingstonei* (Clusiaceae)	Root barks	Antiprotozoal Activity and Cytotoxicity	[105]
129.	Fukugetin (**129**)*	(3 → 8")	*Garcinia gardneriana* (Clusiaceae)	Leaves	Anti-inflammatory activity	[106]
130.	Garciniaflavone A (**130**)	(3' → 8")	*Garcinia subelliptica* (Clusiaceae)	Leaves	—	[76]
131.	Garciniaflavone B (**131**)	(3' → 8")	*Garcinia subelliptica* (Clusiaceae)	Leaves	—	[76]
132.	Garciniaflavone C (**132**)	(3' → 8")	*Garcinia subelliptica* (Clusiaceae)	Leaves	—	[76]
133.	Garciniaflavone D (**133**)	(3' → 8")	*Garcinia subelliptica* (Clusiaceae)	Leaves	—	[76]
134.	Garciniaflavone E (**134**)	(3 → 8")	*Garcinia subelliptica* (Clusiaceae)	Leaves	—	[76]
135.	Garciniaflavone F (**135**)	(3 → 8")	*Garcinia subelliptica* (Clusiaceae)	Leaves	—	[76]
136.	GB-1(2*R*,3*S*,2"*R*,3"*R*) (**136**)*	(3 → 8")	*Garcinia buchananii* (Guttiferae)	Stem barks	Anti-oxidant activities	[93]
			Garcinia kola (Guttiferae)	Dried roots	Antibacterial activities	[45]
137.	GB-1(2*S*,3*R*,2"*R*,3"*R*) (**137**)	(3 → 8")	*Garcinia buchananii* (Guttiferae)	Stem barks	Anti-oxidant activities	[93]
138.	GB1-7"-*O*-β-glucoside (**138**)	(3 → 8")	*Clusia paralicola* (Clusiaceae)	Green fruits	Antioxidant activity	[91]
139.	GB-2 (**139**)*	(3 → 8")	*Garcinia buchananii* (Guttiferae)	Stem barks	Anti-oxidant activities	[94]
			Garcinia preussii (Guttiferae)	Leaves	Antibacterial activity	[107]
			Garcinia kola (Guttiferae)	Seeds	Tyrosinase inhibitor	[108]
140.	GB-2a (I 3-naringenin-II 8-eriodictyol) (**140**)*	(3 → 8")	*Garcinia buchananii* (Guttiferae)	Stem barks	Anti-oxidant activities	[93]
			Garcinia gardneriana (Clusiaceae)	Leaves	Anti-inflammatory	[106]
					Inhibitory effect on melanogenesis	[109]
				Branches	Aromatase (CYP19) inhibition activity	[110]
141.	GB-2 7"-O-β-D-glucopyranoside (**141**)	(3 → 8")	*Garcinia buchananii* (Guttiferae)	Stem barks	Anti-oxidant activities	[111]
			Garcinia gardneriana (Clusiaceae)	Branches	Aromatase (CYP19) inhibition activity	[110]
142.	Genkwanol B (**142**)*	(8 → 3")	*Radix wikstroemiae* (Thymelaeaceae)	Whole plant	Antiviral activity	[113]
143.	Genkwanol C (**143**)*	(8 → 3")	*Radix wikstroemiae* (Thymelaeaceae)	Whole plant	Antiviral activity	[113]

(Table 1) cont.....

144.	Ginkgetin (**144**)*	(3'→8")	*Cephalotaxus koreana* (Cephalotaxaceae)	Leaves and twigs	Osteoblast differentiation	[56]
			Selaginella moellendorffii (Selaginellacea)	Herbs	Cytotoxic activity	[78]
			Torreya nucifera (Taxaceae)	Leaves	SARS-cov 3clpro inhibition	[89]
			Purchased from Shanghai Yuan Ye Biotechnology Co., Ltd. (Shanghai, China)	—	Potential hepatic and renal toxicity	[81]
145.	Heveaflavone (**145**)*	(3'→ 8")	*Selaginella bryopteris* (Selaginellaceae)	Whole plant	Antiplasmodial and leishmanicidal activity	[37]
			Selaginella doederleinii (Selaginellaceae)	Whole plants	Anti-tumour activity	[27]
146.	Hinokiflavone (**146**)*	(4'-O-6")	*Selaginella moellendorffii* (Selaginellacea)	Herbs	Cytotoxic activity and Anti HBV activity	[78]
			Purchased from Extrasynthese (Genay Cedex, France)		Inhibitor of SUMO protease activity	[114]
147.	Holtzinol (**147**)	—	*Ochna holtzii* (Ochnaceae)	Root and Stem barks	Antimicrobial activity	[103]
148.	I-4″,I-7-dimethoxyamentoflavone (**148**)*	(3'→ 8")	*Podocarpus nakaii* (Podocarpaceae)	Twigs	Cytotoxicity activity	[115]
149.	II-3,I-5,II-5,II-7,I-4′,II-4′-hexahydroxy-(I-3,II-8)-flavonylflavanonol (**149**)	(3 → 8")	*Garcinia nervosa* (Guttiferae)	Leaves	Antagonistic activity	[116]
150.	II-7-O-methylrobustaflavone (**150**)	(5'→ 7")	*Araucaria angustifolia* (Araucariaceae)	Leaves	Antiviral activity	[87]
151.	Isochamaejasmenin B (**151**)*	(3 → 3")	*Stellera chamaejasme* (Thymelaeaceae)	Roots	Cytotoxic activity	[100]
152.	Isochamaejasmin (**152**)*	(3 → 3")	*Ormocarpum kirkii* (Papilionaceae)	Roots	Antiplasmodial activity	[23]
153.	Isocryptomerin (**153**)*	(4'- O-6")	*Selaginella tamariscina* (Selaginellaceae)	Whole plants	Matrix metalloproteinase in human skin fibroblasts	[24]
					Neuroprotective effects	[88]
154.	Isoginkgetin (**154**)*	(3' → 8")	*Podocarpus macrophyllus* (Popocarpaceae)	Leaves	Anti-tyrosinase effect	[32]
			Selaginella moellendorffii (Selaginellacea)	Herbs	Cytotoxic activity	[78]
			Purchased from LKT Laboratories	—	Proteasome Inhibitor	[118]
			Purchased from Shanghai Yuan Ye Biotechnology Co., Ltd. (Shanghai, China)	—	Potential hepatic and renal toxicity	[81]
155.	Isomanniflavanone (**155**)	(3 → 6")	*Garcinia buchananii* (Guttiferae)	Stem barks	Anti-oxidant activities	[111, 149]

(Table 1) cont.....

156.	Isoneochamaejasmin A (**156**)*	(3 → 3″)	*Stellera chamaejasme* (Thymelaeaceae)	Roots	Cytotoxic activity	[100]
			Daphne feddei (Thymelaeaceae)	Stem bark	Activities against Nitric Oxide Production	[43]
157.	Isorhamnetin-3-*O*-β-D-gluc*opyranoside*-(4′→*O*→4‴)-galangin-3″-*O*-β-D-glucopyranoside (**157**)	(4′-*O*-4‴)	*Solanum melongena* (Solanaceae)	Aerial parts	—	[119]
158.	Iso-rotundaflavanochalcone (**158**)	(β → 6)	*Boesenbergia rotunda* (Zingiberaceae)	Roots	α-Glucosidase and pancreatic lipase inhibitory activity	[104]
159.	Isosikokianin A (**159**)	(3 → 3″)	*Stellera chamaejasme* (Thymelaeaceae)	Roots	—	[120]
160.	Kolaviron (**160**)*	(3 → 8″)	*Garcinia kola* (Guttiferae)	Seeds	Ethanol induced Oxidative stress	[121]
					Testicular oxidative damage	[122]
					Tyrosinase inhibitor	[108]
					Antimalarial activity	[123]
					Antioxidant activity	[124]
					Ameliorative effect	[125]
					Antioxidant activity	[126]
161.	Lateriflavanone (**161**)	(6 → 8″)	*Garcinia lateriflora* (Clusiaceae)	Stem bark	—	[127]
162.	Linobiflavonoid (**162**)	(3 → 2″)	*Linostoma pauciflorum* (Thymelaeaceae)	Root	—	[128]
163.	Liquiritigeninyl-(I-3,II-3)-naringenin (**163**)	(3 → 3″)	*Ormocarpum kirkii* (Papilionaceae)	Roots	Antiplasmodial activity	[23]
164.	Loniflavone [5,5″,7,7″,3′-pentahydroxy 4′,4‴-biflavonyl ether] (**164**)	(4′-*O*-4‴)	*Lonicera japonica* (Caprifoliaceae)	Leaves	—	[51]
165.	Lophirone A trimethyl ether (**165**)	—	*Ochna holtzii* (Ochnaceae)	Root and Stem barks	Antimicrobial activity	[103]
166.	Lophirone L (**166**)	(3′-*O*-7″)	*Lophira alata* (Ochnaceae)	Leaves	—	[129]
167.	Lophirone M (**167**)	(3′-*O*-7″)	*Lophira alata* (Ochnaceae)	Leaves	—	[129]
168.	Macrophylloflavone (**168**)	(3 → 6″)	*Garcinia macrophylla* (Clusiaceae)	Stem bark	Antimicrobial, antioxidant and antidiabetic	[130]
169.	Malvidin 3-*O*-(6II-*O*-α-rhamnopyranosyl AIV-β-glucopyranoside AII)-5-*O*-β-glucopyranoside AIII) (apigenin 6-C-(2II-*O*-β-glucopyranosyl FIII-β-glucopyra-o-side FII)) malonate AV (AIV-4 →AV-1, FIII-6→AV-3) (**169**)	—	*Oxalis triangularis* (Oxalidaceae)	Leaves		[131]
170.	Manniflavanone (**170**)	(3 → 8″)	*Garcinia buchananii* (Guttiferae)	Stem barks	Anti-oxidant activities	[93-94, 111-112]
					L-type calcium channel inhibitor	[132]
			Garcinia preussii (Guttiferae)	Leaves	Antibacterial activity	[107]
171.	Manniflavanone-7″-*O*-β-D-glucopyranoside (**171**)	(3 → 8″)	*Garcinia buchananii* (Guttiferae)	Stem barks	Anti-oxidant activities	[111]
172.	Mesquitol-(4α,5)-epimesquitol-4β-ol (**172**)	(4 → 5″)	*Acacia nigrescens* (Leguminosae)	Heartwood	—	[48]

(Table 1) cont.....

173.	Morelloflavone (**173**)*	(3 → 8″)	*Garcinia brasiliensis* (Guttiferae)	Fruits	Antioxidant activity	[133]
				Stem bark and roots		[134]
			Garcinia gardneriana (Clusiaceae)	Branches	Aromatase (CYP19) inhibition activity	[110]
			Garcinia lateriflora (Clusiaceae)	Stem bark	Proteasome inhibition and cytotoxicity	[127]
			Garcinia prainiana (Guttiferae)	Stem barks	Antibacterial, antioxidant, Anti-tyrosinase	[57]
174.	Morelloflavone-4‴-*O*-β-D-glycosy (**174**)	(3 → 8″)	*Garcinia brasiliensis* (Guttiferae)	Fruits	Antioxidant activity	[133]
175.	Morelloflavone-7″-*O*-β-D-glucoside (**175**)	(3 → 8″)	*Garcinia brasiliensis* (Guttiferae)	Fruits	Antioxidant activity	[133]
176.	Morusyunnansin C (**176**)	(γ → 5′)	*Morus yunnanensis* (Moraceae)	Leaves	—	[135]
177.	Morusyunnansin D (**177**)	(γ → 5′)	*Morus yunnanensis* (Moraceae)	Leaves	—	[135]
178.	Murrmeranzin (**178**)	(2′-*O*-2‴)	*Murraya paniculata* (Rutaceae)	Aerial parts	—	[136]
179.	Neochamaejasmin B (**179**)*	(3 → 3″)	*Daphne feddei* (Thymelaeaceae)	Stem bark	Activities against Nitric Oxide Production	[43]
			Radix wikstroemiae (Thymelaeaceae)	Whole plant	Antiviral activity	[113]
			Stellera chamaejasme (Thymelaeaceae)	Roots	Cytotoxic activity	[100, 137]
180.	Neochamaejasmin C (**180**)*	(3 → 3″)	*Stellera chamaejasme* (Thymelaeaceae)	Roots	Anti-cancer activity	[99]
181.	Ochnaflavone (**181**)*	(3′-*O*-4‴)	*Lonicera japonica* (Caprifoliaceae)	Whole plants	Phospholipase A$_2$ activity	[138]
					Neuroprotective effects	[88]
					Anti-inflammatory activity	[139]
					Apoptosis in HCT-15 Human Colon Cancer Cells	[140]
					Therapeutic Effect on Fungal Arthritis	[141]
			Ochna pretoriensis (Ochnaceae)	Leaves	Antibacterial and cytotoxic activities	[142]
182.	Oliveriflavone A (**182**)	(4′-*O*-6″)	*Cephalotaxus oliveri* (Taxaceae)	Leaves and twigs	Antioxidant activity	[143]
183.	Oliveriflavone B (**183**)	(3′ → 8″)	*Cephalotaxus oliveri* (Taxaceae)	Leaves and twigs	Antioxidant activity	[143]
184.	Oliveriflavone C (**184**)	(3′ → 8″)	*Cephalotaxus oliveri* (Taxaceae)	Leaves and twigs	Antioxidant activity	[143]
185.	*O*-methylfukugetin (**185**)*	(3′ → 8″)	*Garcinia prainiana* (Guttiferae)	Stem barks	Antibacterial, antioxidant, Anti-tyrosinase activity	[57]
186.	Ormocarpin (**186**)*	(3 → 3″)	*Ormocarpum kirkii* (Papilionaceae)	Roots	Antiplasmodial activity	[23]
187.	Ouratine A (**187**)	(6 → 8″)	*Ouratea nigroviolacea* (Ochnaceae)	Leaves	—	[144]
188.	Ouratine B (**188**)	(6 → 8″)	*Ouratea nigroviolacea* (Ochnaceae)	Leaves	—	[144]

(Table 1) cont.....

189.	Oxytrochalcoflavanone A (**189**)	(β → 6)	*Oxytropis chiliophylla* (Leguminosae)	Aerial part	—	[145]
190.	Oxytrochalcoflavanone B (**190**)	(β → 6)	*Oxytropis chiliophylla* (Leguminosae)	Aerial part	—	[145]
191.	Oxytrodiflavanone A (**191**)	(6 → 4")	*Oxytropis chiliophylla* (Leguminosae)	Aerial part	—	[145]
192.	Paucinervin K (**192**)	(8 → 3")	*Garcinia paucinervis* (Guttiferae)	Leaves	Antioxidant and hypoglycemic activities	[146]
193.	Pierotin A (**193**)	(5-CH$_2$-5")	*Pieris japonica* (Ericaceae)	Leaves	Immunomodulatory activity	[147]
194.	Podocarpusflavone A (**194**)*	(3'→ 8")	*Podocarpus macrophyllus* (Podocarpaceae)	—	β-Secretase (BACE-1) inhibitory effect: Alzheimer	[117]
			Podocarpus nakaii (Podocarpaceae)	Twigs	Cytotoxic activity	[115]
195.	Podocarpusflavone B (**195**)*	(3'→ 8")	*Podocarpus macrophyllus* (Podocarpaceae)		β-Secretase (BACE-1) inhibitory effect: Alzheimer	[117]
196.	Potifulgene (**196**)	(5-O-5")	*Potentilla fulgens* (Rosaceae)	Roots	Antioxidant activities	[148]
197.	Preussianon (**197**)	(8 → 3")	*Garcinia buchananii* (Guttiferae)	Stem barks	Anti-oxidant activities	[149]
			Garcinia preussii (Clusiaceae)	Leaves	—	[107]
198.	Pyranocoumarin dimmer (**198**)	(3'-O-4''')	*Angelica urumiensis* (Apiaceae)	Aerial parts	Antioxidant activities	[150]
199.	Rel-(1-β,2-α-di-(2,4-dihydroxybenzyl)-rel-(3-β, 4-α)-di-(4-hydroxy-ph-nyl)-cyclobutane (**199**)	—	*Agapanthus africanus* (Liliaceae)	Roots	—	[151]
200.	Ridiculflavone A (**200**)	(3 → 6")	*Aristolochia ridicula* (Aristolochiaceae)	Leaves	—	[152]
201.	Ridiculflavone B (**201**)	(3 → 6")	*Aristolochia ridicula* (Aristolochiaceae)	Leaves	—	[152]
202.	Ridiculflavone D (**202**)	(3 → 6")	*Aristolochia ridicula* (Aristolochiaceae)	Leaves	—	[153]
203.	Ridiculflavonylchalcone B (**203**)	—	*Aristolochia ridicula* (Aristolochiaceae)	Leaves	—	[153]
204.	Robustaflavone (**204**)*	(3'→ 6")	*Dietes bicolor* (Iridaceae)	Leaves	Anti-inflammatory activity	[75]
			Selaginella tamariscina (Selaginellaceae)	Whole plants	Matrix metalloproteinase in human skin fibroblasts	[24]
				Aerial parts	Antidiabetic activity	[25]
					CYP2C8 and CYP2C9 enzyme inhibitory activity	[80]
			Selaginella doederleinii (Selaginellaceae)	Whole plants	Anti-tumour activity	[27, 28]
205.	Robustaflavone 4'-methyl ether (**205**)*	(3'→ 6")	*Selaginella doederleinii* (Selaginellaceae)	Whole plant	Cytotoxic activity	[30]
			Selaginella moellendorffii (Selaginellacea)	Herbs	Cytotoxic activity and Anti HBV activity	[78]
206.	Rotundaflavanochalcone (**206**)	(β → 6)	*Boesenbergia rotunda* (Zingiberaceae)	Roots	α-Glucosidase and pancreatic lipase inhibitory activity	[104]

(Table 1) cont.....

207.	Sarcandrone A (**207**)	(4 → 3')	*Sarcandra hainanensis* (Chloranthaceae)	Whole plants	Anti-HIV activity	[63]
208.	Sciadopitysin (**208**)*	(3' → 8")	*Cephalotaxus harringtonia* (Cephalotaxaceae)	—	β-Secretase (BACE-1) inhibitory effect: Alzheimer	[117]
			Cephalotaxus koreana (Cephalotaxaceae)	Leaves and twigs	Osteoblast differentiation	[56]
			Gingko biloba (Ginkgoaceae)	—	Neuroprotective effects	[88]
			Podocarpus macrophyllus (Popocarpaceae)	Leaves	Anti-tyrosinase effect	[32]
			Selaginella bryopteris (Selaginellaceae)	Whole plant	Antiplasmodial and leishmanicidal activity	[37]
			Torreya nucifera (Taxaceae)	Leaves	SARS-cov 3clpro inhibition	[89]
			Purchased from Shanghai Yuan Ye Biotechnology Co., Ltd. (Shanghai, China)	—	Potential hepatic and renal toxicity	[81]
209.	Selariscinin E (**209**)	(5' → 8")	*Selaginella tamariscina* (Selaginellaceae)	Aerial parts	Antidiabetic activity	[25]
					CYP2C8 and CYP2C9 enzyme inhibitory activity	[80]
210.	Sequoiaflavone (**210**)*	(3' → 8")	*Araucaria angustifolia* (Araucariaceae)	Leaves	Antiviral activity	[87]
			Campylospermum excavatum (Ochnaceae)	Leaves	Antiparasitic activities	[66]
			Cunninghamia lanceolata (Cupressaceae)	—	β-Secretase (BACE-1) inhibitory effect: Alzheimer	[117]
			Selaginella bryopteris (Selaginellaceae)	Whole plant	Antiplasmodial and leishmanicidal activity	[37]
211.	Sikokianin A (**211**)*	(3 → 3")	*Stellera chamaejasme* (Thymelaeaceae)	Roots	Cytotoxic activity	[100]
					Antiviral effect	[120]
212.	Sikokianin B (**212**)*	(3 → 3")	*Stellera chamaejasme* (Thymelaeaceae)	Roots	Cytotoxic activity	[100]
			Wikstroemia indica (Thymelaeaceae)	Roots	Anti-inflammatory activity	[154]
			Wikstroemia taiwanensis (Thymelaeaceae)	Stems	Antitubercular activity	[160]
213.	Sikokianin C (**213**)*	(3 → 3")	*Stellera chamaejasme* (Thymelaeaceae)	Roots	Cytotoxic activity	[100]
			Wikstroemia indica (Thymelaeaceae)	Roots	Anti-inflammatory activity	[154]
				Rhizome	Anticancer /cytotoxic activity	[50]
			Wikstroemia taiwanensis (Thymelaeaceae)	Stems	Antitubercular activity	[160]
214.	Sikokianin D (**214**)	(3 → 3")	*Stellera chamaejasme* (Thymelaeaceae)	Roots	Cytotoxic activity	[100]
			Wikstroemia indica (Thymelaeaceae)	Roots	—	[155]
215.	Sophobiflavonoid A (**215**)	(β → 5')	*Sophora flavescens* (Leguminosae)	Roots	Antidiabetic activity	[156]

(Table 1) cont.....

216.	Sophobiflavonoid B (**216**)	(β → 5')	*Sophora flavescens* (Leguminosae)	Roots	—	[156]
217.	Sophobiflavonoid C (**217**)	(β → 5')	*Sophora flavescens* (Leguminosae)	Roots	Antidiabetic activity	[156]
218.	Sophobiflavonoid D (**218**)	(β → 5')	*Sophora flavescens* (Leguminae)	Roots	—	[156]
219.	Sophobiflavonoid E (**219**)	(β → 5')	*Sophora flavescens* (Leguminosae)	Roots	Antidiabetic activity	[156]
220.	Sophobiflavonoid F (**220**)	(β → 3)	*Sophora flavescens* (Leguminosae)	Roots	—	[156]
221.	Sophobiflavonoid G (**221**)	(β → 3)	*Sophora flavescens* (Leguminosae)	Roots	Antidiabetic activity	[156]
222.	Sophobiflavonoid H (**222**)	(β → 3)	*Sophora flavescens* (Leguminosae)	Roots	Antidiabetic activity	[156]
223.	Sparinaritin (**223**)	(3'-O-3''')	*Parinari hypochrysea* (Chrysobalanaceae)	Leaves	—	[157]
224.	Stelleranol (**224**)*	(3 → 8")	*Radix wikstroemiae* (Thymelaeaceae)	Whole plant	Antiviral activity	[113]
225.	Sumaflavone (**225**)*	(3' → 8")	*Selaginella tamariscina* (Selaginellaceae)	Whole plants	Matrix metalloproteinase in human skin fibroblasts	[24]
226.	Taiwaniaflavone (**226**)*	(3 → 3")	*Selaginella tamariscina* (Selaginellaceae)	Whole plants	Matrix metalloproteinase in human skin fibroblasts	[24]
				Aerial parts	Antidiabetic activity	[25]
					CYP2C8 and CYP2C9 enzyme inhibitory activity	[80]
227.	Talbotaflavone (**227**)*	(3 → 8")	*Garcinia lateriflora* (Clusiaceae)	Stem bark	Proteasome inhibition and cytotoxicity	[127]
228.	Tetrahydroamentoflavone (**228**)*	(3' → 8")	*Selaginella bryopteris* (Selaginellaceae)	Whole plant	Antiplasmodial and leishmanicidal activity	[37]
			Selaginella uncinata (Selaginellaceae)	Whole herbs	Protective effect against anoxia	[26]
			Semecarpus anacardium (Anacardiaceae)	Seeds	Inhibitor of xanthine oxidase	[158]
229.	Tetrahydrohinokiflavone (**229**)*	(4'-O-6")	*Selaginella bryopteris* (Selaginellaceae)	Whole plant	Antiplasmodial and leishmanicidal activity	[37]
230.	Tetrahydroisoginkgetin (**230**)	(3' → 8")	*Cycas circinalis* (Cycadaceae)	Leaflets	Antibacterial activity	[36]
231.	Uncinatabiflavone A (**231**)	(3' → 6")	*Selaginella uncinata* (Selaginellaceae)	Whole herbs	—	[159]
232.	Uncinatabiflavone B (**232**)	(3' → 6")	*Selaginella uncinata* (Selaginellaceae)	Whole herbs	—	[159]
233.	Uncinatabiflavone C (**233**)	(3' → 6")	*Selaginella uncinata* (Selaginellaceae)	Whole herbs	—	[159]
234.	Uncinatabiflavone D (**234**)	(3' → 6")	*Selaginella uncinata* (Selaginellaceae)	Whole herbs	Anti-anoxic effect	[159]
235.	Volkensiflavone (**235**)*	(3 → 8")	*Garcinia livingstonei* (Clusiaceae)	Root barks	Antiprotozoal activity and Cytotoxicity	[105]
			Garcinia buchananii (Guttiferae)	Stem bark and roots	Antioxidant activities	[134]
			Garcinia prainiana (Guttiferae)	Stem barks	Antibacterial, Antioxidant, Anti-tyrosinase	[57]

(Table 1) cont.....

No.	Name	Linkage	Source	Part	Activity	Ref.
236.	Wikstaiwanone A (**236**)	(3 → 3″)	*Wikstroemia indica* (Thymelaeaceae)	Rhizome	Anticancer /cytotoxic activity	[50]
			Wikstroemia taiwanensis (Thymelaeaceae)	Stems	—	[160]
237.	Wikstaiwanone B (**237**)	(3 → 3″)	*Wikstroemia indica* (Thymelaeaceae)	Rhizome	Anticancer /cytotoxic activity	[50]
			Wikstroemia taiwanensis (Thymelaeaceae)	Stems	—	[160]
238.	Wikstaiwanone C (**238**)	(3 → 3″)	*Wikstroemia taiwanensis* (Thymelaeaceae)	Stems	—	[160]
239.	Wikstrol A (**239**)*	(3 → 8″)	*Daphne feddei* (Thymelaeaceae)	Stem bark	Activities against Nitric Oxide Production	[43]
			Stellera chamaejasme (Thymelaeaceae)	Roots	Aldose reductase inhibitors	[65]
240.	Aesculitannin B (**240**) #*	—	*Machilus philippinensis* (Lauraceae)	Leaves	α-Glucosidase inhibitory activity	[162]
241.	Alhacidin (**241**) #	—	*Alhagi pseudalhagi* (Fabaceae)	Aerial parts and roots	—	[161]
242.	Alhacin (**242**) #	—	*Alhagi pseudalhagi* (Fabaceae)	Aerial parts and roots	—	[161]
243.	Chalcone-flavone tetramer (**243**) #	—	*Aristolochia ridicula* (Aristolochiaceae)	Leaves	—	[152]
244.	Machiphilitannin A (**244**) #	—	*Machilus philippinensis* (Lauraceae)	Leaves	α-Glucosidase inhibitory activity	[162]
245.	Machiphilitannin B (**245**) #	—	*Machilus philippinensis* (Lauraceae)	Leaves	α-Glucosidase inhibitory activity	[162]
246.	Pavetannin C-1 (**246**) #*	—	*Machilus philippinensis* (Lauraceae)	Leaves	α-Glucosidase inhibitory activity	[162]
247.	Ridiculuflavonylchalcone C (**247**) #	—	*Aristolochia ridicula* (Aristolochiaceae)	Leaves		[153]

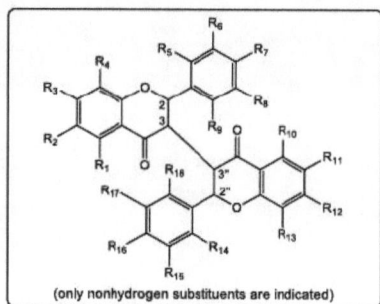

(only nonhydrogen substituents are indicated)

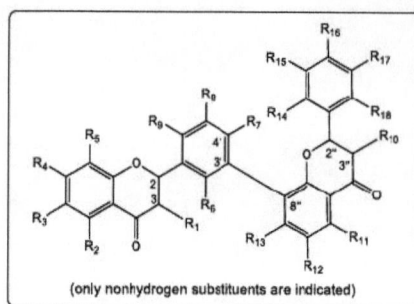

(only nonhydrogen substituents are indicated)

3 $R_3=R_7=R_{12}=R_{16}=OH$

9 $R_1=R_3=R_5=R_7=R_{10}=R_{12}=R_{14}=R_{16}=OH$

10 $R_1=R_5=R_7=R_{10}=R_{12}=R_{14}=R_{16}=OH$; $R_3=\beta$-D-GlcO

26 $R_1=R_3=R_5=R_7=R_{10}=R_{12}=R_{16}=OH$

27 $R_1=R_5=R_7=R_{10}=R_{12}=R_{16}=OH$; $R_3=\beta$-D-GlcO

53 $R_1=R_{10}=OH$; $R_3=R_7=R_{12}=R_{16}=OMe$ (2,3S; 2",3"R)

55 $R_1=R_7=R_{10}=R_{16}=OH$; $R_3=R_{12}=OMe$; (C$_{2-3}$=db)

56 $R_1=R_7=R_{10}=R_{16}=OH$; $R_3=R_{12}=OMe$ (2,3S; 2",3"R)

59 $R_1=R_7=R_{10}=R_{12}=R_{16}=OH$; $R_3=OMe$

60 $R_1=R_7=R_{10}=R_{12}=R_{16}=OH$; $R_3=OMe$ (2,3,3"S; 2"R)

5 $R_2=R_4=R_{11}=R_{13}=R_{16}=OH$; $R_7=OMe$; (C$_{2-3}$=db)

11 $R_2=R_{11}=R_{13}=R_{16}=OH$; $R_4=Me$; $R_4=R_7=OMe$; (C$_{2"-3"}$=db)

12 $R_2=R_4=R_{11}=R_{13}=OH$; Me; $R_7=R_{16}=OMe$; (C$_{2"-3"}$=db)

13 $R_2=R_4=R_7=R_{11}=R_{13}=OH$; $R_{16}=OMe$; (C$_{2"-3"}$=db)

14 $R_2=R_4=R_{11}=R_{13}=R_{16}=OH$; $R_7=OMe$; (C$_{2"-3"}$=db)

16 $R_2=R_4=R_7=R_{11}=R_{13}=R_{16}=OH$; (C$_{2"-3"}$=db)

17 $R_2=R_4=R_7=R_{11}=R_{13}=R_{16}=OH$; (C$_{2-3}$=db)

18 $R_2=R_4=R_{11}=R_{13}=R_{16}=OH$; $R_7=OMe$; (C$_{2"-3"}$=db)

19 $R_2=R_4=R_{11}=R_{13}=R_{16}=OH$; $R_7=OMe$

25 $R_2=R_{11}=R_{13}=OH$; $R_4=R_7=R_{16}=OMe$; (C$_{2"-3"}$=db)

(Fig. 4) contd.....

61 $R_1=R_7=R_{10}=R_{12}=R_{16}=OH$; R_3 ... S; 2"R)

67 $R_1=R_3=R_7=R_{10}=R_{16}=OH$; $R_{12}=\beta$-D-Glc$O$

84 $R_1=R_3=R_7=R_{10}=R_{12}=R_{16}$ ... $_{2\text{-}3}$=db)

85 $R_1=R_7=R_{10}=R_{16}$ ... $_3=R_{12}=\beta$-D-Glc$O$

92 $R_3=R_6=R_7=R_{12}=R_{16}=R_{17}=OH$

100 $R_3=R_7=R_{12}=R_{16}$

101 $R_1=R_3=R_7=R_{12}=R_{16}=OH$

104 $R_1=R_{10}=R_{12}=R_{16}$ ... $_3=R_7=OMe$

105 $R_1=R_3=R_{10}=R_{12}$ ... $_7=R_{16}$ ... S)

106 $R_1=R_3=R_{10}=R_{12}$ ... $_7=R_{16}$ ... R; 3,3"S)

107 $R_1=R_3=R_7=R_{10}=R_{12}=R_{16}$

108 $R_1=R_3=R_7=R_{10}=R_{12}=R_{16}$ ... R ... S)

151 $R_1=R_3=R_{10}=R_{12}$ ... $_7=R_{16}$ ... S; R)

152 $R_1=R_3=R_7=R_{10}=R_{12}=R_{16}$ ... S ... R)

156 $R_1=R_3=R_7=R_{10}=R_{12}=R_{16}$ ... S ... R)

32 $R_2=R_4=R_7=R_{10}=R_{11}=R_{13}=R_{16}=O$ ... $_{2\text{-}3}$ & C_-=db)

33 $R_2=R_7=R_{10}=R_{11}=R_{13}=R_{16}=OH$; R_4 ... $_{2\text{-}3}$ & C_- =db)

35 $R_1=R_{10}=OMe$; $R_2=R_4=R_7=R_{11}=R_{13}=R_{16}$ ... $_{2\text{-}3}$ & $C_{2"\text{-}3"}$=db)

45 $R_2=R_4=R_{11}=R_{16}$ ... $_7=R_{13}$ ... $_{2\text{-}3}$ & C_- =db)

46 $R_2=R_4=R_7=R_{11}=R_{13}$ ... $_{16}$ ... -

50 $R_2=R_4=R_7=R_{11}=R_{13}$ ... $_{16}$ ... $_{2\text{-}3}$ & C_- =db)

54 $R_2=R_{11}$ ... $_4=R_7=R_{13}=R_{16}$ ... $_{2\text{-}3}$ & C_- =db)

62 $R_2=R_7=R_{11}=R_{13}=R_{16}$ ... $_4$ ... $_{2\text{-}3}$ & C_- =db)

64 $R_2=R_{11}=R_{16}$ ... $_4=R_7=R_{13}$ ... $_{2\text{-}3}$ & C_- =db)

83 $R_2=R_7=R_{11}=R_{13}=R_{16}$ ... $_4$ ... $_{2\text{-}3}$ & C_- =db)

91 $R_2=R_4=R_{11}=R_{13}=R_{16}$ ... $_7$ ... $_{2\text{-}3}$ & C_- =db)

102 $R_2=R_7=R_{10}=R_{11}=R_{13}=R_{16}$ ... $_4$ ... $_{2\text{-}3}$=db)

130 $R_2=R_4=R_7=R_{11}=R_{16}$ ... $_{13}=O$- ... $_{2\text{-}3}$ & C_- =db)

131 $R_2=R_4=R_7=R_{11}=R_{16}$ ... $_{13}=O$-(2- ... -1- en-3- ($C_{2\text{-}3}$ & C_- =db)

(Fig. 4) contd.....

159 $R_1=R_3=R_{10}=R_{12}=R_{16}=$OH; $R_7=$OMe (2,3,2"3"R)

163 $R_1=R_3=R_7=R_{10}=R_{12}=R_{16}=$OH (2,2"$S$; 3,3"$R$)

179 $R_1=R_3=R_7=R_{10}=R_{12}=R_{16}=$OH (2,3,3"$S$; 2"$R$)

180 $R_1=R_3=R_{10}=R_{12}=$OH; $R_7=R_{16}=$OMe (2,3,3"S; 2"R)

186 $R_1=R_7=R_{10}=R_{16}=$OH; $R_3=R_{12}=\beta$-D-Glc$O$ (2,2"S; 3,3"R)

211 $R_1=R_3=R_{10}=R_{12}=R_{16}=$OH; $R_7=$OMe (2,3,2"3"S)

212 $R_1=R_3=R_{10}=R_{12}=R_{16}=$OH; $R_7=$OMe (2,3,3"S; 2"R)

213 $R_1=R_3=R_{10}=R_{12}=R_{16}=$OH; $R_7=$OMe (2,3'S; 3,2"R)

214 $R_1=R_3=R_{10}=R_{12}=R_{16}=$OH; $R_7=$OMe (2,3S; 2",3"R)

238 $R_1=R_3=R_{10}=R_{12}=R_{16}=$OH; $R_7=$OMe (2,2"R; 3,3"S)

144 $R_2=R_{11}=R_{13}=R_{16}=$OH; $R_4=R_7=$OMe; (C$_{2-3}$ & C$_{2"-3"}$=db)

145 $R_2=R_7=R_{11}=$OH; $R_4=R_{13}=R_{16}=$OMe; (C$_{2-3}$ & C$_{2"-3"}$=db)

148 $R_2=R_7=R_{11}=R_{13}=$OH; $R_4=$ R$_{16}=$OMe; (C$_{2-3}$ & C$_{2"-3"}$=db)

154 $R_2=R_4=R_{11}=R_{13}=$OH; $R_7=$ R$_{16}=$OMe; (C$_{2-3}$ & C$_{2"-3"}$=db)

183 $R_2=R_4=R_{11}=$OH; $R_3=$Me; $R_7=R_{13}=R_{16}=$OMe; (C$_{2"-3"}$=db)

184 $R_2=R_4=R_{11}=R_{13}=$OH; $R_3=$Me; $R_7=R_{16}=$OMe; (C$_{2"-3"}$=db)

185 $R_2=R_4=R_7=R_{11}=R_{13}=$OH; $R_{16}=$OMe; (C$_{2"-3"}$=db)

194 $R_2=R_4=R_7=R_{11}=R_{13}=$OH; $R_{16}=$OMe; (C$_{2-3}$ & C$_{2"-3"}$=db)

195 $R_2=R_7=R_{11}=R_{13}=$OH; $R_4=R_{16}=$OMe; (C$_{2-3}$ & C$_{2"-3"}$=db)

208 $R_2=R_{11}=R_{13}=$OH; $R_4=R_7=R_{16}=$OMe; (C$_{2-3}$ & C$_{2"-3"}$=db)

210 $R_2=R_7=R_{11}=R_{13}=R_{16}=$OH; $R_4=$OMe; (C$_{2-3}$ & C$_{2"-3"}$=db)

225 $R_2=R_4=R_7=R_{11}=R_{12}=R_{13}=R_{16}=$OH; (C$_{2-3}$ & C$_{2"-3"}$=db)

228 $R_2=R_4=R_7=R_{11}=R_{13}=R_{16}=$OH

230 $R_2=R_4=R_{11}=R_{13}=$OH; $R_7=R_{16}=$OMe

Fig. (4). Chemical structures of biflavonoids with C-C connections.

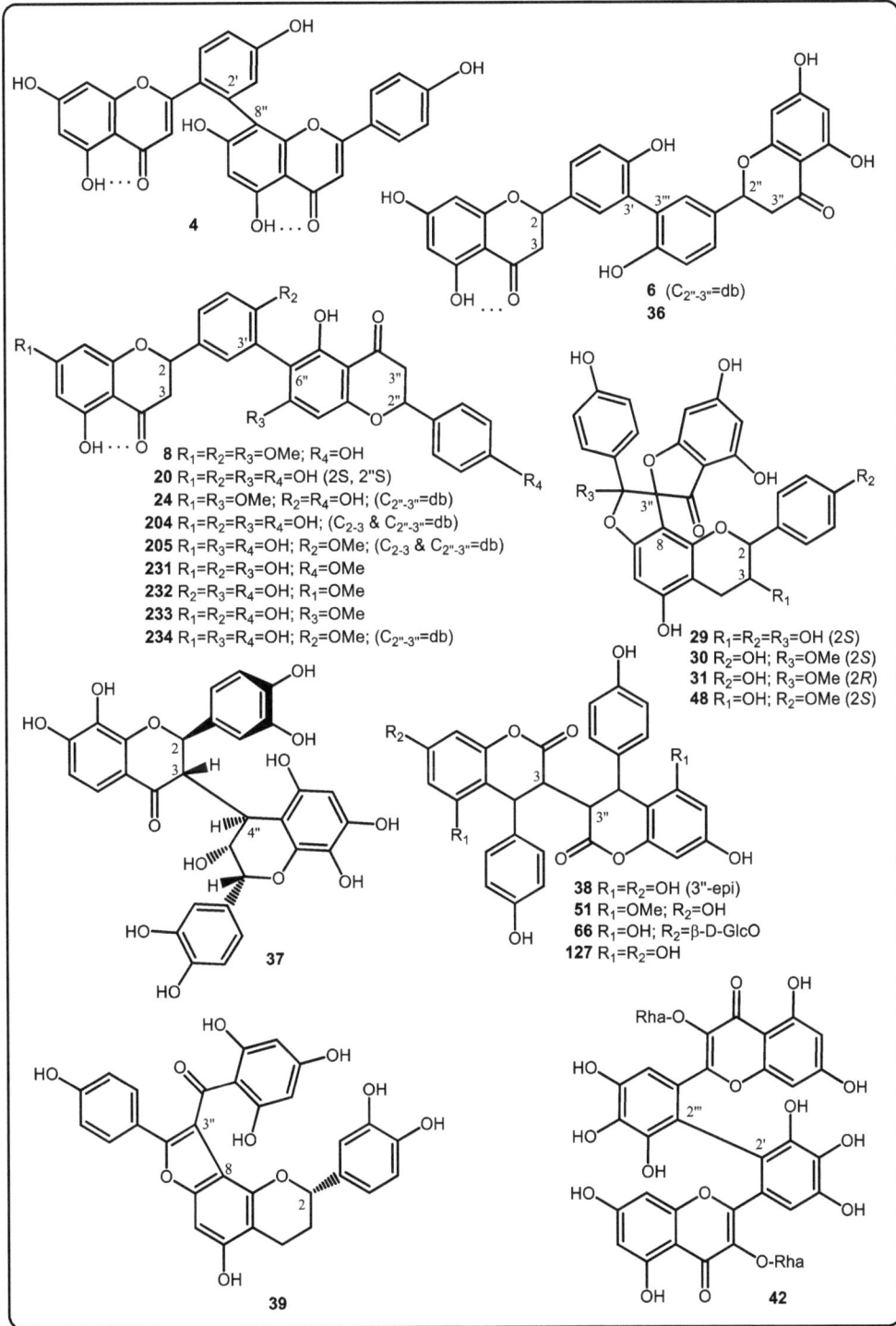

8 R₁=R₂=R₃=OMe; R₄=OH
20 R₁=R₂=R₃=R₄=OH (2S, 2"S)
24 R₁=R₃=OMe; R₂=R₄=OH; (C₂"-₃"=db)
204 R₁=R₂=R₃=R₄=OH; (C₂-₃ & C₂"-₃"=db)
205 R₁=R₃=R₄=OH; R₂=OMe; (C₂-₃ & C₂"-₃"=db)
231 R₁=R₂=R₃=OH; R₄=OMe
232 R₂=R₃=R₄=OH; R₁=OMe
233 R₁=R₂=R₄=OH; R₃=OMe
234 R₁=R₃=R₄=OH; R₂=OMe; (C₂"-₃"=db)

6 (C₂"-₃"=db)
36

29 R₁=R₂=R₃=OH (2S)
30 R₂=OH; R₃=OMe (2S)
31 R₂=OH; R₃=OMe (2R)
48 R₁=OH; R₂=OMe (2S)

37

38 R₁=R₂=OH (3"-epi)
51 R₁=OMe; R₂=OH
66 R₁=OH; R₂=β-D-GlcO
127 R₁=R₂=OH

39

42

(Fig. 5) contd.....

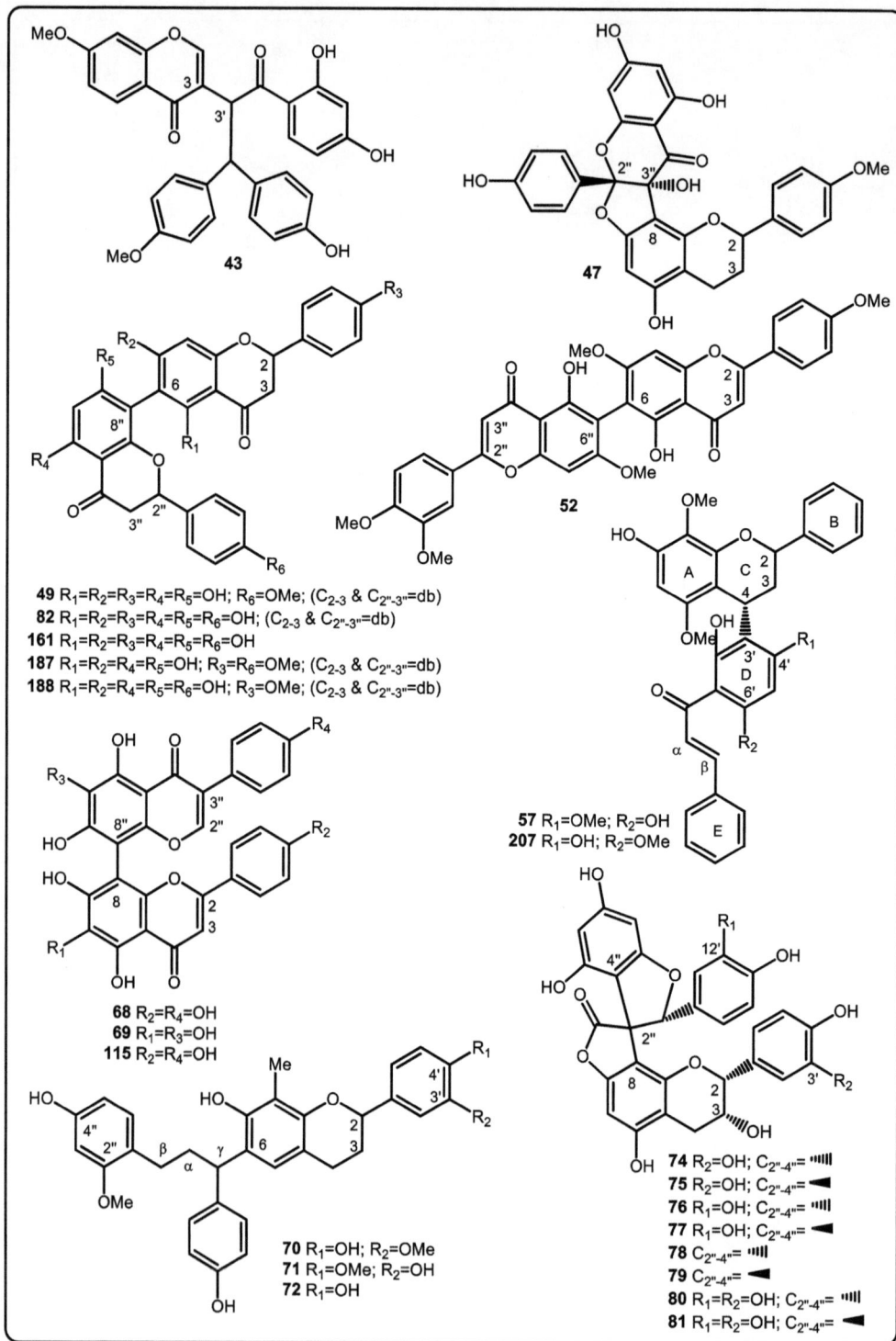

49 $R_1=R_2=R_3=R_4=R_5=OH$; $R_6=OMe$; (C_{2-3} & $C_{2"-3"}$=db)
82 $R_1=R_2=R_3=R_4=R_5=R_6=OH$; ($C_{2-3}$ & $C_{2"-3"}$=db)
161 $R_1=R_2=R_3=R_4=R_5=R_6=OH$
187 $R_1=R_2=R_4=R_5=OH$; $R_3=R_6=OMe$; (C_{2-3} & $C_{2"-3"}$=db)
188 $R_1=R_2=R_4=R_5=R_6=OH$; $R_3=OMe$; (C_{2-3} & $C_{2"-3"}$=db)

68 $R_2=R_4=OH$
69 $R_1=R_3=OH$
115 $R_2=R_4=OH$

70 $R_1=OH$; $R_2=OMe$
71 $R_1=OMe$; $R_2=OH$
72 $R_1=OH$

57 $R_1=OMe$; $R_2=OH$
207 $R_1=OH$; $R_2=OMe$

74 $R_2=OH$; $C_{2"-4"}$= ''''''
75 $R_2=OH$; $C_{2"-4"}$= ◄
76 $R_1=OH$; $C_{2"-4"}$= ''''''
77 $R_1=OH$; $C_{2"-4"}$= ◄
78 $C_{2"-4"}$= ''''''
79 $C_{2"-4"}$= ◄
80 $R_1=R_2=OH$; $C_{2"-4"}$= ''''''
81 $R_1=R_2=OH$; $C_{2"-4"}$= ◄

(Fig. 5) contd.....

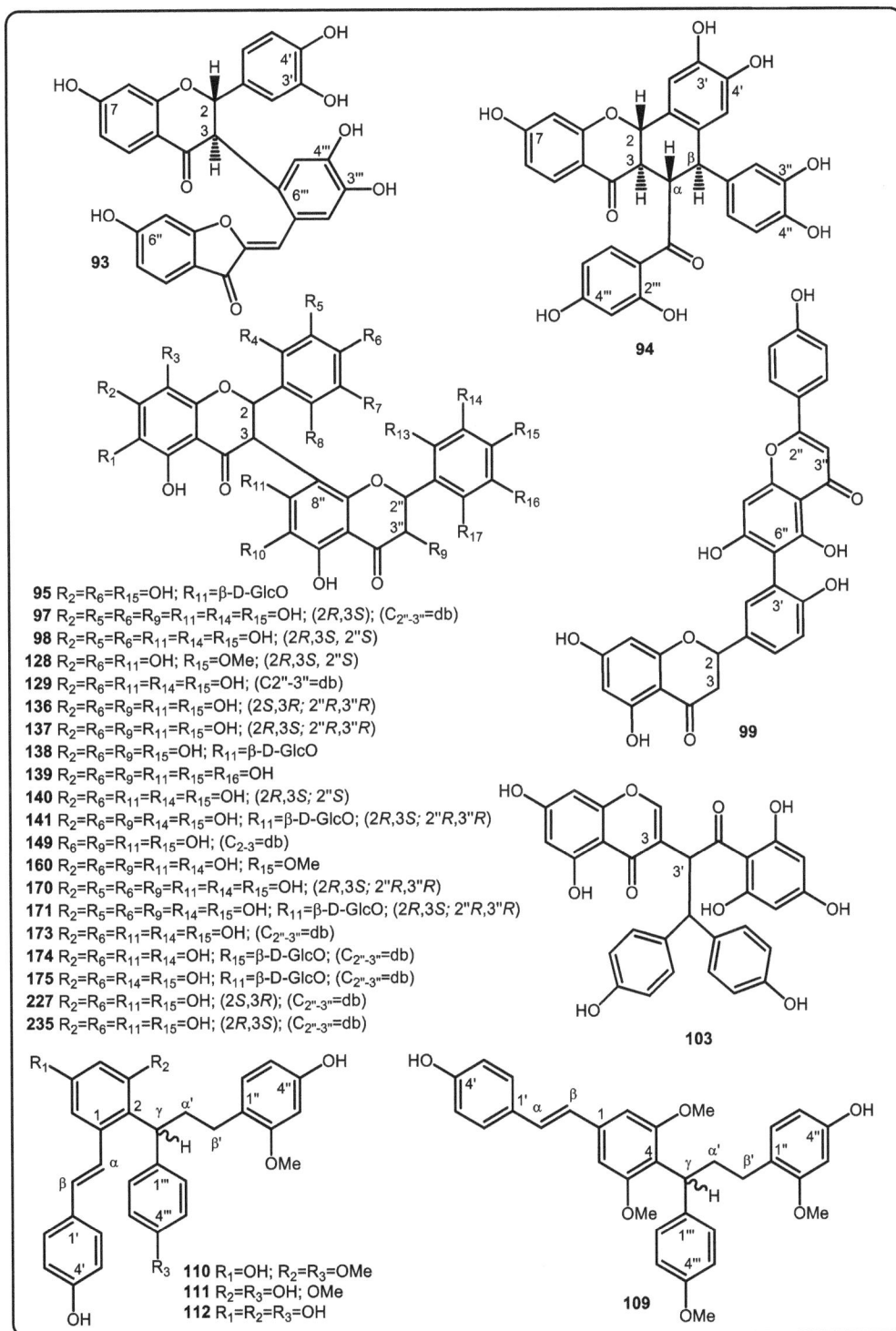

95 $R_2=R_6=R_{15}=OH$; $R_{11}=\beta$-D-GlcO
97 $R_2=R_5=R_6=R_9=R_{11}=R_{14}=R_{15}=OH$; (2R,3S); ($C_{2''-3''}$=db)
98 $R_2=R_5=R_6=R_{11}=R_{14}=R_{15}=OH$; (2R,3S, 2''S)
128 $R_2=R_6=R_{11}=OH$; $R_{15}=OMe$; (2R,3S, 2''S)
129 $R_2=R_6=R_9=R_{11}=R_{14}=R_{15}=OH$; (C2''-3''=db)
136 $R_2=R_6=R_9=R_{11}=R_{15}=OH$; (2S,3R; 2''R,3''R)
137 $R_2=R_6=R_9=R_{11}=R_{15}=OH$; (2R,3S; 2''R,3''R)
138 $R_2=R_6=R_9=R_{15}=OH$; $R_{11}=\beta$-D-GlcO
139 $R_2=R_6=R_9=R_{11}=R_{15}=R_{16}=OH$
140 $R_2=R_6=R_{11}=R_{14}=R_{15}=OH$; (2R,3S; 2''S)
141 $R_2=R_6=R_9=R_{14}=R_{15}=OH$; $R_{11}=\beta$-D-GlcO; (2R,3S; 2''R,3''R)
149 $R_6=R_9=R_{11}=R_{15}=OH$; (C$_{2-3}$=db)
160 $R_2=R_6=R_9=R_{11}=R_{14}=OH$; $R_{15}=OMe$
170 $R_2=R_5=R_6=R_9=R_{11}=R_{14}=R_{15}=OH$; (2R,3S; 2''R,3''R)
171 $R_2=R_5=R_6=R_9=R_{14}=R_{15}=OH$; $R_{11}=\beta$-D-GlcO; (2R,3S; 2''R,3''R)
173 $R_2=R_6=R_{11}=R_{14}=R_{15}=OH$; (C$_{2''-3''}$=db)
174 $R_2=R_6=R_{11}=R_{14}=OH$; $R_{15}=\beta$-D-GlcO; (C$_{2''-3''}$=db)
175 $R_2=R_6=R_{14}=R_{15}=OH$; $R_{11}=\beta$-D-GlcO; (C$_{2''-3''}$=db)
227 $R_2=R_6=R_{11}=R_{15}=OH$; (2S,3R); (C$_{2''-3''}$=db)
235 $R_2=R_6=R_{11}=R_{15}=OH$; (2R,3S); (C$_{2''-3''}$=db)

110 $R_1=OH$; $R_2=R_3=OMe$
111 $R_2=R_3=OH$; OMe
112 $R_1=R_2=R_3=OH$

(Fig. 5) contd.....

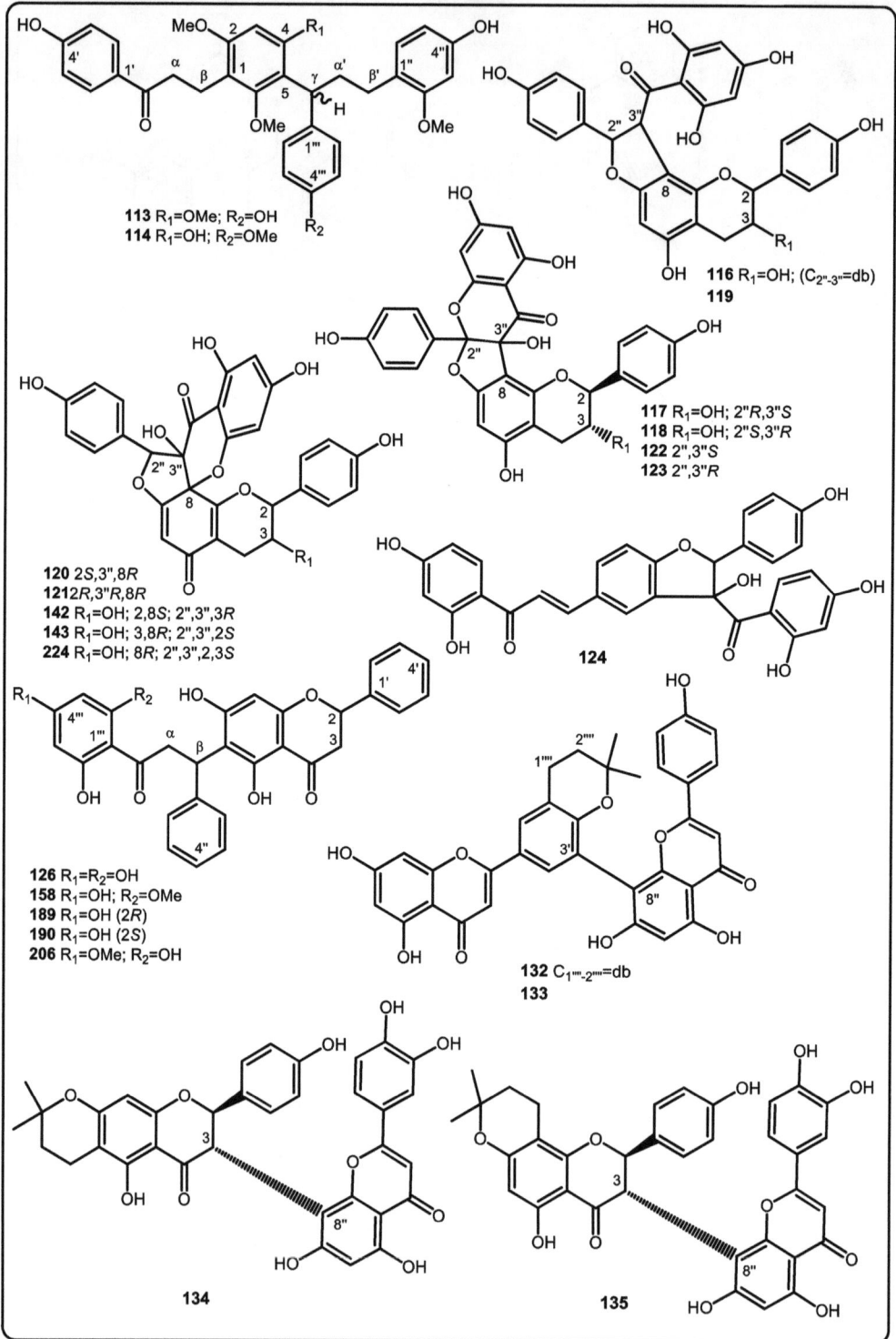

113 R$_1$=OMe; R$_2$=OH
114 R$_1$=OH; R$_2$=OMe

116 R$_1$=OH; (C$_{2''-3''}$=db)
119

117 R$_1$=OH; 2"R,3"S
118 R$_1$=OH; 2"S,3"R
122 2",3"S
123 2",3"R

120 2S,3",8R
121 2R,3"R,8R
142 R$_1$=OH; 2,8S; 2",3",3R
143 R$_1$=OH; 3,8R; 2",3",2S
224 R$_1$=OH; 8R; 2",3",2,3S

124

126 R$_1$=R$_2$=OH
158 R$_1$=OH; R$_2$=OMe
189 R$_1$=OH (2R)
190 R$_1$=OH (2S)
206 R$_1$=OMe; R$_2$=OH

132 C$_{1'''-2''''}$=db
133

134

135

(Fig. 5) contd.....

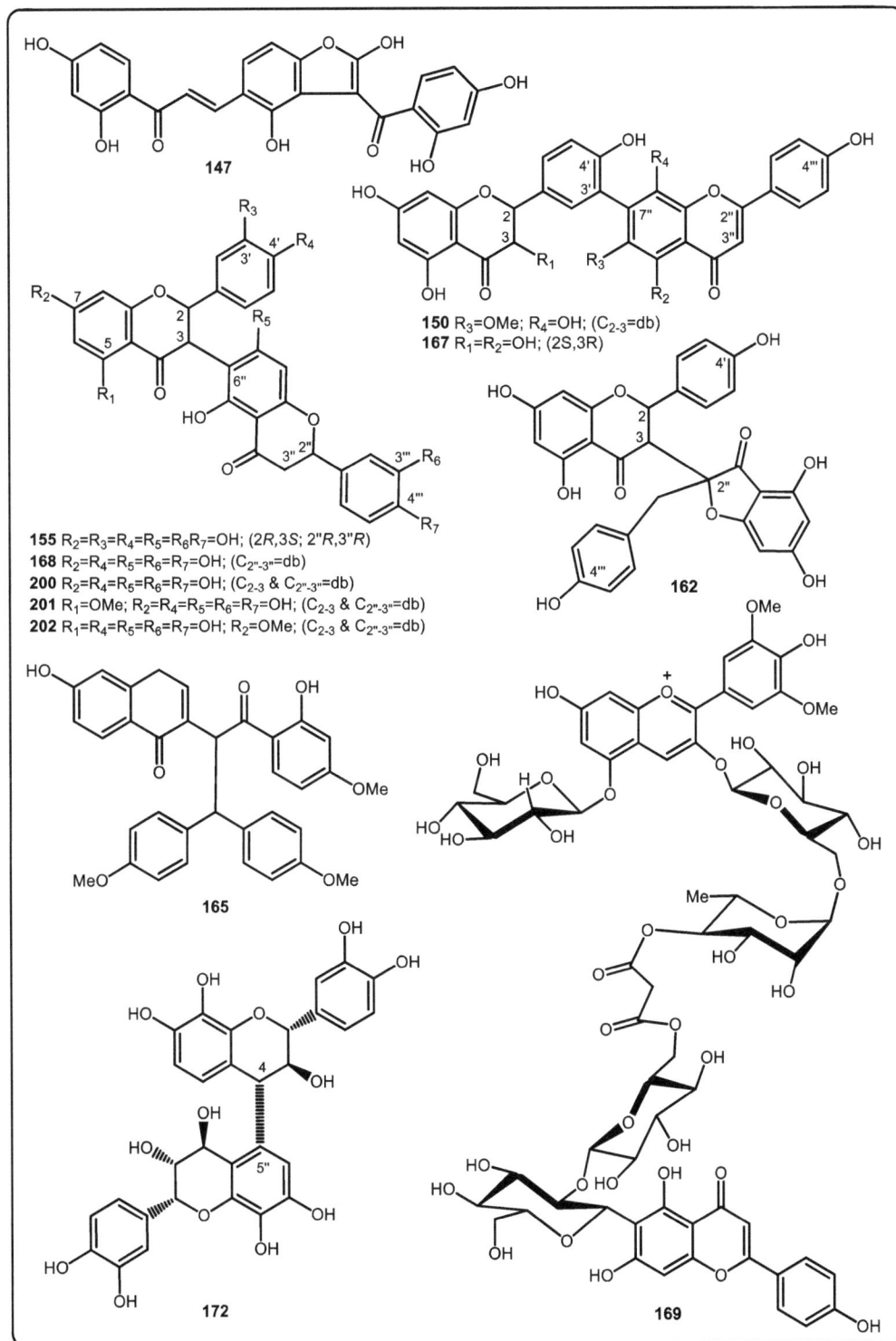

147

150 R$_3$=OMe; R$_4$=OH; (C$_{2-3}$=db)
167 R$_1$=R$_2$=OH; (2S,3R)

155 R$_2$=R$_3$=R$_4$=R$_5$=R$_6$R$_7$=OH; (2R,3S; 2"R,3"R)
168 R$_2$=R$_4$=R$_5$=R$_6$=R$_7$=OH; (C$_{2"-3"}$=db)
200 R$_2$=R$_4$=R$_5$=R$_6$=R$_7$=OH; (C$_{2-3}$ & C$_{2"-3"}$=db)
201 R$_1$=OMe; R$_2$=R$_4$=R$_5$=R$_6$=R$_7$=OH; (C$_{2-3}$ & C$_{2"-3"}$=db)
202 R$_1$=R$_4$=R$_5$=R$_6$=R$_7$=OH; R$_2$=OMe; (C$_{2-3}$ & C$_{2"-3"}$=db)

162

165

172

169

(Fig. 5) contd.....

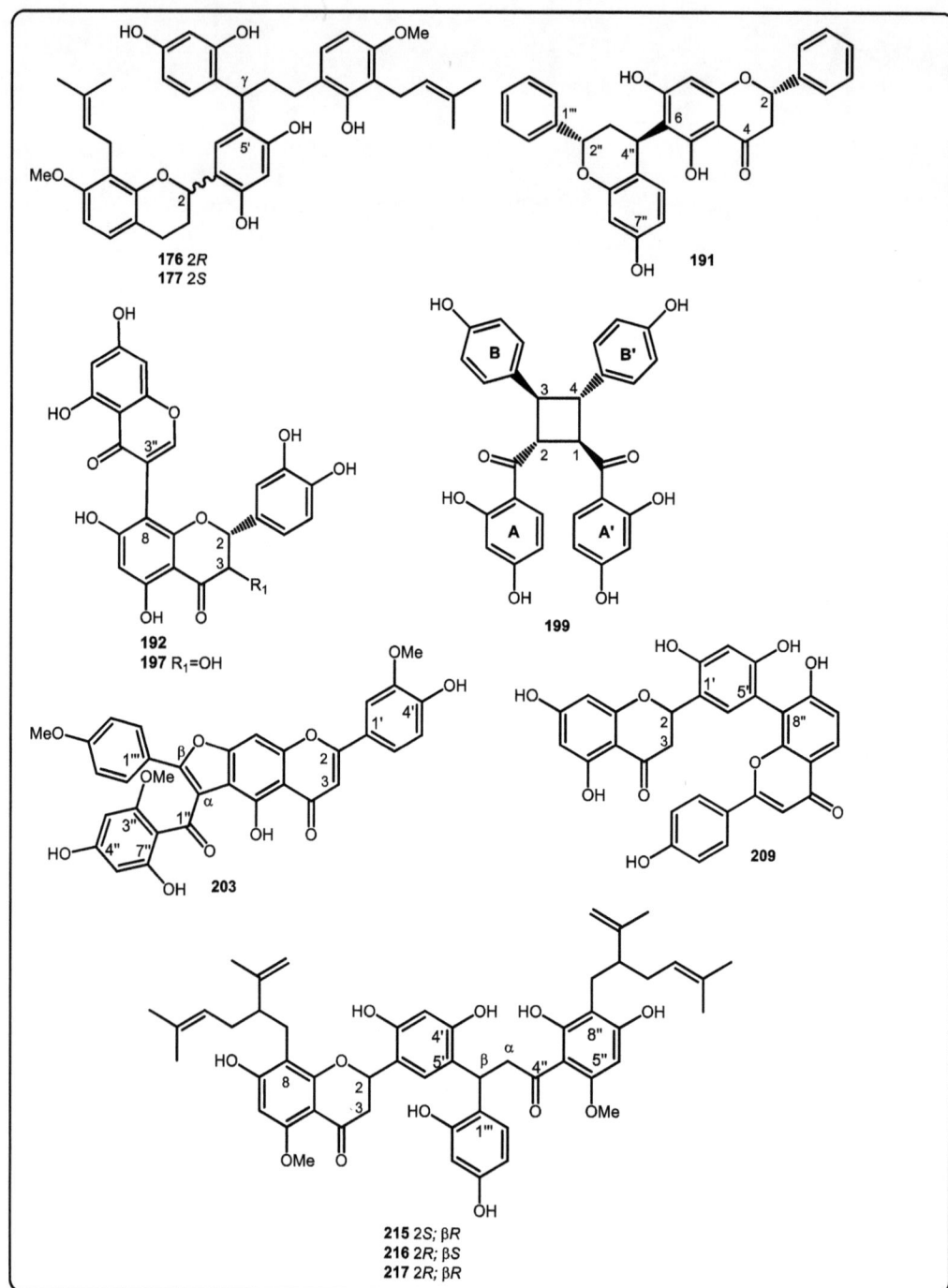

176 2R
177 2S

191

192
197 R$_1$=OH

199

203

209

215 2S; βR
216 2R; βS
217 2R; βR

(Fig. 5) contd.....

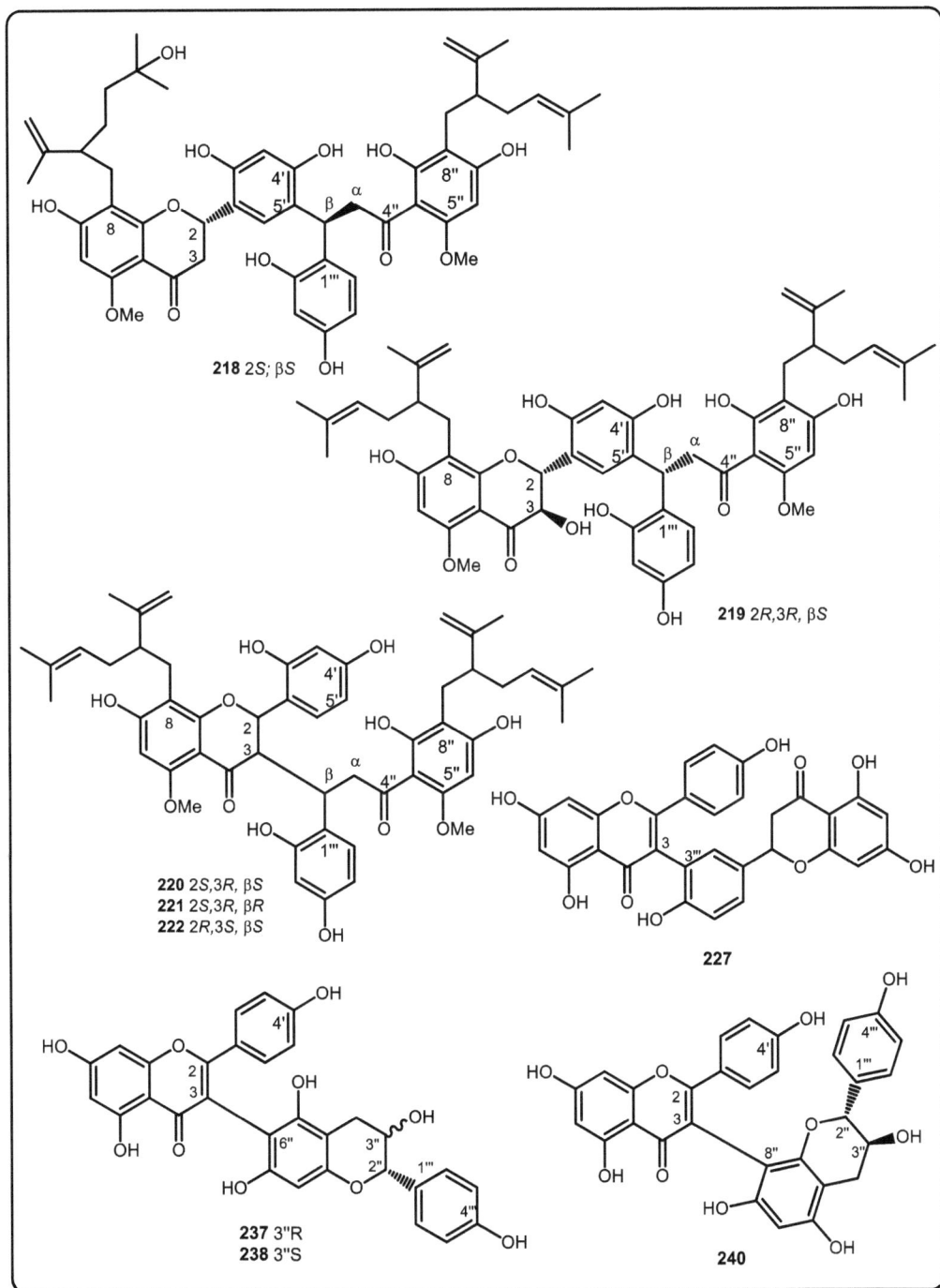

Fig. (5). Chemical structures of biflavonoids with C-CH$_2$-C and C-O-C connections.

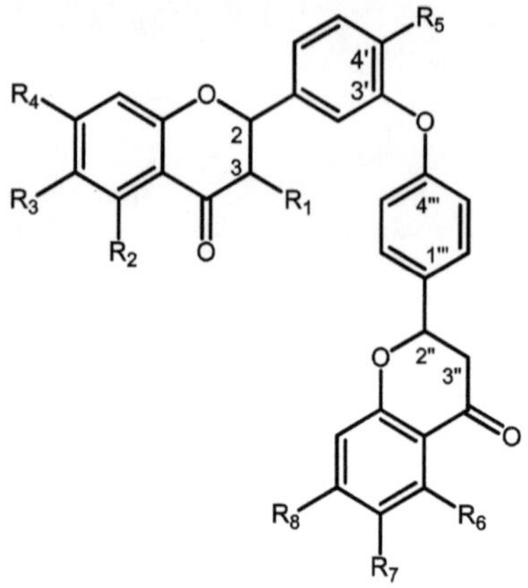

7 $R_2=R_4=R_5=R_6=R_8=OH$; ($C_{2-3}=db$)
15 $R_2=R_4=R_5=R_6=R_8=OH$; $R_3=R_7=Me$; ($C_{2"-3"}=db$)
23 $R_2=R_4=R_5=R_6=OH$; $R_8=OMe$; ($C_{2"-3"}=db$)
41 $R_1=R_2=R_4=R_5=R_6=R_8=OH$; ($C_{2"-3"}=db$)
65 $R_2=R_5=R_6=R_8=OH$; $R_4=OMe$; (C_{2-3} & $C_{2"-3"}=db$)
181 $R_2=R_4=R_5=R_6=R_8=OH$; (C_{2-3} & $C_{2"-3"}=db$)

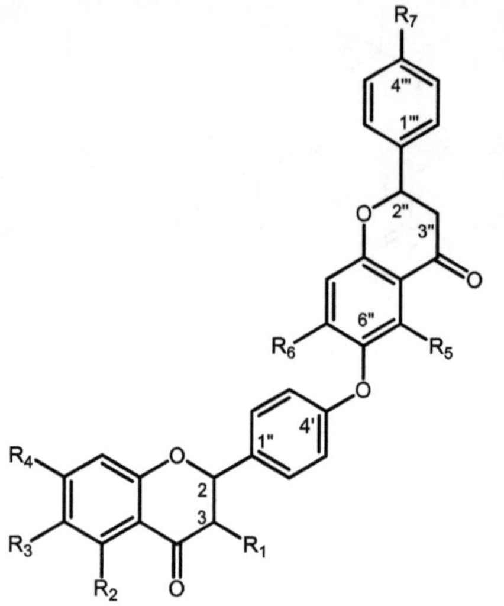

21 $R_2=R_4=R_5=R_6=R_7=OH$; ($C_{2"-3"}=db$)
22 $R_2=R_4=R_5=R_6=R_7=OH$; ($C_{2-3}=db$)
63 $R_2=R_5=R_6=R_7=OH$; $R_4=OMe$; (C_{2-3} & $C_{2"-3"}=db$)
146 $R_2=R_4=R_5=R_7=OH$; $R_6=OMe$; (C_{2-3} & $C_{2"-3"}=db$)
153 $R_2=R_4=R_5=R_7=OH$; $R_6=OMe$; (C_{2-3} & $C_{2"-3"}=db$)
182 $R_2=R_5=R_7=OH$; $R_3=Me$; $R_4=R_6=OMe$ (2,2"S)
229 $R_2=R_4=R_5=R_6=R_7=OH$

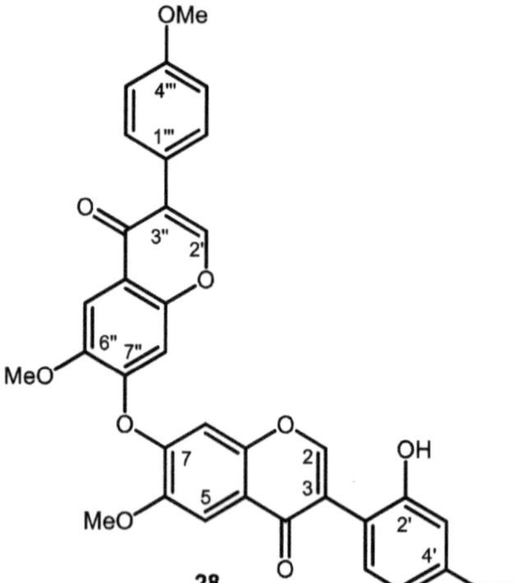

28

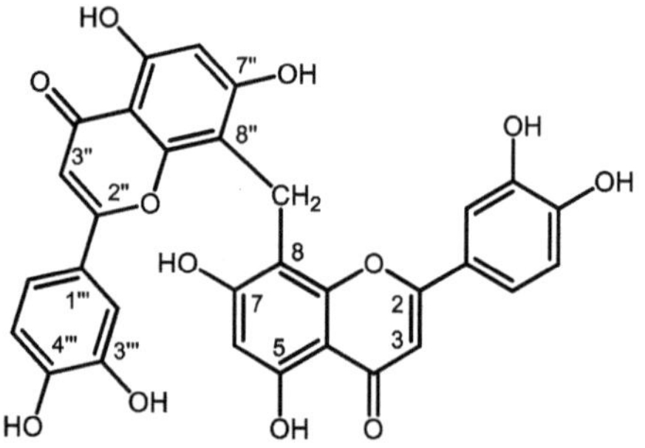

34

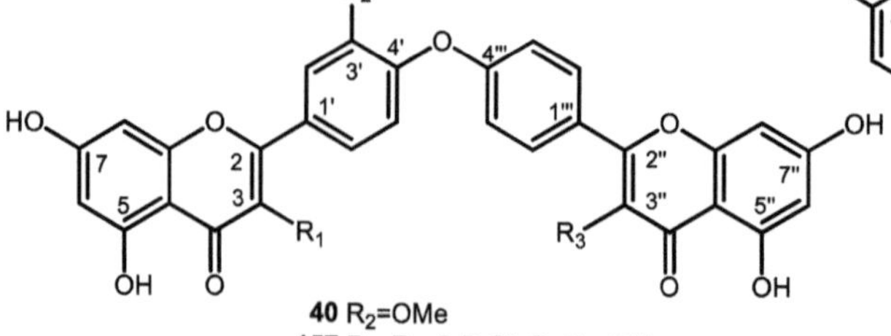

40 $R_2=OMe$
157 $R_1=R_3=\beta$-D-GlcO; $R_2=OMe$
164 $R_2=OH$

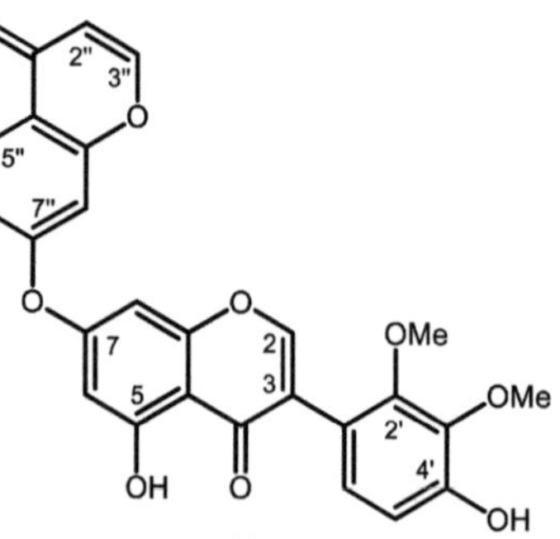

44

(Fig. 6) contd.....

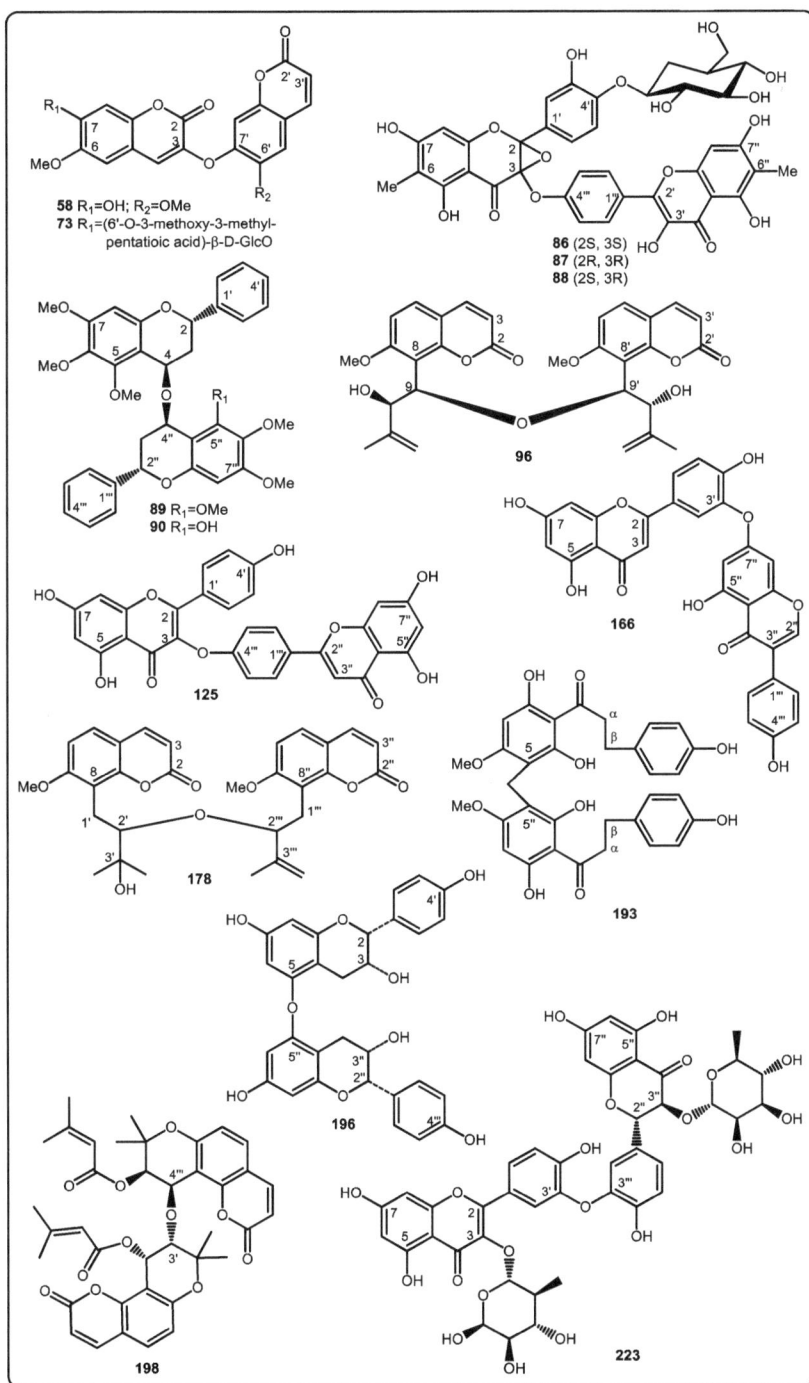

Fig. (6). Chemical structures of polyflavonoids.

BIOLOGICAL AND PHARMACOLOGICAL IMPORTANCE

As per the literature survey, natural biflavonoids are found to exhibit a wide range of biological and pharmacological activities, including anti-microbial and antiviral, cytotoxic and anti-cancer, anti-diabetic, anti-anoxic, antioxidant, Nitric oxide (NO)-inhibitory activity, anti-enzymatic, anti-HIV, anti thrombin, anti-allergic, cytoprotective, neuroprotective and anti-inflammatory activities. In spite of various biological activities, hepatic and renal toxicities are also exhibited by this important class of natural compounds. These activities have been presented below:

Anti-microbial and Antiviral Activity

The biflavanone (**3**) isolated from 80% ethanol extract of the outer bark of *Ochna integerrima* Merr. was found to be the anti-malarial active component showing an IC_{50} value of 0.080 μg/mL against multi-drug resistant strain of *Plasmodium falciparum*; however, the stereoisomer of **3** showed less anti-malarial activity (IC_{50} = 5.2 μg/mL [22]. Compound **3** isolated from another plant source, *Ormocarpum kirkii*, exhibited moderate antiplasmodial activity against *P. falciparum* having an IC_{50} value of 32.3 μM [23]. All the biflavonoids, including compound **3** obtained from methanol extract of dried and peeled roots of *O. kirkii*, were tested *in vitro* for their biological activities in an integrated antimicrobial and antiparasitic screening panel, including *Trypanosoma cruzi, Leishmania infantum, Trypanosoma brucei*, chloroquine-resistant *Plasmodium falciparum* K1, *Staphylococcus aureus, Candida albicans, Trichophyton rubrum, and Aspergillus fumigatus*. Compound **163** showed moderate but non-selective activity. Compound **84** was found to be selectively active against *T. rubrum* (IC_{50} 7.0 ± 6.4 μM). For compound **67**, an IC_{50} value of 19.5 ± 13.9 μM was observed only against *T. rubrum*. 5,5"-Di-*O*-methyldiphysin (**51**) was not selective and showed moderate activity against almost all parasites and bacteria. In contrast, no activity was observed for the mono-glucosylated diphysin (**66**). The known compound (+)-chamaejasmin (**107**) showed better but also non-selective activities against *T. cruzi* (IC_{50} 19.9 ± 8.4 μM) and *P. falciparum* (IC_{50} 15.0 ± 6.2 μM). The diastereomer isochamaejsmin (**152**) revealed a better selectivity index with an IC_{50} value of 7.3 ± 3.8 μM against *P. falciparum*. In contrast, the di-glucosylated analogue (**186**) showed no activity, while compound **3** showed only moderate and non-selective activity. For diphysin (**127**), selective but moderate activity was observed against *P. falciparum* (IC_{50} 39.5 ± 12.3 μM) [23]. Biflavonoids (**16, 18, 19 & 230**) isolated from methanol extract of *Cycas circinalis* exhibited moderate antibacterial activity against *Staphylococcus aureus* (IC_{50} values of 3.9, 9.7, and

8.2 μM, respectively) and methicillin-resistant *S. aureus* (MRSA; IC_{50} values of 5.9, 12.5, and 11.5 μM, respectively) [36]. A number of biflavonoids (**16, 17, 21, 22, 63, 145, 208, 210 & 228**) isolated from the Indian medicinal herb *Selaginella bryopteris* were investigated for their antiprotozoal activity using *in vitro* assays against the K1 strain of *Plasmodium falciparum*, *Leishmania donovani*, *Trypanosoma brucei rhodesiense* and *Trypanosoma cruzi*, and compound **145** was found to be the most active having an IC_{50} value of 0.26 μM [37]. The biflavonoid (**34**) isolated from the roots of *Garcinia kola* exhibited antibacterial activities against vancomycin-resistant *enterococci* (VRE) and methicillin-resistant *Staphylococcus aureus* (MRSA), showing MIC value of 128 and μg/mL 32, respectively [45]. Applying activity-guided fractionation, a research group reported *in vitro* antibacterial activity of the isolated biflavonoids (**38, 55, 56, 107 & 127**) from the aerial parts of *Ormocarpum trichocarpum*, exhibiting MIC values in the range between 4.0 to 136.7 μM against the pathogens *Bacillus subtilis*, *Escherichia coli*, *Klebsiella pneumonia* and *Staphylococcus aureus*. The isolated biflavonoids also showed antiplasmodial activity against the chloroquine-sensitive D10 *Plasmodium falciparum* strain having IC_{50} values in the range of 4.30 to 94.32 μM [49]. Pegnyemb *et al.* have reported biflavonoids **41** and **224** to possess antimicrobial activity against two Gram-positive bacteria, such as *Staphylococcus aureus* and *Bacillus subtilis*, in an agar well diffusion assay using streptomycin as the standard. Compound **42** showed MIC values of 8.51 and 10.05 μg/mL against *S. aureus and B.* subtilis, respectively, whereas compound **224** exhibited MIC values of 12.5 and 8.12 μg/mL, respectively. It was also reported that none of these compounds was active (MIC > 100 μg/mL) against Gram-negative bacterium, *E. coli* [52].

A new biflavonoid compound (**43**) isolated from the ethylacetate extract of *Allexis cauliflora* roots was subjected to evaluation of antibacterial efficacy. The compound showed significant antiplasmodial activity against the chloroquinesensitive *Plasmodium falciparum* strain 3D7 with an IC_{50} value of 10.57±1.44 μM [54]. A research group investigated the antimicrobial activity of a biflavonoid (**44**) isolated from *Uraria picta* using the micro dilution technique. The compound exhibited MIC values against bacteria, such as *S. aurues, B. subtilis, E.coli, P. vulgaris* and *A. nigar*, as 12.5, 25, 50, 12.5 and 25 μg/mL, respectively, and against the fungi, *C. albicans*, as 50 μg/mL [55]. The antibacterial activity of the isolated biflavonoids (**46, 83, 173, 185 & 235**) from *Garcinia prainiana* was tested against Gram-positive bacteria (*B. subtilis* and *S. aureus*) and Gram-negative bacteria (*E. coli* and *Pseudomonas aeruginosa*). The activity was determined qualitatively using the disc diffusion method and quantitatively using minimum inhibitory concentration (MIC). The inhibition zones in the disc diffusion method were in the range of 6.5-10.5 mm [57]. A new biflavonoid (**47**) was isolated from the antiviral fraction of *Wikstroemia indica* and found to be active against the respiratory syncytial virus (RSV). The biflavonoid exhibited potent *in vitro* anti-RSV activity in cytopathic effect (CPE) reduction assay having an IC_{50} value of 2.8µM and selective index (SI) value of 5.4 [58]. The biflavones (**62, 65, 83 & 210**) isolated from *Campylospermum excavatum* were screened for their antiparasitic activity against different *Leishmania* species, such as *L. amazonensis*, *L. donovani* and *L. infantum*. Among the tested biflavones, amentoflavone (**83**) exhibited moderate efficacy against the promastigote form of *L. infantum* with an IC_{50} value of 19.6 µM [66]. Seven new biflavonoid derivatives (**72, 109-114**) were isolated from *Dracaena cochinchinensis*, and the isolates were tested for antibacterial activities against *Helicobacter pylori* (ATCC43504). The new flavonoid derivatives **113** and **114** were found to be most efficacious against *H. pylori* (ATCC43504) with MIC values of 29.5 and 29.5 µM, respectively [70]. Amentoflavone (**83**) isolated from *Hypericum connatum* was found to exhibit antiviral activity inhibiting the cytopathic effect (CPE) and reducing the viral titer of HSV-1 DNA viral strains KOS and VR733 (ATCC) at a dose of 0.078 µg/mL [77]. Amentoflavone (**83**) has also been found to exhibit potent antifungal activity against a number of pathogenic fungal strains, such as *C. albicins, Saccharomyces cerevisiae* and *Trichosporon beigelli*, with MIC values of 5.0, 50 and 5.0-10.0 µg/mL, respectively [79]. Two biflavonoids, beilschmieflavonoid A (**89**) and beilschmieflavonoid B (**90**), found from the stem bark of *Beilschmiedia zenkeri*, were evaluated *in vitro* for their antibacterial activity against three strains of bacteria, *Pseudomonas agarici, Bacillus subtilis*, and *Streptococcus minor*, and for their antiplasmodial activity against *Plasmodium falciparum*, chloroquine-resistant strain W2. Their activities were found to be moderate compared to the reference drugs, ampicillin and gentamicin. Only biflavonoid (**90**) exhibited weak antibacterial activity against *S. minor* (MIC 197.5 µM) while both the biflavonoids remained inert towards antiplasmodial activity [86]. Four biflavonoids (**83, 91, 144 & 208**) were isolated and evaluated for SARS-CoV 3CLpro inhibition using fluorescence resonance energy transfer analysis. Of these compounds, the biflavone, amentoflavone (**83**), showed to have the most potent 3CLpro inhibitory effect with an IC_{50} value of 8.3 µM [89]. The isolated biflavonoids (**124, 147 & 165**) from *Ochna holtzii* showed varying degrees of antibacterial activities against the two gram-positive and two gram-negative bacteria, such as *S. aureus, P. aeruginosa, B. subtilis* and *B. typhi*, as well as against the diploid fungus, *C. albicans* [103]. Dehydrolophirone C (**124**) and lophirone A trimethyl ether (**165**) showed strong activities against these tested bacteria as well as against *C. albicans* (Table **2**).

Table 2. Antimicrobial activities of biflavonoids isolated from *Ochna holtzii.*

Biflavonoids	Zone of Inhibition (mm)				
	S. aureus	*P. aeruginosa*	*B. subtilis*	*S. typhi*	*C. albicans*
Dehydrolophirone C (**124**)	21	24	23	15	18
Holtzinol (**147**)	16	14	16	12	10
Tri-*O*-methyllophirone A (**165**)	23	20	24	14	16

A new biflavonoid (**128**), isolated from the root bark of *Garcinia livingstonei*, was investigated for antiparasitic activity against *Plasmodium falciparum, Leishmania infantum, Trypanosoma brucei brucei*, and *T. cruzi.* This biflavonoid (**128**) showed moderate activity against *P. falciparum* having an IC_{50} value of 6.7 μM [105]. The antibacterial activities of the isolated compounds, GB-2 (**139**) and manniflavanone (**170**), from *Garcinia preussii*, were examined against *E. coli, P. aeruginosa, S. aureus*, and *E. faecalis.* Their MIC values were found to be moderate compared to those of amentoflavone and 4'-methoxyamentoflavone [107]. Four biflavonoids (**142-143, 179 & 224**) isolated from *Radix Wikstroemiae* were subjected to assessment of *in vitro* antiviral activity against the respiratory syncytial virus (RSV) using cytopathic effect (CPE) reduction assay and the MTT. Compounds **142-143 & 224** showed similar *in vitro* antiviral activity against RSV with IC_{50} values of 9.6, 6.6, 10.2 μM and SI values of 11.0, 21.9, 15.8, respectively, but compound **179** was unable to show anti-RSV effect in its maximal non-cytotoxic concentration (MNCC), the highest concentration tested in the CPE reduction assay [113]. The isolated bioflavonoids (**103, 159 & 211**) from *Stellera chamaejasme* were tested for their anti-HBV (infection with hepatitis B virus) activities *in vitro.* The known compounds, sikokianin A (**211**) and chamaechromone (**103**), at a dose of 0.2 mmol/ml, exhibited potent antiviral activities by inhibiting HBsAg secretion by 71.9 and 34.0, respectively [120]. Sikokianin A (**211**) at a non-cytotoxic concentration of 0.2 mmol/ml inhibited HBsAg secretion by more than 50% in comparison to the positive control, lamivudine (29.6% at 1.0 mmol/ml). Kolaviron (**160**), a biflavonoid fraction from *Garcinia kola* seeds, was found to be active against *Plasmodium berghei* infection in Swiss albino mice. This biflavonoid, especially at 200 mg/kg, has been found to possess high antimalarial activities in *P. berghei*-infected mice, in addition to its known antioxidant properties [123]. Macrophylloflavone (**168**), isolated from *Garcinia macrophylla*, exhibited significant antibacterial activity against *E. coli* ATCC 25922 and *S. aureus* ATCC 25923 with cephazolin as a positive control [130].

A research group reported that ochnaflavone (**181**) may be regarded as an ideal immunologically evaluated agent for treating arthritis due to *Candida albicans* involving T-cell immunoregulation [141]. Two antibacterial biflavonoids, ochnaflavone (**181**) and ochnaflavone 7-*O*-methyl ether (**65**), isolated from *Ochna pretoriensis*, were evaluated for antibacterial activity using bioautography and serial microplate dilution methods against four nosocomial bacterial pathogens, namely *Escherichia coli, Staphylococcus aureus, Enterococcus faecalis* and *Pseudomonas aeruginosa*. The most sensitive organism to both biflavonoids was *P. aeruginosa* with an MIC value of 31.3 µg/mL. Ochnaflavone was found to have more efficacy than its methoxy derivative against the other pathogens tested [142]. Shikokianin B (**212**) and Shikokianin C (**213**), isolated from *Wikstroemia taiwanensis*, were evaluated for their *in vitro* antitubercular activity against *M. tuberculosis* H37Rv with the clinically used drug ethambutol as a positive control [160]. Results showed that both **212** and **213** exhibited MIC values of about 15 µg/mL compared to the positive control used (MIC value 6.25 µg/mL).

Cytotoxic and Anti-cancer Activity

The biflavonoids isolated from methanol extract of dried and peeled roots of *Ormocarpum kirkii* were tested for *in vitro* cytotoxicity using MRC-5 cells. 5,5''-Di-*O*-methyldiphysin (**51**) & (+)-chamaejasmin (**107**) was found to exhibit high cytotoxicity having CC_{50} value of 11.7 ± 6.2 µM & 18.3 ± 10.6 µM, respectively, whereas compounds **84, 152** and **163** exhibited comparatively low cytotoxicity [23].

Six biflavonoids isolated from dichloromethane extract of *Selaginella doederleinii* exhibited anti-proliferation effect against the five human cancer cell lines, *viz.* human lung-cancer cell lines (A549 and PC-9), human acute promyelocytic leukaemia cell line (HL60), human erythroleukemia cell line (K562) and human nasopharyngeal carcinoma line (CNE2) [27, 28]. Cytotoxicities of the isolated flavonoids against five human cancer cell lines after 48 h exposure at dosages ranging from 3.125 to 50 µg/mL are shown in the following table (Table **3**) using doxorubicin as a positive control at dosages in the range from 0.313 to 5 µg/mL. From the table, it can be observed that amentoflavone (**83**) has exhibited cytotoxicity against the five human cancer cell lines, suggesting amentoflavone to be one of the main anti-tumour active components in *S. doederleinii*; 2'', 3''-dihydro-3', 3'''-biapigenin (**6**), heveaflavone (**145**) and 7, 4', 7'', 4'''- tetra-*O*-methyl-amentoflavone (**54**) have shown strong cytotoxicity to human lung cancer cell lines (A549 and PC-9), and hence, may be regarded as the main active constituents for the therapeutic effect of *S. doederleinii* on nasopharyngeal carcinoma. In addition, robustaflavone (**204**) exhibited cytotoxicity (IC_{50}<50 µg/mL) against human cancer cell lines, PC-9, HL60 and CNE2. The research group concluded that these six compounds should be considered as the markers of quality control for the plant *S. doederleinii* [27, 28].

Table 3. The inhibition effects of the six compounds on human cancer cell lines.

Cell lines	IC_{50} values of the compounds (μg/ML)					
	83	204	6	36	145	54
A549	36.3 ± 5.3	> 50	42.0 ± 1.2	19.3 ± 2.3	> 50	> 50
PC-9	6.41 ± 1.9	37.4 ± 10.0	8.12 ± 1.0	49.7 ± 0.37	6.74 ± 2.1	9.46 ± 2.8
K562	5.25 ± 0.87	> 50	39.29 ± 2.2	> 50	> 50	> 50
HL60	46.3 ± 4.3	48.0 ± 5.6	> 50	> 50	46.0 ± 4.6	49.2 ± 1.9
CNE2	17.3 ± 1.7	42.8 ± 0.2	> 50	> 50	15.8 ± 2.9	> 50

The biflavonoid (**7**), isolated from leaves of *Luxemburgia nobilis*, was evaluated for cytotoxicity against Ehrlich carcinoma and human K562 leukemia cells in a 45-hour cell culture [29]. The biflavonoid exhibited concentration-dependent inhibition of Ehrlich and K562 cell growth. In comparison to the reference drugs used (quercetin and etoposide), the compound has been found to be significantly active against Ehrlich cells (IC_{50} = 17.2 μM) but moderately active against K562 cells (IC_{50} = 89 μM). A new biflavanone (**8**), together with a known biflavonoid, robustaflavone (**204**), isolated from the whole plant of *Selaginella doederleinii*, exhibited cytotoxic activity against the three human cancer cell lines, HCT116, NCI-H358, and K562. Compound **8** showed IC_{50} values of 19.1, 23.5 and 28.8 μM, respectively, whereas compound **204** exhibited IC_{50} values as 15.6, 20.1, and 22.5 μM, respectively [30]. A number of biflavonoids (**16, 17, 21, 22, 63, 145, 208, 210 & 229**) isolated from the Indian medicinal herb *Selaginella bryopteris* were investigated for their cytotoxic activity on rat skeletal myoblast cell line (L-6 cells), and the biflavonoid **21** was found to be most active against *Leismania* having IC_{50} value of 1.6 μM; compound **145** remained almost inactive here (IC_{50} > 150μM) [37]. Two new biflavonoids, 2'-hydroxygenkwanol A (**29**) and 4'-methylgenkwanol A (**48**), isolated from the aerial parts of *Daphne linearifolia* Hart, were investigated for their anti-cancer activity against Hsp90, one of the most promising targets for the modern anti-cancer therapy by means of surface plasmon resonance technique; biflavonoid **29** was found to be an active compound as it significantly interacted with the protein [42]. The isolated biflavonoid, biisokaempferide (**35**), from *Nanuza plicata*, was found to be cytotoxic as reported by Pinto *et al*. The investigators studied cytotoxicity in cultures of human glioblastoma GL-15 cells and reported 36.5 μmol L^{-1} as an effective concentration, which killed 50% of cells after 72 h. They also noticed changes in cellular morphology, including retraction and degradation of cytoplasm, when cells were treated at a concentration of 20 μmol L^{-1} of the compound (**35**) for 72 h [47].

Eight isolated biflavonoids **39, 116-119, 213, 237-238**, from *Wikstroemia indica* were evaluated for their cytotoxicity against three cancer cell lines, Hep3B, HepG2 and CNE2, respectively [50]. It was found that compound **39** showed moderate toxicity against HepG2 and CNE2 cells with IC_{50} values of 65.5 ± 11.4 and 53.6 ± 10.1 µM, respectively, whereas compounds **119** and **213** showed significant activity against CNE2 cell having IC_{50} values of 13.8 ± 3.5 and 11.6 ± 4.2 µM, respectively [50]. The other biflavonoids (**116, 236** and **237**) remained inactive against the tested cell lines, having an IC_{50} value greater than 100 µM.

Six isolated biflavonoids from *Cephalotaxus koreana* showed cytotoxicity on osteoblast differentiation as revealed by measuring the ALP activity in primary cultures of mouse osteoblasts. Compounds **39, 54, 64** and **208** were found to significantly increase ALP activity at concentrations in the range from 1.0 to 20.0 µM. However, compounds **45** and **144** did not show any cytotoxicity at a concentration of 20.0 µM as measured by MTT assay [56].

A bis-coumarin derivative (**58**) isolated from *Erycibe hainanesis* was found to exhibit D-galactosamine-induced cytotoxicity in WB-F344 rat hepatic epithelial stemlike cells and showed significant hepatoprotective activitiy at a concentration of 1×10^{-4} M [64].

The isolated spiro-biflavonoids, abiesinols **A–F** (**74 – 79**) from *Abies sachalinensis*, were screened for anti-tumor-initiating activity. As a primary screening test for anti-tumor-initiating activity, **74 – 79** were found to exhibit inhibitory effects on the activation of NOR 1, a nitric oxide (NO) donor. Again, abiesinol A (**75**), bearing a spiro-biflavonoid skeleton, showed remarkable anti-tumor-initiating activity in the *in vivo* two-stage mouse skin carcinogenesis test using peroxynitrite (PN) as the initiator and 12-*O*-tetradecanoylphorbol-13-acetate (TPA) as the promoter [72].

The biflavonoids (**83, 144, 146 & 154**) isolated from *Selaginella moellendorffii* exhibited selective cytotoxicity against the three human cancer cell lines, such as A549, BGC-823 and BEL-7402 [78].

Two biflavonoids, chamaejasmenin B (**105**) and neochamaejasmin C (**180**), isolated from the root of *Stellera chamaejasme* L exerted potent anti-proliferative effects against eight human solid tumor cell lines, *viz.* human liver carcinoma cell lines (HepG2 and SMMC-7721), a human non-small cell lung cancer cell line (A549), human osteosarcoma cell lines (MG63, U2OS, and KHOS), a human colon cancer cell line (HCT-116) and a human cervical cancer cell line HeLa, using SRB cytotoxicity assay [99]. The anti-proliferative effects of the compounds were measured in terms of DNA damage and were detected by immunofluorescence and Western blotting. Apoptosis and cell cycle distribution were assessed using flow cytometry analysis. The expression of the related proteins was examined with Western blotting analysis. Chamaejasmenin B (the IC_{50} value ranging from 1.08 to 10.8 μmol/L) was found to be slightly more potent than neochamaejasmin C (the IC_{50} value ranging from 3.07 to 15.97 μmol/L). These two compounds were found to induce prominent expression of the DNA damage marker γ-H2AX as well as apoptosis. Moreover, treatment of the cells with these two compounds was found to cause prominent G0/G1 phase arrest [99].

The same research group reported cytotoxic activities of ten biflavones isolated from the same plant against Bel-7402 and A549 cell lines using vincristine as the positive control. The results showed that seven biflavones exhibited significant cytotoxic activities against these two human cancer cell lines with IC_{50} values ranging from 1.05 to 9.31 μM for Bel-7402 and 0.75 to 7.91 μM for A549, respectively, as shown in Table **4**. Chamaejasmenin E (**106**), sikokianin D (**214**), isochamaejasmenin B (**151**) and chamaejasmenin B (**105**) showed higher cytotoxic activities than vincristine against Bel-7402 cell line, while only sikokianin D (**214**) showed higher cytotoxic activities than vincristine against A549 cell line [100]. Obviously, sikokianin D (**214**) possessed the most potent cytotoxic activities against both Bel-7402 and A549 cell lines with IC_{50} values of 1.29 ± 0.21 and 0.75 ± 0.25 μM, respectively. Based on their results, it seemed that for this type of biflavones, 4'-OCH_3 contributed more to cytotoxic activity than 4'-OH and other groups because compounds without 4'-OCH_3 (**108**, **156** & **179**) were the least active. The contributions of 4'''-OH and 4'''-OCH_3 were nearly the same, since no obvious difference could be observed between IC_{50} values of compounds with 4'''-OCH_3 (**105**, **106** & **151**) and compounds with 4'''-OH (**211**, **212** & **213**), except for **214**. The relatively higher cytotoxic activities of **214** may be attributed to the absolute configuration of C-3'', because among the four compounds with both 4'-OCH_3 and 4'''-OH (**211-214**), only **214** had a 3''R configuration. Certainly, these interesting structure-function relationships of biflavanones need to be further evaluated in the future [100].

Table 4. Cytotoxic activities of ten biflavones against two human tumor cell lines.

Compounds	Cell lines (IC_{50}, μM)	
	Bel-7402	**A549**
Chamaejasmenin E (**106**)	1.17 ± 0.07	4.71 ± 0.35
Chamaejasmin D (**108**)	31.85 ± 0.85	43.81 ± 3.30
Sikokianin D (**214**)	1.29 ± 0.21	0.75 ± 0.25
Isochamaejasmenin B (**151**)	2.70 ± 0.26	4.55 ± 0.12
Chamaejasmenin B (**105**)	1.05 ± 0.40	3.60 ± 0.42
Sikokianin C (**213**)	6.47 ± 0.15	3.46 ± 0.10

(Table 4) cont.....

Sikokianin A (211)	9.31 ± 0.93	7.91 ± 0.56
Sikokianin B (212)	8.42 ± 0.32	5.53 ± 0.17
Isoneochamaejasmin A (156)	46.77 ± 0.70	56.67 ± 1.41
Neochamaejasmin B (179)	55.13 ± 0.31	56.63 ± 1.99
Vincristine (positive control)	4.35 ± 0.10	1.05 ± 0.13

Chamaejasmin A (**107**) has been reported to possess anti-cancer properties relating to β -TB depolymerization inhibition. For this purpose, the anticancer activity of **107** was studied by evaluating its *in vitro* cytotoxicity against several cell lines (CAL-27, UMSCC-1, UMSCCG19, HEP-2 and Vero cells) using the 3-(4,5)- dimethylthiazoly1)-3,5-diphenytetrazolium bromide assay. Results indicated that chamaejasmin A (**107**) exhibited more significant anticancer activity against HEP-2 cells, with IC_{50} value of 3.48 μM. Besides, western blot analysis showed this biflavonoid to be able to increase the expression of β-tubulin (TB), but not α-TB, and intake of chamaejasmin A through gavage resulting in β -TB depolymerization inhibition in HEP-2 tumors [101]. The biflavonoids (**140-141 & 173**) isolated from *Garcinia gardneriana* may have the prospect to be anticancer agents as these flavonoids exhibited *in vitro* aromatase modulatory effect. All three biflavonoids were able to significantly inhibit the enzyme having IC_{50} values ranging from 1.35 to 7.67 μM [110]. Bioassay-guided fractionation of the EtOH extract of the dried twigs of *Podocarpus nakaii* Hayata (Podocarpaceae) has afforded four [3′→8″]-biflavonoid derivatives, amenotoflavone (**83**), podocarpusflavone-A (**194**), II-4″,I-7-dimethoxyamentoflavone (**148**), and heveaflavone (**145**). Compounds **194** and **148** showed significant inhibitions against DLD, KB, MCF-7, and HEp-2 tumor cell lines (ED_{50} ca. 4.56-16.24 μg/mL) and induced cell apoptosis in MCF-7 mainly *via* sub-G1/S phase arrest. Furthermore, these compounds exhibited moderate Topoisomerase I inhibitory activity as well [115]. Isoginkgetin (**154**), a naturally derived biflavonoid, was found to sensitize cells undergoing nutrient starvation to apoptosis, induced lysosomal stress, and activated the lysosome biogenesis of gene *TFEB*. Isoginkgetin treatment may also lead to the accumulation of aggregates of polyubiquitinated proteins that colocalized strongly with the adaptor protein p62, the 20S proteasome, and the endoplasmic reticulum-associated degradation (ERAD) protein UFD1L. This biflavonoid was found to directly inhibit the chymotrypsin-like, trypsin-like, and caspase-like activities of the 20S proteasome and impaired NF-*k*B signaling, suggesting that the molecule may display its biological activity in part through proteasome inhibition. Moreover, isoginkgetin was found effective at killing multiple myeloma (MM) cell lines *in vitro* and displayed a higher rate of cell death induction than the clinically approved proteasome inhibitor, bortezomib. Isoginkgetin may be accounted for cancer cell death by disturbing protein homeostasis, and hence, leading to an excess of protein cargo that places a burden on the lysosomes/autophagic machinery [118]. A research group investigated the effect of ochnaflavone on the growth inhibitory activity in cultured human colon cancer cell line, HCT-15. This biflavonoid was found to inhibit the proliferation of the cancer cells with an IC_{50} value of 4.1 μM by arresting cell cycle progression in the G2/M phase as well as induction of apoptosis in such cancer cell [140]. Two biflavonoids, ochnaflavone (**181**) and ochnaflavone 7-*O*-methyl ether (**65**), isolated from *Ochna pretoriensis*, were examined for their toxic effects in the MTT toxicity assay using monkey kidney vero cells and Ames genotoxicity test using *Salmonella typhimurium* strain TA98 [142]. Ochnaflavone (**181**) showed more efficacy (LC_{50} value 125.9 μg/mL) than its methoxy derivative (LC_{50} value 162.0 μg/mL). A biflavonoid (**193**) from *Pieris japonica* was found to exhibit significant immunomodulatory activity by inhibiting the proliferation of murine B cells [147].

Anti-diabetic Activity

Five known biflavonoids (**4, 115, 204, 209 & 226**) isolated from methanol extract of the aerial parts of *Selaginella tamariscina* exhibited antidiabetic activity. All isolates exhibited potent inhibitory effects on the Protein Tyrosine phosphatase 1B (PTP1B) enzyme with IC_{50} values ranging from 4.5 ± 0.1 to 9.6 ± 0.3 μM. Furthermore, the isolates (**3–7**) showed profound stimulatory effects on 2-NBDG uptake in 3T3-L1 adipocyte cells. This result showed these biflavonoids to be lead molecules for the development of antidiabetic drugs in the future [25]. Six biflavonoids (**59, 60, 103, 105, 107 & 239**) isolated from *Stellera chamaejasme* showed significant inhibition activity against aldose reductase having IC_{50} values of 4.1, 2.9, 7.4, 5.9, 1.8 and 27.7 μM, respectively. The better activity of the biflavanones **59, 60, 105** and **107** compared to chromone derivatives **103** and flavan biflavonoids **239** is due to the more number of OH functions present in biflavanones [65]. It has been reported that the roots of *Boesenbergia rotunda* may be used for functional food for controlling after-meal blood glucose levels on the basis of the observation that the three new biflavonoids (**126, 158 & 206**) showed stronger inhibitory activity (>90% inhibition at 20 μg/mL with IC_{50} value of 1.3–3.4 μM) against α-glucosidase than the drug acarbose (IC_{50} value 1.2 μM) and moderate pancreatic lipase inhibitory effect than the drug orlistat [104]. Macrophylloflavone (**168**) isolated from *Garcinia macrophylla* exhibited significant anti-type 2 diabetes mellitus activity using metformin as a positive control. *In vivo* treatment with this biflavonoid reduced blood glucose levels in diabetic rats to the normal level [130]. A biflavonoid (**192**) isolated from *Garcinia paucinervis* was assayed for its α-glycosidase inhibitory effect. The biflavonoid exhibited potent activity showing IC_{50} value of 12.48±4.60 μM [146]. Biflavonoid compounds **215, 217, 219, 221-222**, isolated from the roots of *Sophora* *flavescens*, were evaluated for their *in vitro* inhibitory activity in antidiabetic bioassay on human recombinant PTP1B at a concentration of 10 μM, and they exhibited significant activity showing effective inhibitory ratios of 95.7%, 96.0%, 96.6%, 94.1% and 93.0%, respectively. Biflavonoids **215** & **217** exhibited IC_{50} values as 0.33 and 0.35 μM, respectively [156].

The inhibitory effects of the polyflavonoids **240, 244-246** (isolated from the leaves of *Machilus philippinensis*) against α-glucosidase type IV from *Bacillus stearothermophilus* were assayed, and from the results, aescultitannin B (**240**) was found to be the most potent with an IC_{50} value of 3.5 μM. Compounds **244-246** exhibited moderate activity having IC_{50} values of 313, 184 and 105 μM, respectively [162].

Anti-anoxic Activity

Seven 3′,8″-linked biflavonoids (**5, 16-20** & **83**) isolated from the 60% ethanol extract of the dried whole herbs of *S. unicinata* were evaluated for their anti-anoxic activity [26]. These isolated biflavonoids included (2″S)-2″,3′--dihydroamentoflavone-4′-methyl ether (**5**), (2S)-2,3-dihydroamentoflavone (**16**), (2″S)-2″,3″-dihydroamentoflavone (**17**), 2,3-dihydroamentoflavone-4′-methyl ether (**18**), (2S,2″S)-2,3,2″,3″-tetrahydroamentoflavone- 4′-methyl ether (**19**), (2S,2″S)-tetrahydroamentoflavone (**20**), and amentoflavone (**83**). The protective effect against anoxia of the compounds was evaluated in the PC12 cells assay, and all seven compounds showed protective effects, with compound **17** showing the most potent activity [26]. The anti-anoxic activity of two biflavonoids (**20** & **234**) of *Selaginella uncinata* was evaluated by using the anoxic PC12 cell assay. Compound **20** displayed a potent anti-anoxic effect, whereas compound **234** showed a moderate effect [159].

Anti-oxidant Activity

The biflavonoid **12** isolated from *Podocarpus macrophyllus* was screened to evaluate the free radical and melanin synthesis in human epidermal melanocytes (HEMn) using Western blot analysis of tyrosinase-related proteins and quantitative real-time PCR. In the melanin synthesis assay, the compound (**12**) showed a potent anti-tyrosinase effect with an IC_{50} value of 0.098 mM and also significantly decreased both protein and mRNA levels of the tyrosinase-related protein-2 (TRP-2) [32]. The isolated biflavonoid (**42**) from *Baeckea frutescens* exhibited sigmoidal dose-response inhibition of copper-induced LDL oxidation with IC_{50} value of 0.95 μM. This biflavonoid containing two pyrogallol units showed three times stronger activity than the known antioxidant BHT [53]. A new biflavonoid compound (**43**), isolated from the ethylacetate extract of *Allexis cauliflora* roots, was found to exhibit weak antioxidant activity against DPPH radicals [54]. All the isolated biflavonoids from *Garcinia prainiana* were evaluated for their antioxidant activity by using DPPH radical scavenging assay and their efficacies were determined at scavenging concentration to obtain 50% of the maximum scavenging capacity (SC_{50}) of DPPH by the most abundant compounds (**46, 83, 173, 185 & 235**). The reduction of DPPH radicals could be observed by absorbance decrement at 517 nm, and it was visually noticeable as discoloration from purple to yellow. Meanwhile, all biflavonoids exhibited antioxidant activity with the SC_{50} value ranging from 110 – 15.7 µg/mL. Morelloflavone (**173**) exhibited the strongest antioxidant activity (SC_{50} 15.7 µg/mL) among all biflavonoids, comparable to the standard vitamin C (SC50 11.9 µg/mL). A large number of phenolic groups contributed to its strong antioxidant activity and it acted as a hydrogen donor to scavenge the DPPH radical [57]. The antioxidant activities of the isolated biflavonoids (85-87) from *Baeckea frutescens* were tested in an *in vitro* DPPH radical scavenging activity assay and compared with those of reference antioxidant quercetin (IC_{50}, 18.2 µM). All isolated compounds displayed strong antioxidant activities in the IC_{50} value range of 11.8–16.1 µM [85]. Biflavonoids (**92-94**) isolated from *Butea monosperma* were tested for antioxidant activity using the DPPH free-radical scavenging assay. Biflavonoid **94** showed significant radical scavenging efficacy with an IC_{50} value of 1.7 µg/mL, while biflavonoid (**93**) showed moderate activity having IC_{50} value close to 9.8 µg/mL [90].

Two 3,8"-biflavonoids (**95 & 138**), isolated from the green fruits of *Clusia paralicola*, exhibited moderate antioxidant activity in DPPH, ABTS, and β-carotene/linoleic acid assays [91]. Stark *et al.* [93] investigated antioxidant activity using hydrogen peroxide scavenging, oxygen radical absorbance capacity (ORAC), and trolox equivalent antioxidant capacity (TEAC) assays of the isolated biflavonoids (**97, 136-137, 140 & 170**) from the stem bark extract of the *Garcinia buchananii* tree. All these tested natural products exhibited extraordinarily high antioxidative power, especially **170** with an EC_{50} value of 3.0 µM, 4.00 mmol TE/mmol, and 10.30 µmol TE/ µmol, respectively (Table **5**).

Table 5. Antioxidant activities of isolated biflavonoids (97, 136-137, 140 & 170) from *Garcinia buchananii*.

Structure Number	EC_{50} value in H_2O_2 assay (µM)	µmol TE/µmol assay for ORAC assay	mmol TE/mmol assay for ABTS assay
97	3.70	7.20	3.61
136	10.90	8.34	1.84
137	7.80	7.46	1.84

(Table 5) cont.....

140	5.10	5.50	1.59
170	3.0	10.30	4.00

Stark *et al.,* in another investigation, reported antioxidant efficacies of the isolated biflavonoids (**97, 139 & 170**) from the same plant against H_2O_2 scavenging and ORAC [94]. The biflavonoids **139 & 170** exhibited strong antioxidative power with EC_{50} values of 2.2 and 2.8 µM, respectively, and 12.10 and 13.73 µmol TE/ µmol, respectively (Table **6**). These two findings indicated *G. buchananii* bark extract to be a rich and natural source of antioxidants.

Table 6. Antioxidant activities of isolated biflavonoids (97, 139 & 170) from *Garcinia buchananii.*

Structure Number	EC_{50} in H_2O_2 assay (µM)	µmol TE/µmol assay for ORAC assay
97	14.40	10.50
139	2.20	12.10
170	2.80	13.73

Two new biflavonoids, daphnogirins A (**122**) and B (**123**), obtained from the roots of *Daphne giraldii*, exhibited significant anti-oxidant activity. The working curves of fluorescein oxidation were used as an index of time resistance for the oxidative reaction. Quenching curves of disodium fluorescein illustrated the ability of the sample to absorb the peroxyl radical compared to that of the standard trolox [102]. Two biflavonoids, (2*R*,3*S*,2″*R*,3″*R*)-GB-2 7″-*O*-β-D-glucopyranoside (**141**) and 2R,3S,2″R,3″R)-manniflavanone-7″-O-β-D-glucopyranoside (**171**) isolated from *Garcinia buchananii* showed high anti-oxidative capacity in the H_2O_2 scavenging, hydrophilic Trolox equivalent antioxidant capacity (H-TEAC) and hydrophilic oxygen radical absorbance capacity (H-ORAC) assays, as shown in the following table (Table **7**). These two biflavonoids have been found to be less potent than their aglycons (**139 & 170**) with an EC_{50} value of 10.6 and 9.7 µM (H_2O_2 scavenging), 3.40 and 3.98 mmol TE/mmol (H-TEAC), and 9.27 and 7.74 µmol TE/µmol (HORAC), respectively [111, 149].

Table 7. Anti-oxidant activities of isolated compounds from *Garcinia buchananii.*

Compound	H-TEAC mmol TE/mmol	H-ORAC mmol TE/mmol	H_2O_2 EC_{50} µM
141	3.40 ± 0.08	9.27 ± 0.06	10.6 (9.5–11.8)
171	3.98 ± 0.19	7.74 ± 0.12	9.7 (8.7–10.8)
170	5.58 ± 0.3	13.73 ± 0.43	2.8 (2.4–3.2)
139	2.38 ± 0.26	12.10 ± 0.26	2.2 (1.9–2.6)

Kolaviron (**160**), a biflavonoid complex from *Garcinia kola* seeds, was found to reduce *in vivo* oxidative stress in the liver of Wistar albino rats following chronic ethanol administration [121]. Kolaviron was also found to exhibit an ameliorative effect on the di-n-butylphthalate (DBP)-induced testicular damage in rats. Administration of DBP to rats at a dose of 2 g/kg for 9 days significantly decreased the relative testicular weights compared to the controls, while the weights of other organs remained unaffected [122]. Inhibitory effects of kolaviron (**160**) were investigated on benzoyl peroxide (BPO)-induced free radical generation in rat's skin, and experimental results showed that kolaviron significantly inhibited the adverse effects of BPO induced free radical generation [124]. Kolaviron (**160**) exhibited a protective effect against scopolamine-induced memory impairment/oxidative stress which is associated with *Alzheimer's* disease. Kolaviron was found to possess cognition-enhancing effect as evident from the enhanced antioxidant defense and cholinergic systems [125]. Kolaviron (**160**) was also found to protect the male reproductive system from oxidative damage by anti-tuberculosis drugs *via* the antioxidative mechanism. This biflavonoid at 10, 20, 50 and 100 μg/mL dose exhibited strong reducing potential and effectively scavenged DPPH and OH radicals in a concentration-dependent manner. Moreover, it significantly inhibited LPO in rats' liver homogenate [126].

Macrophylloflavone (**168**), isolated from *Garcinia macrophylla*, exhibited significant antioxidant activity in 2,2 diphenyl-1-picrylhydrazyl (DPPH) assay with ascorbic acid as the positive control [130]. Morelloflavone (**173**) and its two glycosylated derivatives (**174-175**) isolated from the epicarp of *Garcinia brasiliensis* exhibited antioxidant activity in the DPPH assay using ascorbic acid and BHT as standards. Morelloflavone (**173**) showed the greatest activity with an IC_{50} value of 49.50 mM, followed by biflavonoid glycosides (**174 & 175**) with IC_{50} values of 62.6 and 52.4 mM, respectively [133]. Morelloflavone (**173**) and volkensiflavone (**235**) isolated from *Garcinia buchananii* showed moderate to strong H_2O_2 scavenging, Trolox equivalent antioxidant capacity (H/L-TEAC), and hydrophilic and lipophilic oxygen radical absorbance capacity (H/L-ORAC), as well as *in vitro* antioxidant activities [134].

A research group investigated the *in vitro* protective effects of ochnaflavone (**181**), a group IIA secretory phospholipase A2 (sPLA2-IIA) inhibitor, on the progression of carbon tetrachloride (CCl_4)-induced acute liver injury in rat liver microsomes. When rat liver was incubated at 37 °C in the presence of CCl_4, the level of phosphatidylethanolamine (PE) degradation was found to increase significantly in a dose-dependent manner with an IC_{50} value of 3.45mM compared to the control used. Ochnaflavone (**181**) was also found to inhibit lipid peroxidation in a dose-dependent manner with an IC_{50} value of 7.16 mM. This result suggested that ochnaflavone may prevent the progression of CCl_4-induced

PE hydrolysis by inhibiting the endogenous sPLA2 activity [138]. Three biflavonoids, named oliveriflavones A-C (**182–184**), isolated from the endangered plant *C. oliveri*, were assessed for antioxidant activities in DPPH and hydroxyl assays. All these compounds exhibited significant DPPH scavenging activity with IC_{50} values less than 2.0 µM, and hydroxyl scavenging activity with IC_{50} values less than 5.0 µM [143]. A biflavonoid (**192**) isolated from *Garcinia paucinervis* was assayed for its antioxidant activities using DPPH and ABTS radical scavenging capacities. The biflavonoid exhibited potent activities in both cases showing IC_{50} values of 3.52±.96 µM against ABTS and 77.85±1.77 µM against DPPH [146]. Antioxidant activities of an isolated biflavonoid compound, potifulgene (**196**), from the roots of *Potentilla fulgens*, were evaluated for *in vitro* activity using ABTS, DPPH, and FRAP assays, and scavenging potential has been measured in terms of TEAC (mM Trolox equivalent/mg extract). The biflavonoid (**196**) showed notable TEAC values as 6.85±0.38, 4.24 ± 0.41, and 5.35 ± 0.53 in ABTS, DPPH, and FRAP assays, respectively [148].

Two isolated biflavonoids (**155 & 197**) from the stem bark of *Garcinia buchananii* exhibited strong antioxidant activity in H_2O_2 scavenging, oxygen radical absorbance capacity (ORAC), and Trolox equivalent antioxidant capacity (TEAC) assays [149]. These natural products exhibited significant *in vitro* antioxidative potencies in the tested assays. The biflavonoid **155** showed EC_{50} value of 17.5 µM (H_2O_2 scavenging), 1.48/2.92 mmol TE/mmol (H/L-TEAC), and 4.38/6.96 mmol TE/mmol (H/L-ORAC), whereas biflavonoid **197** exhibited EC_{50} value of 8.5 µM (H_2O_2 scavenging), 3.50/4.95 mmol TE/mmol (H/L-TEAC), and 7.54/14.56 mmol TE/mmol (H/L-ORAC) [149]. A pyranocoumarin dimer (**198**) isolated from the aerial parts of *Angelica urumiensis* exhibited moderate antioxidant activity in DPPH radical scavenging assay having an IC_{50} value of 170 µg/mL [150].

Nitric Oxide (NO) InhibitoryActivity

Biflavonoids (**30, 31, 120, 122, 156, 179 & 239**) isolated from dried stem barks of *Daphne feddei* were tested for inhibitory activities against lipopolysaccharide (LPS)-induced nitric oxide (NO) production in RAW 264.7 macrophages and it was found that the isolated compounds showed varying degrees of inhibitory activities at the tested concentrations of 25, 50, 75 and 100 mg/mL, respectively [43].

Anti-enzymatic Activity

UV irradiation regulates the synthesis of MMP in human skin *in vivo*, and MMP-mediated collagen destruction accounts for the connective tissue damage that occurs during aging [24]. Two known biflavonoids, sumaflavone (**225**) and amentoflavone (**83**), isolated from ethylacetate soluble fraction of whole plants of *Selaginella tamariscina* exhibited significant MMP-1 inhibitory activity in primary human dermal fibroblasts after UV irradiation having IC_{50} values of 0.78 µM and 1.8 µM, respectively, using retinoic acid as the positive control (IC_{50}=10 µM). This result demands that sumaflavone and amentoflavone could be regarded as potential preventive or therapeutic agents for skin aging [24].

Biflavonoids (**46, 81, 173, 185** & **235**) isolated from *Garcinia prainiana* were found to have tyrosinase inhibitory activity employing L-DOPA as the substrate. The inhibition concentration to obtain 50% of the inhibition activity (IC_{50}) of tyrosinase by compounds was determined. The isolated biflavonoids showed strong anti-tyrosinase inhibitory activity [57]. Morelloflavone (**173**) exhibited higher inhibitory activity with IC_{50} value of 34.0 µg/mL than other biflavonoids, suggesting the catechol moiety in the ring B to play a key role in enhancing the tyrosinase inhibitory activity. In addition, biflavonoids (**83**) and (**185**) showed weaker activity compared to other compounds owing to methoxylation of the hydroxyl groups [57]. From the n-butanol fraction of the crude extracts of the nuts of *Cupressus sempervirens*, several compounds were isolated and screened for their efficacies to inhibit differentiation of murine bone marrow cells (BMCs) to osteoclasts. Only cupressuflavone (**70**) was found to significantly inhibit differentiation of BMCs to tartrate-resistant acid phosphatase (TRAP) positive cells when cultured in the presence of receptor activator of nuclear factor kappa B ligand (RANKL) and macrophage-colony stimulating factor (M-CSF). The investigators also observed that compound **70** inhibited adipocyte differentiation and stimulated osteoblast functions. Therefore, compound **70** may be regarded as a novel phytochemical that prevents estrogen deficiency-induced bone loss [67].

Biflavonoids **83** and **204** isolated from *Dietes bicolor* exhibited anti-inflammatory activity by inhibiting superoxide anion generation with an IC_{50} value of 1.0 µM as well as elastase release with IC_{50} values of 0.75 and 0.45 µM, respectively. This activity was further justified by virtual docking of the isolated biflavonoids to the binding sites in the human neutrophil elastase (HNE) crystal structure. It was concluded that the biflavonoids bound directly to HNE and then inhibited its enzymatic activity based on the CDOCKER algorithm [75]. A research group reported that amentoflavone (**83**) isolated from *Garcinia subelliptica* significantly inhibited hypoxia-inducible factor-1 in human embryonic kidney 293 cells under hypoxic conditions. The treatment of cells with **83** significantly reduced the luciferase activity at a concentration of 100 *µ*M [76].

Another research group [82] evaluated the inhibitory potential of five biflavonoids isolated from *Selaginella tamariscina* against nine P450 activities (P450s1A2,

2A6, 2B6, 2C8, 2C9, 2C19, 2D6, 2E1, and 3A) in human liver microsomes (HLMs) using cocktail incubation and liquid chromatography-tandem mass spectrometry (LC–MS/MS). The most strongly inhibited P450 activity was CYP2C8-mediated amodiaquine N-dealkylation with IC_{50} value in the range of 0.019~0.123µM. Moreover, the biflavonoids, selariscinin E (**209**), amentoflavone (**83**), robustaflavone (**204**), cupressuflavone (**115**), and taiwaniaflavone (**226**), were found to non-competitively inhibit CYP2C8 activity with respective Ki values of 0.018, 0.083, 0.084, 0.103, and 0.142 µM. Besides, selariscinin E (**209**) exhibited efficacy against six UGT isoforms (UGTs1A1, 1A3, 1A4, 1A6, 1A9 & 2B7) showing weaker inhibition (IC50 > 1.7 µM) [80].

A research group [82] showed the first binding model of amentoflavone (**83**) with few selected human proteins (α-glucosidase, tyrosinase and 15-lipoxygenase) as validated therapeutic targets by means of computational procedures. Interference of amentoflavone with the metal ions within the active site of tyrosinase and lipoxygenase was noticed as part of its inhibitory mechanism against the proteins. The inhibitory potential of the biflavonoid against 15-lipoxygenase was observed with an IC_{50} value of 0.04 µM [82]. It was observed that amentoflavone stably occupied the active sites of all the proteins with lesser ΔG values and engaged one of its monoflavonoid subunits for penetration into the binding pocket, preventing substrate access, binding and conversion. The polyhydroxyl groups of the biflavonoid participated critically in the formation of hydrophilic interaction, whereas the aromatic rings enjoyed hydrophobic interactions with residues side chain and π-π stacking with the phenolic rings of aromatic amino acids. The resulting data established amentoflavone as a useful candidate in the treatment of diabetes, inflammation and hyperpigmentation disorders [82].

The biflavonoid (**85**), isolated from *Aster yomena,* was screened for the inhibitory activity of IL-6 production in the TNF-a stimulated MG-63 cell. The compound exhibited moderate inhibitory activity with 42.8% inhibition [83]. Biflavonoid (**139**) isolated from *Garcinia kola* was found to have potent tyrosinase inhibition activity (IC_{50} 582µM) compared to reference, kojic acid (IC_{50} 130µM), as assessed in a 96-well microplate format using Spectra Max 340 microplate reader [108]. The biflavonoid, GB-2a (**140**), has been reported to promote inhibition of tyrosinase activity and reduce melanin biosynthesis in B16F10 cells. The experimental results revealed that the biflavonoid, without reducing cell *via*bility, significantly inhibited the melanin content. It also exhibited high antityrosinase activity in the mushroom tyrosinase assay [109]. The biflavonoid, hinokiflavone (**146**), may act as an inhibitor of splicing *in vitro* and a modulator of alternative splicing in cells. It was found to inhibit *in vitro* splicing by blocking spliceosome assembly, and hence, prevent the formation of the B complex. Cells treated with hinokiflavone thus modified subnuclear organization specifically of splicing factors required for a complex formation [114]. A new biflavonoid (**149**) from leaves of *Garcinia nervosa* var. *pubescens* King was evaluated for its ability to inhibit platelet-activating factor (PAF) receptor binding to rabbit platelets using 3H-PAF as a ligand. The biflavonoid exhibited significant inhibition with an IC_{50} value of 28.0 μM [116].

Several amentoflavone-type biflavonoids (**11, 16, 22, 45, 54, 83, 91, 144-145, 154, 194, 208, 210**), isolated from different natural sources, were found to have β-secretase (BACE-1) inhibitory activity. It was reported that BACE-1 inhibitor could be an effective and safe therapeutic strategy for Alzheimer's disease (AD), the most common form of dementia characterized by accumulation and deposition of amyloid β (A β) peptides [117]. Among the tested biflavonoids, 2,3-dihydro-6-methylginkgetin (**11**) and 2,3-dihydroamentoflavone (**16**) exhibited significant inhibitory effects with IC_{50} values of 0.35 and 0.75 μM, respectively. As per the investigators, potent inhibitory effects of these amento-biflavonoids (**11 & 16**) are due to the presence of flavanone moiety [117]. Two biflavonoids, morelloflavone (**173**) and talbotaflavone (**227**), isolated from *Garcinia lateriflora*, were found to inhibit proteasome activity using bortezomib as the positive control [127]. The biflavonoid **173** exhibited more activity (IC_{50} 1.3 μM) than the biflavonoid **227** (IC_{50} 4.4 μM). It was reported that neochamaejasmin B (**179**), isolated from *Stellera chamaejasme* L., could inhibit P-glycoprotein (P-gp) mediated cellular efflux both in a competitive and a non-competitive manner. Moreover, the mechanism of reversing P-gp-mediated multi-drug resistance of NCB adds a new mechanism to Langdu's antitumor activity [137]. Tetrahydroxyamentoflavone (**228**), isolated from *Semecarpus anacardium* L. seed, was found to inhibit xanthine oxidase (XO), the overexpression of which leads to inflammation and gout. The biflavonoid **228** exhibited an IC_{50} value of s 92 nM, whereas the standard drug, allopurinol, exhibited an IC_{50} value of 100 nM [158].

Anti-HIV Activity

Compounds **57** and **207**, isolated from *Sarcandra hainanensis*, were examined for their HIV-1 integrase (IN) inhibition activities applying microplate screening method using magnetic beads and baicalein as the standard with an IC_{50} value of 1.06μ M in the test. Compounds **57** and **206** exhibited weak inhibition activities for the integrase strand transfer reaction *in vitro* with IC_{50} values of 25.27and 18.05 μ M, respectively [63].

The isolated biflavonoid (**103**) from *Stellera chamaejasme* was evaluated for anti-HIV-1 activity against the NL4-3 virus in MT4 lymphocytes [98]. The anti-HIV EC90 value was found to be 4.21 μM, respectively, whereas the biflavonoid exhibited low cytotoxicity (IC_{50} value 17.5 μM).

Anti-thrombin Activity

Chemical studies on the constituents of *Dracaena cochinchinensis* led to the discovery of eight new flavonoid derivatives (**72, 109-114**). All isolates were tested for thrombin inhibitory effects. The seven isolated new flavonoid derivatives (**72, 109-114**) were observed to exhibit moderate thrombin inhibitory activity [70].

Anti-allergic Activity

Biflavonoidsnds **83** and **204** isolated from *Dietes bicolor* exhibited anti-allergic activity by inhibiting antigen-induced β-hexosaminidase release at 45.7% and 46.3%, respectively, at a dose of 400 μM [75].

Cytoprotective Activity

The cytoprotective activities of the isolated biflavonoids (**86-88**) from *Baeckea frutescens* were tested using the PC12 cells stressed by H_2O_2. When the cell survival (%) of the control group was 40%, the cytoprotection (%) of the test compounds (**86-88**) (at a dose of 10 μM) was 34.8%, 36.0% and 31.8%, respectively, displaying significant cytoprotective effects in this assay compared to the control [85].

Neuroprotective Activity

Agathisflavone (**82**) and amentoflavone (**83**) competitively inhibited the binding of 3H-Ro 15-1788 with a *K*i value of 28 and 37 nM, respectively. These two biflavonoids were found to fit into a pharmacophore model for ligands binding to the GABAA receptor benzodiazepine site and reflected the affinities of the compounds in the [3H]-flumazenil binding assay [74]. Amentoflavone (**83**), bilobetin (**91**), ginkgetin (**144**), isoginkgetin (**154**), ochnaflavone (**181**), and sciadopitysin (**208**) were found to have neuroprotective activity on oxidative stress-induced and amyloid β peptide-induced cell death in neuronal cells [88]. Out of the tested biflavonoids, amentoflavone (**83**), ginkgetin (**144**) and isoginkgetin (**154**) showed profound neuroprotection efficacies against cytotoxic insults induced by oxidative stress and amyloid β, and established their therapeutic potentiality against neurodegenerative diseases, including ischemic stroke and Alzheimer's disease [88].

The biflavonoid, CGY-1 (**102**), isolated from *Cardiocrinum giganteum* exhibited neuroprotective activity on a scopolamine-induced memory deficit model [97]. To justify such potential of the biflavonoid, behavioral experiments (Morris water maze, the Y-maze and the fear conditioning test) were performed. The results suggested that oral administration of CGY-1 (20 and 40 mg/kg) and donepezil improved the percentage of spontaneous alternation, shortened the escape latency, and increased the freezing times, respectively. CGY-1 was found to decrease the levels of reactive oxygen species and malondialdehyde and to increase the activities of superoxide dismutase and glutathione peroxidase in the hippocampus. Moreover, CGY-1 (**102**) increased the activities of choline acetyltransferase and acetylcholine in the hippocampus and decreased the activity of acetylcholinesterase. It was also established that the expressions of neurotrophic factors, brain-derived neurotrophic factor and nerve growth factor were upregulated in the hippocampus after CGY-1 treatment. In conclusion, CGY-1 is expected to be a promising candidate for the treatment of cognitive dysfunction [97].

Anti-inflammatory Activity

The isolated biflavonoids (**129 & 139**) from the *Garcinia gardneriana* were examined for anti-inflammatory activity in the carrageenan-induced oedema. The results demonstrated that both fukugetin and GB- 2a (i.p., 30 min before) were capable of preventing oedema formation. Only GB-2a (**139**) was found to cause a dose-dependent inhibition, with an estimated mean ID_{50} value of 78.36 (47.25–129.98) mg/kg, whereas fukugetin (**139**) was found to reduce oedema formation by only 38±4% [106]. Two biflavonoids (**212-213**) from *Wikstroemia indica* exhibited significant cytotoxic effects against MTT assay by inhibiting NO production at a dose of 100μM [154].

Miscellaneous Activity

(2*R*,3*S*,2"*R*,3"*R*)-Manniflavanone (**170**) isolated from stem bark extract of *Garcinia buchananii* was found to relax the smooth muscle by inhibiting L-type Ca^{2+} channels which have been found to have the potential for use in therapies of gastrointestinal smooth muscle spasms and arrhythmia [132].

Hepatic and Renal toxicity

The five biflavonoids from *Ginkgo biloba* have been found to exert potential hepatic and renal toxicity. The investigators studied the *in vitro* and *in vivo* toxicological effects of the biflavonoids, *i.e.* amentoflavone (**83**), sciadopitysin

(**208**), ginkgetin (**144**), isoginkgetin (**154**), and bilobetin (**91**), from *Ginkgo biloba*. In the *in vitro* cytotoxicity test, the five biflavonoids were found to reduce cell *via*bility in a dose-dependent manner in normal human hepatocytes (L-02) as well as human renal tubular epithelial cells (HK-2), thereby indicating to have potential liver and kidney toxicity. In the *in vivo* experiments, after intragastrical administration of these biflavonoids at 20 mg.kg^{-1}d^{-1} for 7 days, serum biochemical analysis and histopathological examinations were performed [81]. The activity of alkaline phosphatase was found to be significantly increased after all the biflavonoid administrations, and widespread hydropic degeneration of hepatocytes was observed in ginkgetin or bilobetin-treated mice. Moreover, all the five biflavonoids were found to induce acute kidney injury in treated mice, and the main pathological lesions were ascertained to the tubule, glomeruli, and interstitium injuries. These biflavonoids may be more toxic to the kidney than the liver, as revealed from *in vitro* and *in vivo* results. The increased TUNEL-positive cells were detected in kidney tissues of biflavonoids-treated mice, followed by elevated expression of proapoptotic protein BAX and unchanged levels of antiapoptotic protein BCL-2, indicating apoptosis to be involved in biflavonoids-induced nephrotoxicity [81].

SYNTHESIS OF BIFLAVONOIDS

Structurally, biflavonoids are polyphenolic molecules comprised of two identical or non-identical flavonoid units joined together in a symmetrical or unsymmetrical manner through an alkyl or an alkoxy-based linker of varying length (Fig. 7). Large numbers of variations are possible in the parent flavonoid units coupled with the large number of permutations in the position and nature of the inter-flavonoid linkage, which introduce significant structural diversity in biflavonoids. Apart from the presence of variable functional groups in variable positions, *e.g.* hydroxy, methoxy, keto or double bond, and chiral centres on the flavonoid, scaffold increases the structural variability of bioflavonoids to a large extent.

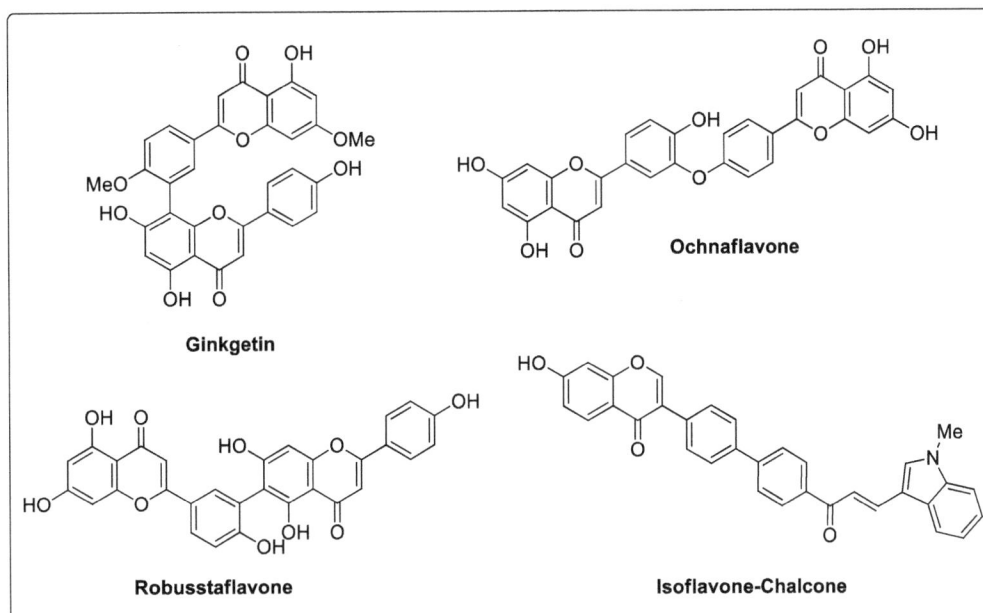

Fig. (7). Different structural units of biflavonoids.

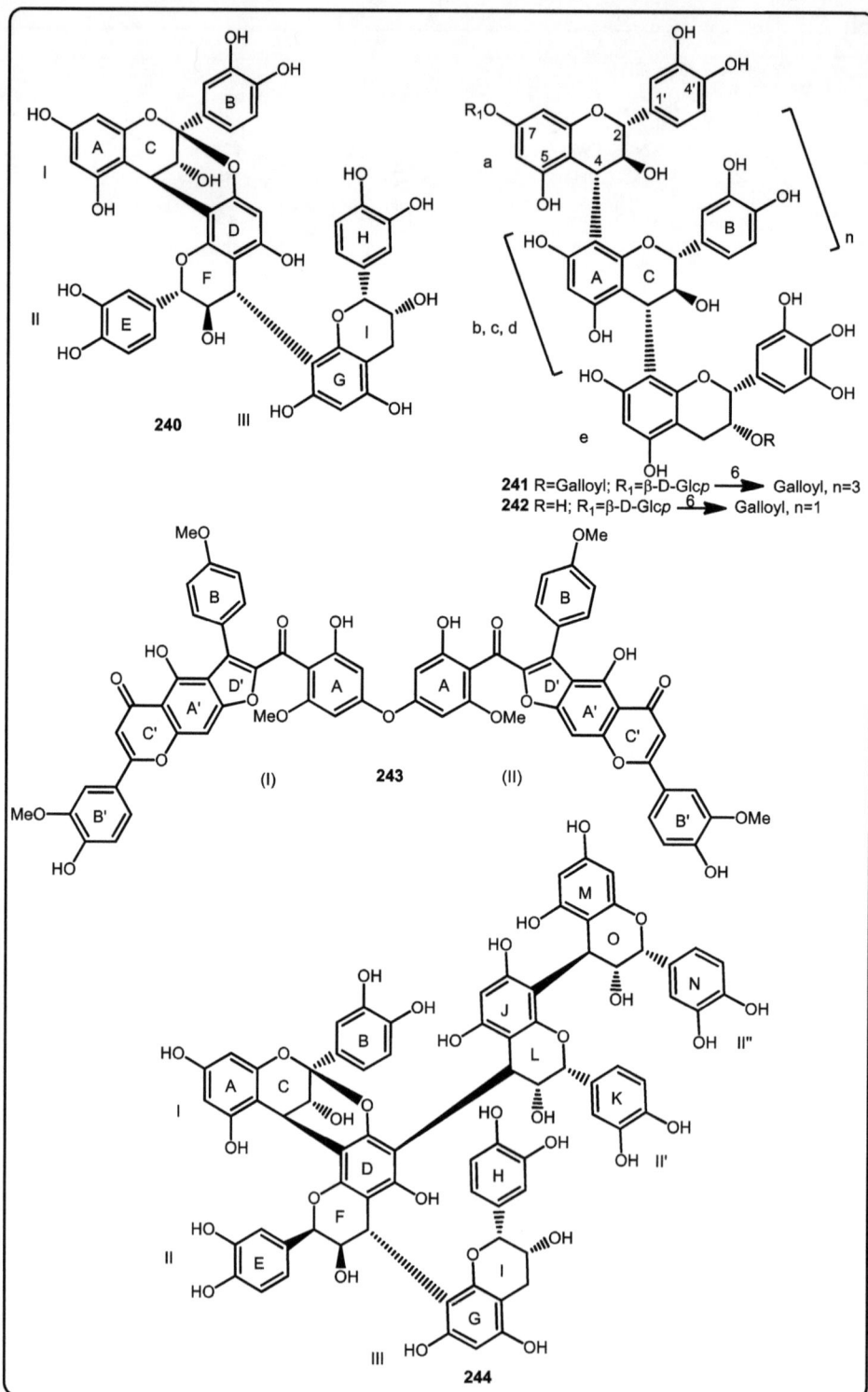

241 R=Galloyl; R$_1$=β-D-Glc*p* $\xrightarrow{6}$ Galloyl, n=3
242 R=H; R$_1$=β-D-Glc*p* $\xrightarrow{6}$ Galloyl, n=1

240

243

244

(Fig) contd.....

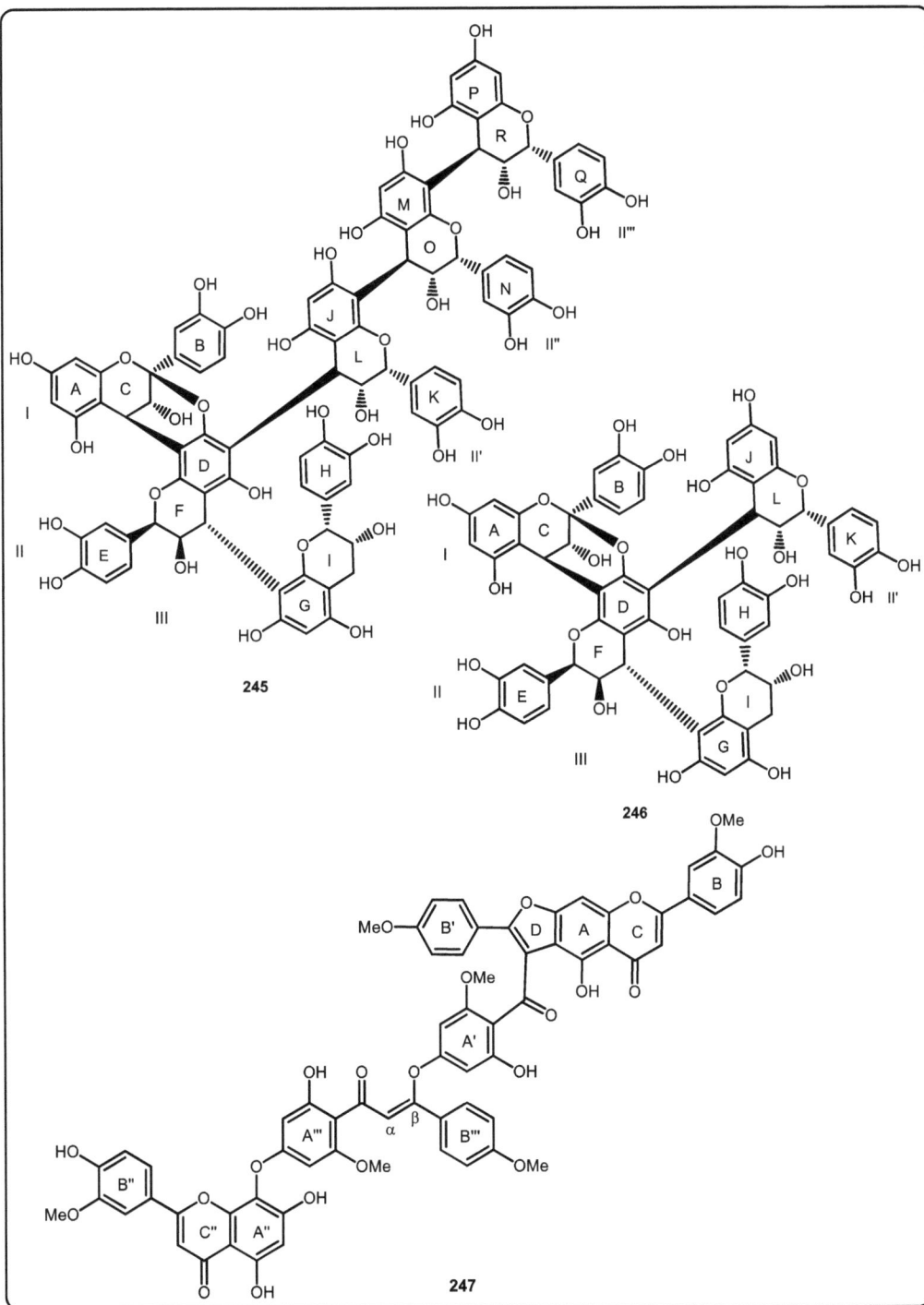

245

246

247

db=double bond; Glc =glucopyranosyl; Rha=rhamnopyranosyl.

Thus, the synthesis of biflavonoids remains a challenging task for organic chemists. Different synthetic strategies that have been reported for the synthesis of structurally different biflavonoids are presented below.

Heerden *et al.* proposed the synthesis of ochnaflavone biflavonoid by a three-step synthetic protocol Scheme. (**1**) [163]. A simple base promoted aromatic nucleophilic substitution between **181a** and **181b** results in diaryl ether unit **181c**, which is then subjected to aldol reaction resulting in chalcone unit **181d**. The chalcone unit then undergoes cyclization in the presence of I_2 in pyridine to give **181e**, which upon demethylation by BBr_3, produces ochnaflavone (**181**) in 60% yield.

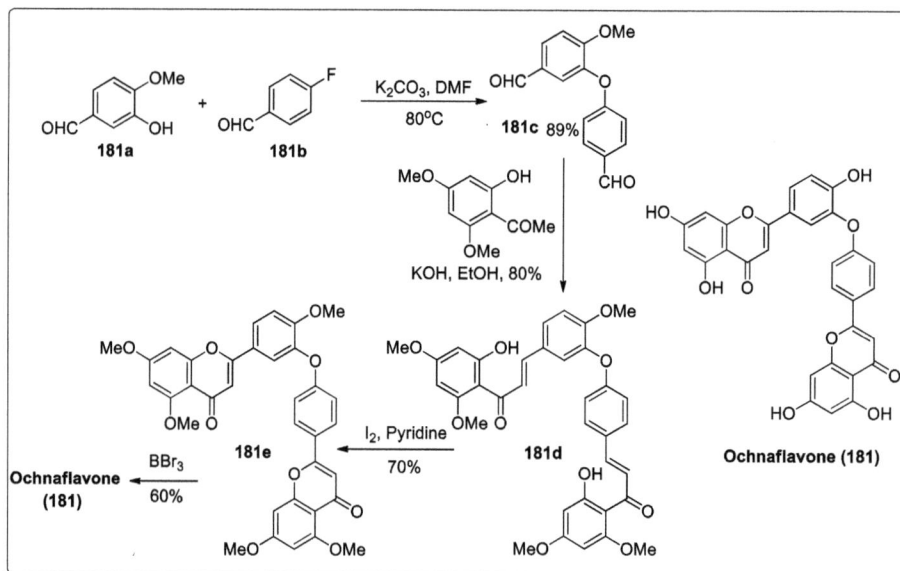

Scheme (1). Synthesis of ochnaflavone (**181**).

Suzuki-Miyaura cross-coupling reaction was found to be a striking protocol for the synthesis of different symmetrical and unsymmetrical biflavonoids. Spring and coworkers utilized this methodology for the successful synthesis of isoflavone-aurone biflavonoid **248** Scheme. (**2**) [163]. The authors performed Pd-catalysed Suzuki Miyaura cross-coupling reaction between isoflavone boronate ester (**248a**) and bromoaurone (**248b**) to synthesize the desired bioflavonoid (**248**). Boronate ester unit **248a** synthesis was started from acylation of resorcinol **P** by **Q** to form **R** in the presence of BF_3. Treatment of **R** with methylsulfonyl chloride produced **S** which upon Pd-catalysed Miyaura borylation by B_2pin_2 furnished the desired isoflavone boronate ester **248a**. Authors have performed a

5-step synthesis for producing bromoaurone unit starting from phloroglucinol (**A**) which is commercially available. Treatment of **A** with chloroacetonitrile in the presence of ZnCl$_2$ produced imine intermediate **B**. Hydrolysis of **B** under acidic conditions provided **C**, which on treatment with methanolic sodium methoxide, produced **D**. Methylation of free hydroxyl groups in **D** produced benzofuranone **E** and condensation was performed with bromobenzaldehyde **F** to give **248b**, *i.e.* bromoaurone.

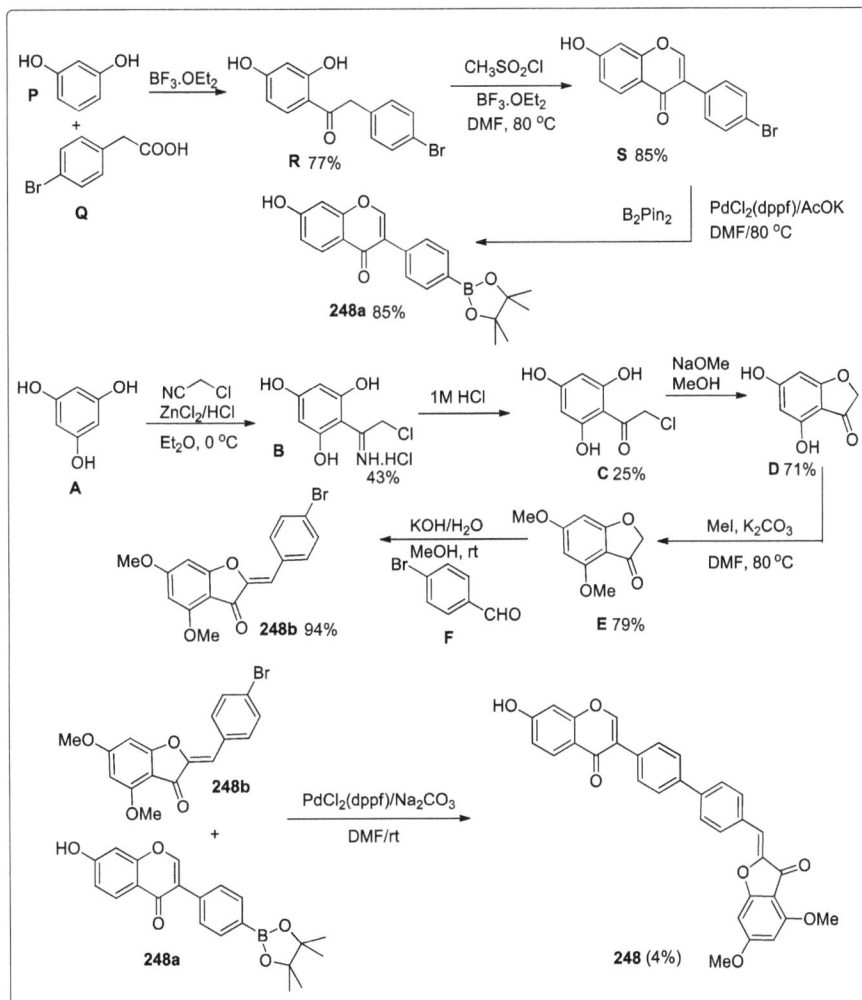

Scheme (2). Synthesis of isoflavone-aurone biflavonoid (**248**).

The same group also reported the synthesis of heterocycle-based Isoflavone-chalcone biflavonoid **249** Scheme. (**3**) [163]. Authors have performed the preparation of indole bromochalcone **249e** from indole in three steps. Performing

Vilsmeier-Haack in indole (**249a**) produces **249b**. N-methylation of **249b** produced **249c,** which was allowed to react with 4-bromo-acetophenone (**249d**) in a basic medium to obtain the desired bromochalcone by aldol reaction. The indole-based bromochalcone **249e** was subjected to Suzuki-Miyaura coupling with isoflavone boronate easter **248a** to give the desired bioflavonoid **249**.

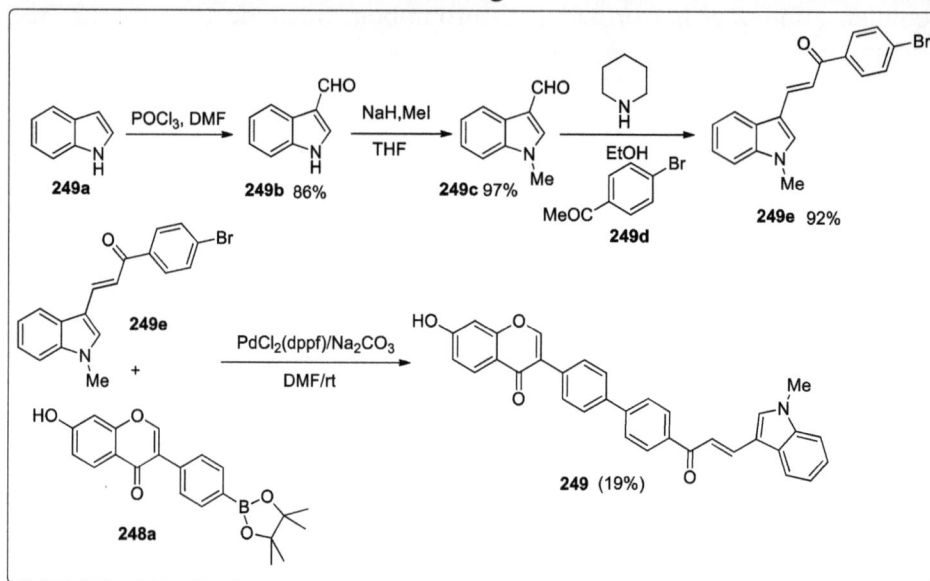

Scheme (3). Synthesis of indole based isoflavone-chalcone bioflavonoid (**249**).

The authors also synthesized isoflavone-flavonol bioflavonoid **250** by performing Pd-catalysed Suzuki-Miyaura coupling of isoflavone boronate ester **248a** with brormoflavonol **250** Scheme. (**4**) [164]. Aldol condensation of trimethoxybenzaldehyde **250a** and bromoacetophenone **250b** gave bromochalcone **250c**, which was converted to the required bromoflavonol coupling partner **250d** by an Algar-Flynn-Oyamada (AFO) oxidation.

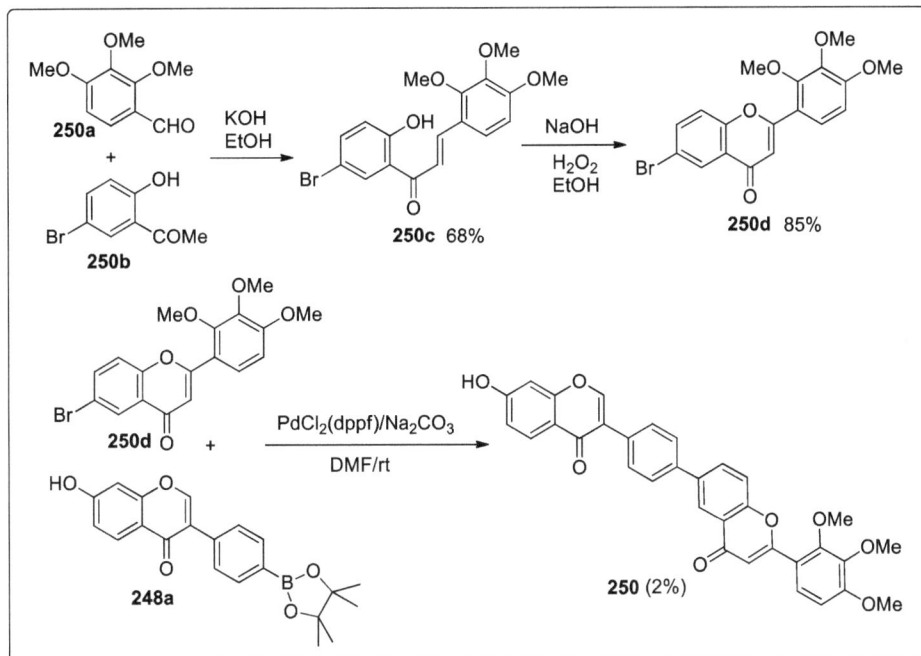

Scheme (4). Synthesis of isoflavone-flavonol bioflavonoid (**250**).

The authors also synthesized methylenedioxy-bridged bidihydrochalcone Scheme. (**5**) [165] from acetophenone **251b,** which was prepared by performing Fries rearrangement of **251a** in the presence of Eaton's reagent. Base-catalysed Claisen-Schmidt reaction of **251c** and **251b** furnished chalcone which upon hydrogenation produced dihydro chalcone **251e**. Methylation of **251e** produced the desired product **251**.

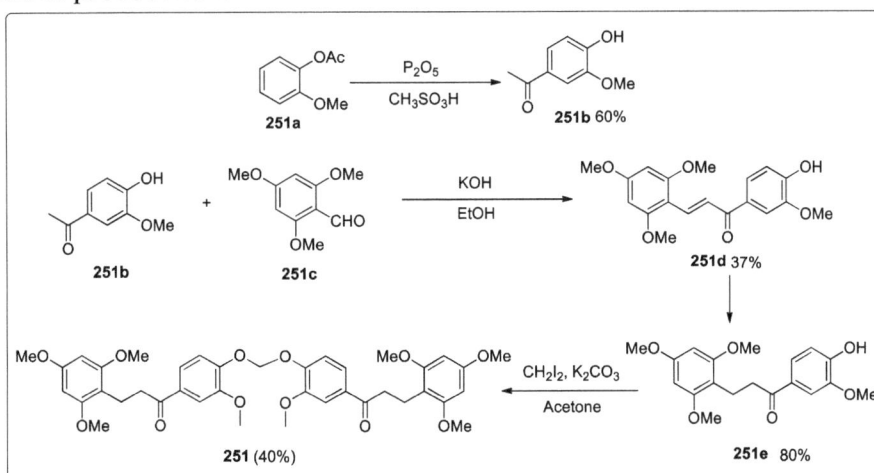

Scheme (5). Synthesis of methylenedioxy-bridged bidihydrochalcone (**251**).

Spring *et al.* synthesized triflavone 40, triaurone triflavone **252** and triaurone **253** starting from common starting material trichalcone **252c**, which was synthesized by aldol condensation of trialdehyde **252a** and acetophenone **252b** Scheme. **(6)** [166].

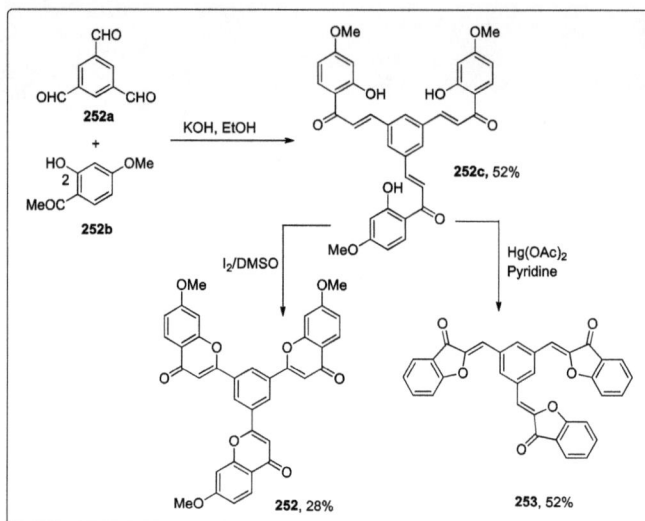

Scheme (6). Synthesis of triflavone (**252**) and triaurone (**253**).

Mathai and coworkers first introduced the synthesis of biflavonones by utilizing a 1,1'-biphenyl skeleton. 4,4'-Dimethoxy-3,3'-diformyl-1,1'-biphenyl (**254a**) was condensed with 2-hydroxyaceto-phenone (**254b**) in the presence of ethanolic KOH to give the bichalconyl derivative **254c**, which on refluxing with SeO_2 in amyl alcohol gave the symmetrical 3',3'-biflavonyl derivative **254** Scheme. **(7)** [167].

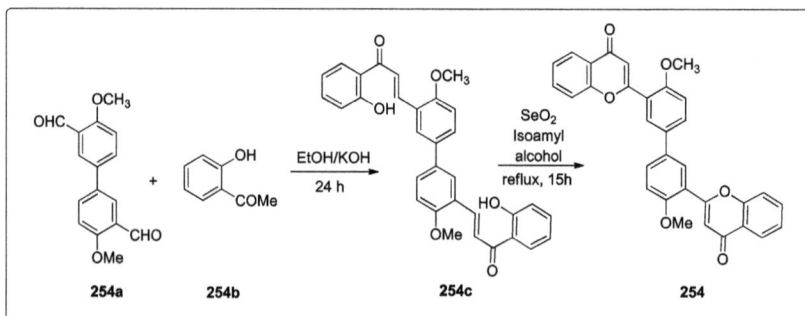

Scheme (7). Synthesis of 1,1'-biaryl based biflavone (**254**).

Enantioselective synthesis of biflavonoids has also been reported [168]. Atropisomerism of the biflavone moiety is the main reason for the chirality of bioflavonoids. As shown in Scheme. (8), chiral tetra-ether **255c** was first prepared through the sequential introduction of 2-iodo-3,5-dimethoxyphenol moieties on the erythrityl skeleton **255b**. In this process, the second Mitsunobu reaction (conversion of **255b** to **255c**) is low-yielding because of steric hindrance. Treatment of **255c** with BuLi, followed by the addition of CuCN/TMEDA, led to the *in situ* formation of a higher order cyanocuprate intermediate, which gave **255g** upon exposure to dryness starting from **255d** in four steps. Diacetate **255j**, synthesized from **255g**, underwent a $TiCl_4$-promoted Friedel–Crafts rearrangement to afford **255k** in 94% yield. Following aldol reaction with p-anisaldehyde, bichalcone **255l** was obtained in 80% yield, which was cyclized to biflavonoid **255** using I_2/DMSO in 60% yield.

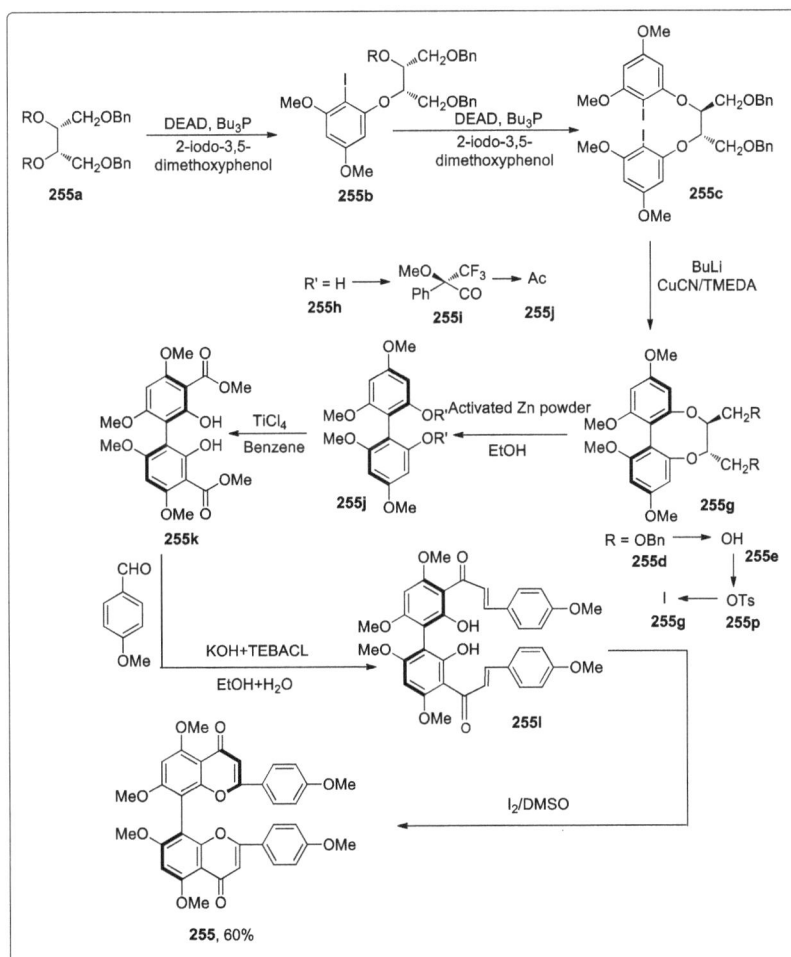

Scheme (8). Synthesis of biflavonoid **255**.

A similar approach has been applied to synthesize biflavonoids **256** and **257** in four steps from benzyl 4-iodo-3,5-dimethoxyphenyl ether (**256a**), as shown in Scheme. (**9**. Compound **256a** was subjected to the Ullmann coupling to give 4,4'-(dibenzyloxy)-2,2',6,6'-tetramethoxy-1,1'-biphenyl (**256b**), which *via* Hoesch reaction yielded 4,4'-dihydroxy-3,3'-diacetyl-2,2',6,6'-tetramethoxybiphenyl (**256c**). Aldol condensation with p-anisaldehyde, followed by oxidative cyclization with SeO$_2$, gave I-6,II-6-biapigenin **256**. In contrast, bichalcone **256c** in refluxing alcoholic H$_3$PO$_4$ for three weeks gave 6,6"-binarigenin hexamethyl ether **257** [169].

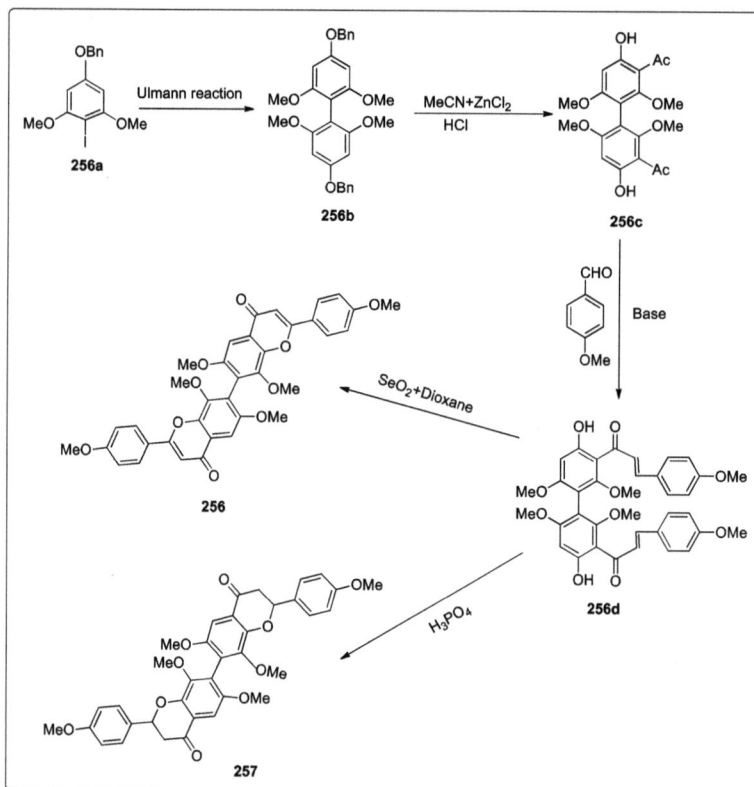

Scheme (9). Synthesis of Biflavonoids **256** and **257**.

Pd-catalysed C-C cross-coupling reaction was found to be a powerful tool for the synthesis of biflavonoids. Stille and co-workers have synthesized bioflavonoids by performing Stille coupling of flavone triflates **258a** with distannes to produce biflavonoid **258** (Scheme. (**10**) [170].

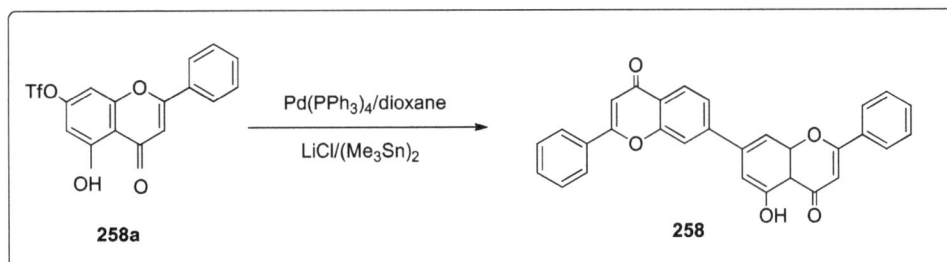

Scheme (10). Synthesis of biflavonoid (**258**) *via* Stille coupling.

Synthesis of biflavonoids was also achieved *via* Pd-catalyzed Suzuki Coupling. J.P. Fleury *et al.* reported the synthesis of Biflavonoid **259** by utilizing Pd-catalyzed Suzuki coupling Scheme. (**11**) [171]. At first, boronic acid **259b** was prepared from **259a** using B(OMe)₃ in the presence of BuLi. Then, **259b** was subjected to Suzuki coupling with **259c** to give **259**.

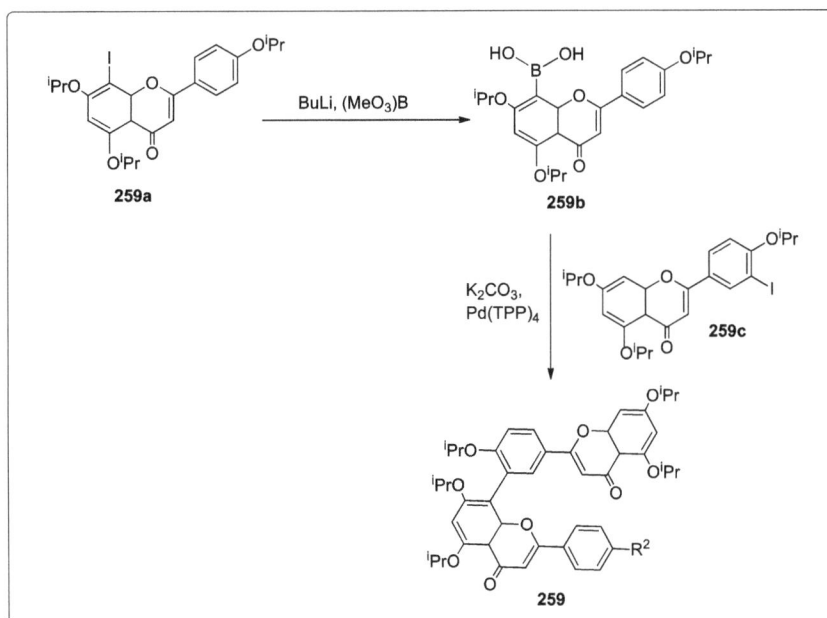

Scheme (11). Synthesis of Bioflavonoid (**259**) by Pd-catalyzed Suzuki Coupling.

The same group has reported the synthesis of bioflavonoid by an alternative protocol utilizing Suzuki coupling [171]. Firstly, iodoflavone **260b** was subjected to Suzuki coupling with aryl boronic acid **260a** to form unit **260c** Scheme. (**12**), which then underwent lewis acid catalysed acylation *via* para methoxy cinnamic acid **260d** to form **260e**. Finally, **260e** underwent oxidative cyclization to produce the desired bioflavonoid **260**.

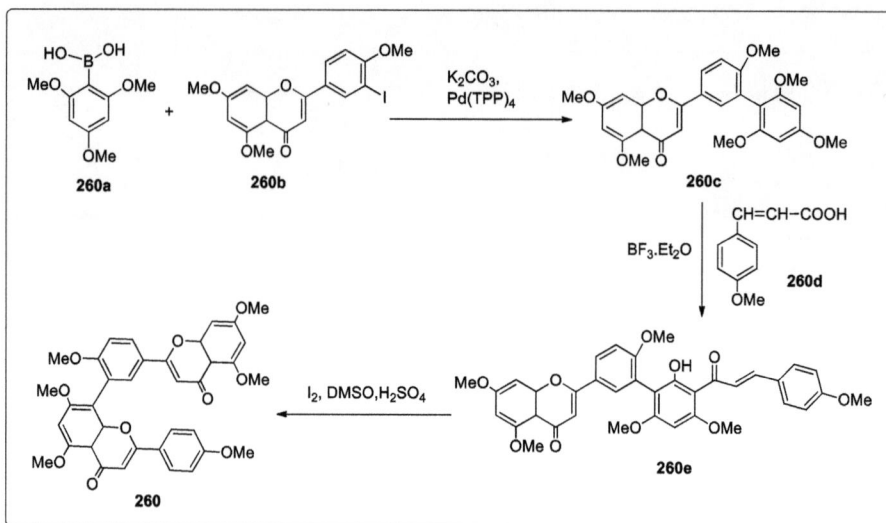

Scheme (12). Synthesis of Biflavonoid (**260**) by alternative Suzuki Coupling.

Zhang and co-workers attempted the synthesis of Robustaflavone (**204**) by applying Suzuki coupling Scheme. (**13**) [172]. At first, **204a** was iodinated by TlOAc catalysed regioselective iodization to form **204b**. In a separate reaction, boronate ester derivative **204d** of iodoflavone **204c** was synthesized. The Suzuki coupling between **204b** and **204d** furnished desired bioflavonoid **204**.

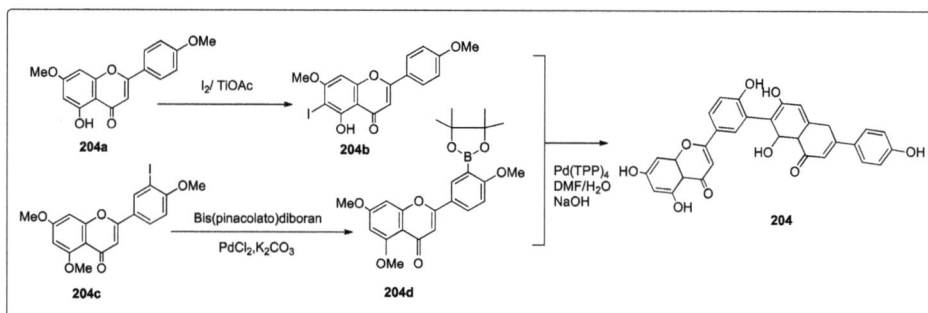

Scheme (13). Synthesis of Robustaflavone (**204**) by applying Suzuki Coupling.

Haddon and co-workers reported the strategy of oxidative coupling of monoflavonoids for the synthesis of biflavonoids. Apegenin **261a** was subjected to oxidative coupling in the presence of basic potassium ferricyanide to form two biflavonoids **261** and **262** Scheme. (**14**) [173]. The authors reported that the two flavone units were joined *via* the radical mechanism.

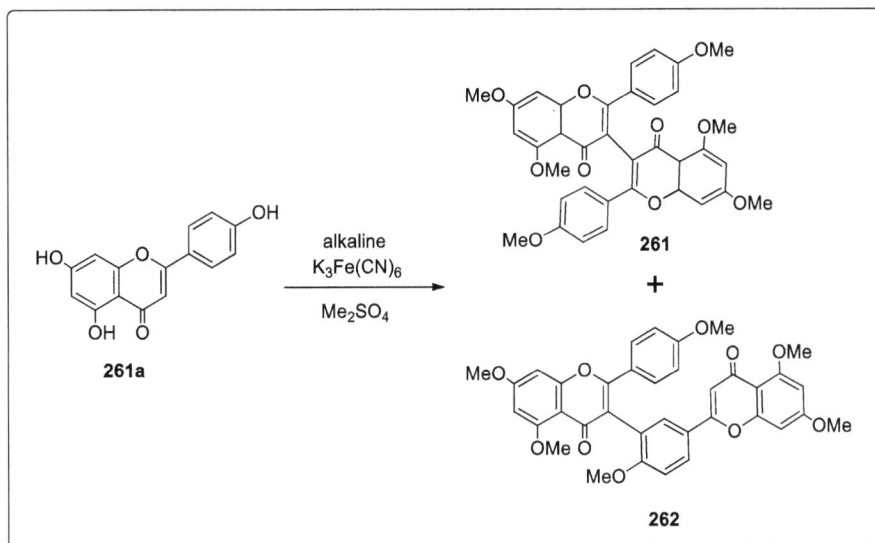

Scheme (14). Synthesis of Biflavonoids (**261** & **262**) by oxidative coupling of monoflavonoid.

Nakazawa *et al.* reported Cu catalysed Ullman coupling-based synthesis of biflavonoids (**263** & **264**) starting from monoflavones **263b** Scheme. (**15**) and **263c** Scheme. ((**16**), which underwent C-O coupling with **263a** bearing iodoarene with $-NO_2$ substituent at ortho position w.r.t the iodo group [174].

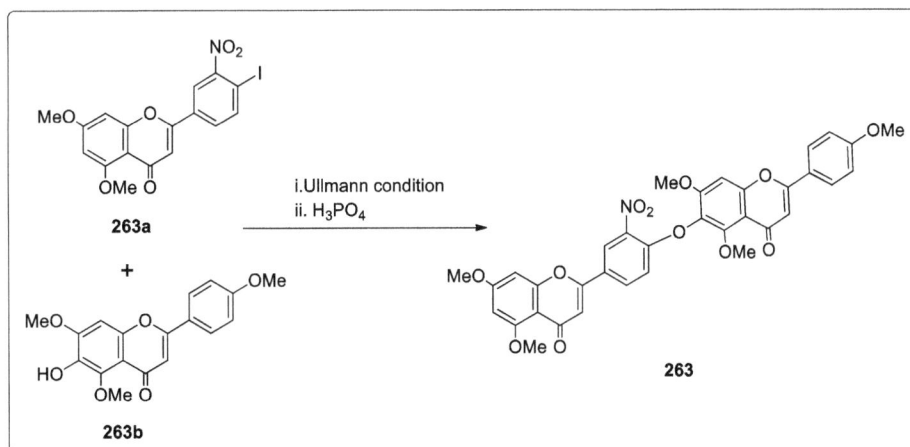

Scheme (15). Synthesis of biflavonoid (**263**)*via* Ullmann Coupling.

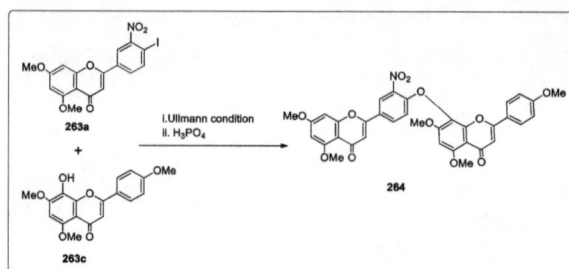

Scheme (16). Synthesis of biflavonoid (**264**) *via* Ullmann Coupling.

Chen *et al.* reported the electrochemical reduction of flavone **265a** under H-type cell and glass-filter diaphragm equipped with a series of electrodes and supporting electrolytes, including H_2SO_4 and TsOH, which yielded two types of dimers, racemic and mesoforms of 2,2'-biflavanone **265** and **266** with **265b** as the side product Scheme. (**17**) [175]. The reaction proceeded *via* a radical mechanism.

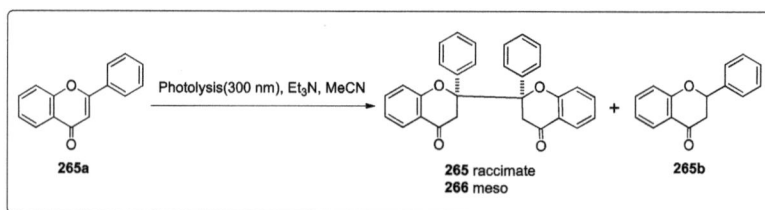

Scheme (17). Synthesis of Biflavonoid under electrochemical reduction.

Li and co-workers have successfully introduced Pd–catalyzed hydrogenation of biflavones for the synthesis of biflavanones Scheme. (**18**) [176]. Pd-catalysed hydrogenation of biflavone **267a** under glacial AcOH medium for 4 hrs at 80°C furnished biflavanone **267b**. However, prolonging the reaction for 12 hrs resulted in **267**.

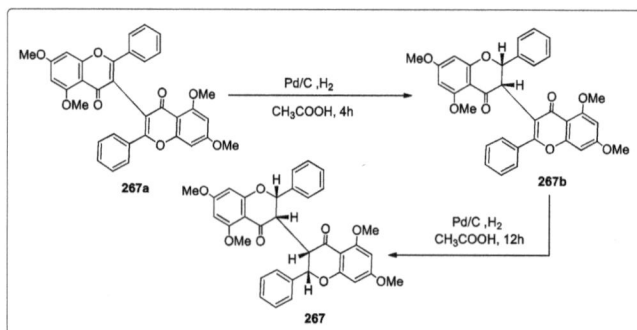

Scheme (18). Synthesis of Biflavanone from Biflavone (**267**) *via* Pd-catalyzed hydrogenation.

db=double bond; Glc =glucopyranosyl; Rha=rhamnopyranosyl.

CONCLUSION

This chapter focuses on the natural abundance of recently reported biflavonoids in the plant kingdom on one hand, and on the other, it deals with the pharmacological efficacies along with notable biological activities of this group of naturally occurring secondary metabolites. Moreover, synthetic strategies of this important group of natural constituents have been discussed. We have reported in this chapter the progress of research on natural biflavonoids from the period of 2005 to early 2020. A wide range of biological and pharmacological properties, including anti-microbial and antiviral, cytotoxic and anti-cancer, anti-diabetic, anti-anoxic, antioxidant, NO-inhibitory activity, anti-enzymatic, anti-HIV, anti-thrombin, anti-allergic, cytoprotective, neuroprotective and anti-inflammatory activities, as exhibited by the naturally occurring bioflavonoids are discussed in detail. Such efficacies as exhibited by this group of phytochemicals have already created a stir in the scientific community at large and attracted the present-day researchers to undertake systematic studies on biflavonoids in more depth so that mankind is benefited from the outcome of such research. We surely expect that this overview will boost the progress of research on naturally occurring flavonoids in the near future.

CONSENT FOR PUBLICATION

Not applicable.

CONFLICT OF INTEREST

The author declares no conflict of interest, financial or otherwise.

ACKNOWLEDGEMENTS

DK thanks the WBDST-BT [Memo No. 43(sanc)/ST/P/S&T/15G-21/2018, dated 30/01/2019)] for financial support.

REFERENCES

[1]   Verma, A.K.; Pratap, R. The biological potential of flavones. *Nat. Prod. Rep.,* **2010**, *27*(11), 1571-1593.
[http://dx.doi.org/10.1039/c004698c] [PMID: 20877900]

[2]   Grotewold, E., Ed. *The science of flavonoids*; Springer: New York, **2006**.
[http://dx.doi.org/10.1007/978-0-387-28822-2]

[3]   Alzand, K.I.; Mohamed, M.A. Flavonoids: Chemistry, biochemistry and antioxidant activity. *J. Pharm. Res.,* **2012**, *5*, 4013-4020.

[4]   Samanta, A.; Das, G.; Das, S.K. Roles of flavonoids in plants. *Int. J. Pharm. Pharm. Sci.,* **2011**, *6*(1), 12-35.

[5]   Pandey, R.P.; Sohng, J.K. Genetics of Flavonoids.*Natural Products-Phytochemistry, Botany, Metabolism of Alkaloids, Phenolics and Terpenes*; Ramawat, G.K.; Mérillon, M.J., Eds.; Springer-Verlag Berlin Heidelberg: Germany, 2013, pp. 1617-1645.
[http://dx.doi.org/10.1007/978-3-642-22144-6_52]

[6]   Andersen, O.M.; Markham, K.R. *Flavonoids: chemistry, biochemistry and applications*; CRC Press: US, 2005.
[http://dx.doi.org/10.1201/9781420039443]

[7]   Gontijo, V.S.; Dos Santos, M.H.; Viegas, C., Jr Biological and Chemical Aspects of Natural Biflavonoids from Plants: A Brief Review. *Mini Rev. Med. Chem.,* 2017, *17*(10), 834-862.
[http://dx.doi.org/10.2174/1389557517666161104130026] [PMID: 27823559]

[8]   Wang, G.; Yao, S.; Cheng, L.; Luo, Y.; Song, H. Antioxidant and anticancer effection of the volatile oil from various habitats of *Selaginella doederleinii* Hieron. *Technol. Health Care,* 2015, *23* Suppl. 1, S21-S27.
[http://dx.doi.org/10.3233/thc-150924] [PMID: 26410323]

[9]   Suzart, L.R.; Daniel, J.F.S.; de Carvalho, M.G.; Kaplan, M.A.C. Biodiversidade flavonoídica e aspectos farmacológicos em species dos gêneros *ouratea* e *luxemburgia* (ochnaceae). *Quim. Nova,* 2007, *30*(4), 984-987.
[http://dx.doi.org/10.1590/S0100-40422007000400038]

[10]   Rahman, M.; Riaz, M.; Desai, U.R. Synthesis of biologically relevant biflavanoids--a review. *Chem. Biodivers.,* 2007, *4*(11), 2495-2527.
[http://dx.doi.org/10.1002/cbdv.200790205] [PMID: 18027351]

[11]   Rana, A.C.; Gulliya, B. Chemistry and Pharmacology of Flavonoids- A Review. *Indian J. Pharm. Educ. Res.,* 2019, *53*(1), 8-20.
[http://dx.doi.org/10.5530/ijper.53.1.3]

[12]   Jash, S.K.; Brahmachari, G. Recent progress in the research of naturally occurring flavonoids: A look through. *Signpost Open Access J. Org. Biomol. Chem.,* 2013, *1*, 65-168.

[13]   Wang, T.Y.; Li, Q.; Bi, K.S. Bioactive flavonoids in medicinal plants: Structure, activity and biological fate. *Asian J. Pharm. Sci.,* 2018, *13*(1), 12-23.
[http://dx.doi.org/10.1016/j.ajps.2017.08.004] [PMID: 32104374]

[14]   Miki, K.; Nagai, T.; Suzuki, K.; Tsujimura, R.; Koyama, K.; Kinoshita, K.; Furuhata, K.; Yamada, H.; Takahashi, K. Anti-influenza virus activity of biflavonoids. *Bioorg. Med. Chem. Lett.,* 2007, *17*(3), 772-775.
[http://dx.doi.org/10.1016/j.bmcl.2006.10.075] [PMID: 17110111]

[15]   Agrawal, P.K. *Carbon-13 of Flavonoids*; Elsevier: New York, 1989, p. 564.

[16]   Jash, S.K.; Gorai, D.; Mandal, L.C.; Roy, R. Nuclear magnetic resonance spectroscopic behaviour of some selective natural flavonoids: A look through. *Mini Rev. Org. Chem.,* 2020, *17*(2), 185-196.
[http://dx.doi.org/10.2174/1570193X16666181224110603]

[17]   Carvalho, M.G.; Alves, C.C.F.; Silva, K.G.S.; Werle, A.A.; Eberlin, M.N. Luxenchalcone, a new bichalcone and other constituents from *Luxemburgia octandra. J. Braz. Chem. Soc.,* 2004, *15*, 146-149.
[http://dx.doi.org/10.1590/S0103-50532004000100023]

[18]   Drewes, S.E.; Hudson, N.A.; Bates, R.B.; Linz, G.S. The flavonoids: Advances in research since 1980. *Tetrahedron Lett.,* 1984, *25*, 105.
[http://dx.doi.org/10.1016/S0040-4039(01)91161-X]

[19]   Moreira, I.C.; Sobrinho, D.C.; de Carvalho, M.G.; Braz-Filho, R. Isoflavanone dimers hexaspermone A, B and C from *Ouratea hexasperma. Phytochemistry,* 1994, *35*, 1567-1572.
[http://dx.doi.org/10.1016/S0031-9422(00)86895-8]

[20]   Daniel, J.F. de S.; de Carvalho, M.G.; Cardoso, R.D.S.; Agra, M. de F.; Eberlin, M.N. Others flavonoids from *Ourtea hexasperma* (Ochnaceae). *J. Braz. Chem. Soc.,* **2005**, *16*, 634-638.
[http://dx.doi.org/10.1590/S0103-50532005000400022]

[21]   Miyaichi, Y.; Hanamitsu, E.; Kizu, H.; Tomimori, T. Studies on the constituents of Scutellaria species (XXII). Constituents of the roots of Scutellaria amabilis HARA. *Chem. Pharm. Bull. (Tokyo),* **2006**, *54*(4), 435-441.
[http://dx.doi.org/10.1248/cpb.54.435] [PMID: 16595941]

[22]   Ichino, C.; Kiyohara, H.; Soonthornchareonnon, N.; Chuakul, W.; Ishiyama, A.; Sekiguchi, H.; Namatame, M.; Otoguro, K.; Omura, S.; Yamada, H. Antimalarial activity of biflavonoids from *Ochna integerrima. Planta Med.,* **2006**, *72*(7), 611-614.
[http://dx.doi.org/10.1055/s-2006-931569] [PMID: 16732520]

[23]   Dhooghe, L.; Maregesi, S.; Mincheva, I.; Ferreira, D.; Marais, J.P.J.; Lemière, F.; Matheeussen, A.; Cos, P.; Maes, L.; Vlietinck, A.; Apers, S.; Pieters, L. Antiplasmodial activity of (I-3,II--)-biflavonoids and other constituents from *Ormocarpum kirkii. Phytochemistry,* **2010**, *71*(7), 785-791.
[http://dx.doi.org/10.1016/j.phytochem.2010.02.005] [PMID: 20189612]

[24]   Lee, C-W.; Choi, H-J.; Kim, H-S.; Kim, D-H.; Chang, I-S.; Moon, H.T.; Lee, S.Y.; Oh, W.K.; Woo, E.R. Biflavonoids isolated from *Selaginella tamariscina* regulate the expression of matrix metalloproteinase in human skin fibroblasts. *Bioorg. Med. Chem.,* **2008**, *16*(2), 732-738.
[http://dx.doi.org/10.1016/j.bmc.2007.10.036] [PMID: 18029185]

[25]   Nguyen, P-H.; Ji, D-J.; Han, Y-R.; Choi, J-S.; Rhyu, D-Y.; Min, B-S.; Woo, M-H. Selaginellin and biflavonoids as protein tyrosine phosphatase 1B inhibitors from *Selaginella tamariscina* and their glucose uptake stimulatory effects. *Bioorg. Med. Chem.,* **2015**, *23*(13), 3730-3737.
[http://dx.doi.org/10.1016/j.bmc.2015.04.007] [PMID: 25907369]

[26]   Zheng, J-X.; Zheng, Y.; Zhi, H.; Dai, Y.; Wang, N-L.; Fang, Y-X.; Du, Z-Y.; Zhang, K.; Li, M-M.; Wu, L-Y.; Fan, M. New 3′,8″-linked biflavonoids from Selaginella uncinata displaying protective effect against anoxia. *Molecules,* **2011**, *16*(8), 6206-6214.
[http://dx.doi.org/10.3390/molecules16086206] [PMID: 21788929]

[27]   Li, S.; Zhao, M.; Li, Y.; Sui, Y.; Yao, H.; Huang, L.; Lin, X. Preparative isolation of six anti-tumour biflavonoids from *Selaginella doederleinii* Hieron by high-speed counter-current chromatography. *Phytochem. Anal.,* **2014**, *25*(2), 127-133.
[http://dx.doi.org/10.1002/pca.2478] [PMID: 24115163]

[28]   Chen, B.; Wang, X.; Lin, D.; Xu, D.; Li, S.; Huang, J.; Weng, S.; Lin, Z.; Zheng, Y.; Yao, H.; Lin, X. Proliposomes for oral delivery of total biflavonoids extract from *Selaginella doederleinii*: formulation development, optimization, and *in vitro-in vivo* characterization. *Int. J. Nanomedicine,* **2019**, *14*, 6691-6706.
[http://dx.doi.org/10.2147/IJN.S214686] [PMID: 31692515]

[29]   Oliveira, M.C.; de Carvalho, M.G.; Grynberg, N.F.; Brioso, P.S. A biflavonoid from *Luxemburgia nobilis* as inhibitor of DNA topoisomerases. *Planta Med.,* **2005**, *71*(6), 561-563.
[http://dx.doi.org/10.1055/s-2005-864159] [PMID: 15971129]

[30]   Lee, N.Y.; Min, H.Y.; Lee, J.; Nam, J.W.; Lee, Y.J.; Han, A.R.; Wiryawan, A.; Suprapto, W.; Lee, S.K.; Seo, E.K. Identification of a new cytotoxic biflavanone from *Selaginella doederleinii. Chem. Pharm. Bull. (Tokyo),* **2008**, *56*(9), 1360-1361.
[http://dx.doi.org/10.1248/cpb.56.1360] [PMID: 18758121]

[31]   Liang, S.; Shen, Y-H.; Tian, J-M.; Feng, Y.; Xiong, Z.; Zhang, W-D. Five New Biflavonoids from *Daphne aurantiaca. Helv. Chim. Acta,* **2011**, *94*(7), 1239-1245.
[http://dx.doi.org/10.1002/hlca.201000382]

[32]   Cheng, K.T.; Hsu, F.L.; Chen, S.H.; Hsieh, P.K.; Huang, H.S.; Lee, C.K.; Lee, M.H. New constituent from *Podocarpus macrophyllus* var. macrophyllus shows anti-tyrosinase effect and regulates tyrosinase-related proteins and mRNA in human epidermal melanocytes. *Chem. Pharm. Bull. (Tokyo),*

2007, *55*(5), 757-761.
[http://dx.doi.org/10.1248/cpb.55.757] [PMID: 17473463]

[33]   Das, B.; Mahender, G.; Koteswara Rao, Y.; Prabhakar, A.; Jagadeesh, B. Biflavonoids from *Cycas beddomei*. *Chem. Pharm. Bull. (Tokyo)*, **2005**, *53*(1), 135-136.
[http://dx.doi.org/10.1248/cpb.53.135] [PMID: 15635250]

[34]   Yao, X.; Wang, N.; Fan, M.; Zheng, J.; Wu, L.; Liu, H.; Ding, A.; Gao, H.; Dai, Y. Application of flavone derivatives as antioxidation and anti-hypoxia drug or food and their preparation. *Faming Zhuanli Shenqing Gongkai Shuomingshu*, **2009**.

[35]   Xu, J.C.; Liu, X.Q.; Chen, K.L. A new biflavonoid from Selaginella labordei Hieron. ex *Christ. Chin. Chem. Lett.*, **2009**, *20*, 939-941.
[http://dx.doi.org/10.1016/j.cclet.2009.03.046]

[36]   Moawad, A.; Hetta, M.; Zjawiony, J.K.; Jacob, M.R.; Hifnawy, M.; Marais, J.P.J.; Ferreira, D. Phytochemical investigation of *Cycas circinalis* and *Cycas revoluta* leaflets: moderately active antibacterial biflavonoids. *Planta Med.*, **2010**, *76*(8), 796-802.
[http://dx.doi.org/10.1055/s-0029-1240743] [PMID: 20072955]

[37]   Kunert, O.; Swamy, R.C.; Kaiser, M.; Presser, A.; Buzzi, S. A.V.N.; Rao, A.; Schühly, W. Antiplasmodial and leishmanicidal activity of biflavonoids from Indian *Selaginella bryopteris*. *Phytochem. Lett.*, **2008**, *1*, 171-174.
[http://dx.doi.org/10.1016/j.phytol.2008.09.003]

[38]   Das, B.; Mahender, G.; Rao, Y.K.; Thirupathi, P. A new biflavonoid from *Cycas beddomei*. *Indian J. Chem.*, **2006**, *45B*, 1933-1935.

[39]   Reddy, B.A.K.; Reddy, N.P.; Gunasekar, D.; Blond, A.; Bodo, B. Biflavonoids from *Ochna lanceolata*. *Phytochem. Lett.*, **2008**, *1*, 27-30.
[http://dx.doi.org/10.1016/j.phytol.2007.12.005]

[40]   Han, A-R.; Lee, N-Y.; Nam, J-W.; Wiryawan, A.; Seo, E-K. Identification of a New Biflavonoid from *Selaginella doederleinii* Hieron. *Bull. Korean Chem. Soc.*, **2013**, *34*(10), 3147-3149.
[http://dx.doi.org/10.5012/bkcs.2013.34.10.3147]

[41]   Falcão, M.J.C.; Pouliquem, Y.B.M.; Lima, M.A.S.; Gramosa, N.V.; Costa-Lotufo, L.V.; Militão, G.C.; Pessoa, C.; de Moraes, M.O.; Silveira, E.R. Cytotoxic flavonoids from *Platymiscium floribundum*. *J. Nat. Prod.*, **2005**, *68*(3), 423-426.
[http://dx.doi.org/10.1021/np049854d] [PMID: 15787450]

[42]   Malafronte, N.; Vassallo, A.; Dal Piaz, F.; Bader, A.; Braca, A.; De Tommasi, N. Biflavonoids from *Daphne linearifolia* Hart. *Phytochem. Lett.*, **2012**, *5*, 621-625.
[http://dx.doi.org/10.1016/j.phytol.2012.06.008]

[43]   Liang, S.; Tang, J.; Shen, Y.H.; Jin, H.Z.; Tian, J.M.; Wu, Z.J.; Zhang, W.D.; Yan, S.K. Biflavonoids from *Daphne feddei* and their inhibitory activities against nitric oxide production. *Chem. Pharm. Bull. (Tokyo)*, **2008**, *56*(12), 1729-1731.
[http://dx.doi.org/10.1248/cpb.56.1729] [PMID: 19043248]

[44]   Chen, Y.G.; Yu, L.L.; Huang, R.; Liu, J.C.; Lv, Y.P.; Zhao, Y. 3"-hydroxyamentoflavone and its 7--methyl ether, two new biflavonoids from *Aristolochia contorta*. *Arch. Pharm. Res.*, **2005**, *28*(11), 1233-1235.
[http://dx.doi.org/10.1007/BF02978204] [PMID: 16350847]

[45]   Han, Q.B.; Lee, S.F.; Qiao, C.F.; He, Z.D.; Song, J.Z.; Sun, H.D.; Xu, H-X. Complete NMR assignments of the antibacterial biflavonoid GB1 from *Garcinia kola*. *Chem. Pharm. Bull. (Tokyo)*, **2005**, *53*(8), 1034-1036.
[http://dx.doi.org/10.1248/cpb.53.1034] [PMID: 16079543]

[46]   Zhao, C.C.; Shao, J.H.; Li, X.; Kang, X.D.; Zhang, Y.W.; Meng, D.L.; Li, N. Flavonoids from *Galium verum* L. *J. Asian Nat. Prod. Res.*, **2008**, *10*(7-8), 613-617.

[PMID: 18636371]

[47]   Pinto, M.E.F.; Da Silva, M.S.; Schindler, E.; Filho, J.M.B. El- Bacha, R.D.S.; Castello-Branco, M.V.S.; De Fatima Agra, M.; Tavares, J.F. 3′,8-biisokaempferide, a cytotoxic biflavonoid and other chemical constituents of nanuza Plicata (velloziaceae). *J. Braz. Chem. Soc.,* **2010**, *21*(10), 1819-1824. [http://dx.doi.org/10.1590/S0103-50532010001000005]

[48]   Howell, H.; Malan, E.; Brand, D.J.; Kamara, B.I.; Benuidenhoudt, B.C.B.; Marais, C.; Steenkamp, J.A. Two new promelacacinidin dimers, including a novel flavanone-flavanol dimer characterized by a unique C(3)-C(4) linkage, from the heartwood of *Acacia nigrescens. Chem. Nat. Compd.,* **2007**, *43*(5), 533-538. [http://dx.doi.org/10.1007/s10600-007-0184-0]

[49]   Chukwujekwu, J.C.; de Kock, C.A.; Smith, P.J.; van Heerden, F.R.; van Staden, J. Antiplasmodial and antibacterial activity of compounds isolated from *Ormocarpum trichocarpum. Planta Med.,* **2012**, *78*(17), 1857-1860. [http://dx.doi.org/10.1055/s-0032-1315386] [PMID: 23059633]

[50]   Shao, M.; Huang, X-J.; Liu, J-S.; Han, W-L.; Cai, H-B.; Tang, Q-F.; Fan, Q. A new cytotoxic biflavonoid from the rhizome of *Wikstroemia indica. Nat. Prod. Res.,* **2015**, •••, 1-6. [PMID: 26252201]

[51]   Kumar, N.; Singh, B.; Bhandari, P.; Gupta, A.P.; Uniyal, S.K.; Kaul, V.K. Biflavonoids from *Lonicera japonica. Phytochemistry,* **2005**, *66*(23), 2740-2744. [http://dx.doi.org/10.1016/j.phytochem.2005.10.002] [PMID: 16293275]

[52]   Pegnyemb, D.E.; Mbing, J.N.; de Théodore Atchadé, A.; Tih, R.G.; Sondengam, B.L.; Blond, A.; Bodo, B. Antimicrobial biflavonoids from the aerial parts of *Ouratea sulcata. Phytochemistry,* **2005**, *66*(16), 1922-1926. [http://dx.doi.org/10.1016/j.phytochem.2005.06.017] [PMID: 16083925]

[53]   Kamiya, K.; Satake, T. Chemical constituents of Baeckea frutescens leaves inhibit copper-induced low-density lipoprotein oxidation. *Fitoterapia,* **2010**, *81*(3), 185-189. [http://dx.doi.org/10.1016/j.fitote.2009.08.021] [PMID: 19699785]

[54]   Amang A Ngnoung, G.A. Nganso Ditchou Yves Oscar, Meli Lannang and Mala Opono M.T.G. New biflavonoid from the roots of *Allexis cauliflora* (Violaceae) and evaluation of antibacterial activities. *Int. J. Curr. Adv. Res.,* **2018**, *7*(9B), 15375-15378.

[55]   Rahman, M.M.; Gibbons, S.; Gray, A.I. Isoflavanones from Uraria picta and their antimicrobial activity. *Phytochemistry,* **2007**, *68*(12), 1692-1697. [http://dx.doi.org/10.1016/j.phytochem.2007.04.015] [PMID: 17540419]

[56]   Lee, M.K.; Lim, S.W.; Yang, H.; Sung, S.H.; Lee, H.S.; Park, M.J.; Kim, Y.C. Osteoblast differentiation stimulating activity of biflavonoids from Cephalotaxus koreana. *Bioorg. Med. Chem. Lett.,* **2006**, *16*(11), 2850-2854. [http://dx.doi.org/10.1016/j.bmcl.2006.03.018] [PMID: 16574412]

[57]   On, S.; Aminudin, N.; Ahmad, F.; Sirat, H.M.; Taher, M. Chemical Constituents from Stem Bark of *Garcinia prainiana* and Their Bioactivities. *Intern. J. Pharmacog. Phytochem. Res.,* **2016**, *8*(5), 756-760.

[58]   Huang, W-H.; Zhou, G-X.; Wang, G-C.; Chung, H.Y.; Ye, W-C.; Li, Y-L. A new biflavonoid with antiviral activity from the roots of *Wikstroemia indica. J. Asian Nat. Prod. Res.,* **2012**, *14*(4), 401-406. [http://dx.doi.org/10.1080/10286020.2011.653963] [PMID: 22375879]

[59]   Ndongo, J.T.; Shaaban, M.; Mbing, J.N.; Bikobo, D.N.; Atchadé, Ade.T.; Pegnyemb, D.E.; Laatsch, H. Phenolic dimers and an indole alkaloid from *Campylospermum flavum* (Ochnaceae). *Phytochemistry,* **2010**, *71*(16), 1872-1878. [http://dx.doi.org/10.1016/j.phytochem.2010.08.006] [PMID: 20822781]

[60]   Al-Shagdari, A.; Alarcón, A.B.; Cuesta-Rubio, O.; Piccinelli, A.L.; Rastrelli, L. Biflavonoids, main

constituents from *Garcinia bakeriana* leaves. *Nat. Prod. Commun.,* **2013**, *8*(9), 1237-1240.
[http://dx.doi.org/10.1177/1934578X1300800913] [PMID: 24273855]

[61]   Rodrigues, J.; Rinaldo, D.; dos Santos, L.C.; Vilegas, W. An unusual C6-C6" linked flavonoid from Miconia cabucu (Melastomataceae). *Phytochemistry,* **2007**, *68*(13), 1781-1784.
[http://dx.doi.org/10.1016/j.phytochem.2007.04.020] [PMID: 17540417]

[62]   Yamaguchi, L.F.; Vassão, D.G.; Kato, M.J.; Di Mascio, P. Biflavonoids from Brazilian pine *Araucaria angustifolia* as potentials protective agents against DNA damage and lipoperoxidation. *Phytochemistry,* **2005**, *66*(18), 2238-2247.
[http://dx.doi.org/10.1016/j.phytochem.2004.11.014] [PMID: 16153416]

[63]   Cao, C.M.; Peng, Y.; Xu, L.J.; Wang, Y.J.; Yang, J.S.; Xiao, P.G. Two flavonoid dimers from *Sarcandra hainanensis* (PEI) SWAMY et BAILEY. *Chem. Pharm. Bull. (Tokyo),* **2009**, *57*(7), 743-746.
[http://dx.doi.org/10.1248/cpb.57.743] [PMID: 19571424]

[64]   Song, S.; Li, Y.; Feng, Z.; Jiang, J.; Zhang, P. Hepatoprotective constituents from the roots and stems of *Erycibe hainanesis. J. Nat. Prod.,* **2010**, *73*(2), 177-184.
[http://dx.doi.org/10.1021/np900593q] [PMID: 20092289]

[65]   Feng, B.; Wang, T.; Zhang, Y.; Hua, H.; Jia, J.; Zhang, H.; Pei, Y.; Shi, L.; Wang, Y. Aldose Reductase Inhibitors from *Stellera chamaejasme. Pharm. Biol.,* **2005**, *43*(1), 12-14.
[http://dx.doi.org/10.1080/13880200590903246]

[66]   Njock, G.B.B.; Grougnet, R.; Efstathiou, A.; Smirlis, D.; Genta-Jouve, G.; Michel, S.; Mbing, J.N.; Kritsanida, M. A Nitrile Glucoside and Biflavones from the Leaves of *Campylospermum excavatum* (Ochnaceae). *Chem. Biodivers.,* **2017**, *14*(11), e1700241.
[http://dx.doi.org/10.1002/cbdv.201700241] [PMID: 28695668]

[67]   Siddiqui, J.A.; Swarnkar, G.; Sharan, K.; Chakravarti, B.; Sharma, G.; Rawat, P.; Kumar, M.; Khan, F.M.; Pierroz, D.; Maurya, R.; Chattopadhyay, N. 8,8"-Biapigeninyl stimulates osteoblast functions and inhibits osteoclast and adipocyte functions: Osteoprotective action of 8,8"-biapigeninyl in ovariectomized mice. *Mol. Cell. Endocrinol.,* **2010**, *323*(2), 256-267.
[http://dx.doi.org/10.1016/j.mce.2010.03.024] [PMID: 20380869]

[68]   Dinda, B.; Mohanta, B.C.; Arima, S.; Sato, N.; Harigaya, Y. Flavonoids from the Stem-bark of *Oroxylum indicum. Nat. Prod. Sci.,* **2007**, *13*, 190-194.

[69]   Dai, H-F.; Wang, H.; Liu, J.; Wu, J.; Mei, W-L. Two new biflavonoids from the stem of *Dracaena cambodiana. Chem. Nat. Compd.,* **2012**, *48*(3), 376-378.
[http://dx.doi.org/10.1007/s10600-012-0256-7]

[70]   Zhu, Y.; Zhang, P.; Yu, H.; Li, J.; Wang, M.W.; Zhao, W. Anti-Helicobacter pylori and thrombin inhibitory components from Chinese dragon's blood, *Dracaena cochinchinensis. J. Nat. Prod.,* **2007**, *70*(10), 1570-1577.
[http://dx.doi.org/10.1021/np070260v] [PMID: 17883259]

[71]   Yang, Q.Y.; Tian, X.Y.; Fang, W.S. Bioactive coumarins from *Boenninghausenia sessilicarpa. J. Asian Nat. Prod. Res.,* **2007**, *9*(1), 59-65.
[http://dx.doi.org/10.1080/10286020500382397] [PMID: 17365191]

[72]   Wada, S.; Hitomi, T.; Tokuda, H.; Tanaka, R. Anti-tumor-initiating effects of spiro-biflavonoids from *Abies sachalinensis. Chem. Biodivers.,* **2010**, *7*(9), 2303-2308.
[http://dx.doi.org/10.1002/cbdv.201000147] [PMID: 20860032]

[72a] Wada, S.; Hitomia, T.; Tokuda, H.; Tanaka, R. Phenolic Compounds Isolated from the Bark of *Abies sachalinensis. Helv. Chim. Acta,* **2009**, *92*, 1610-1620.
[http://dx.doi.org/10.1002/hlca.200900032]

[73]   Djova, S.V.; Nyegue, M.A.; Messi, A.N.; Afagnigni, A.D.; Etoa, F-X. Phenolic Compounds Isolated from the Bark of Abies sachalinensis. In: *Helv, Chim, Acta*; , **2019**; 92, pp. 1610-1620.

[http://dx.doi.org/10.1155/2019/8908343]

[74]   Svenningsen, A.B.; Madsen, K.D.; Liljefors, T.; Stafford, G.I.; van Staden, J.; Jäger, A.K. Biflavones from Rhus species with affinity for the GABA(A)/benzodiazepine receptor. *J. Ethnopharmacol.*, **2006**, *103*(2), 276-280.
[http://dx.doi.org/10.1016/j.jep.2005.08.012] [PMID: 16168585]

[75]   Ayoub, I.M.; Korinek, M.; Hwang, T-L.; Chen, B-H.; Chang, F-R.; El-Shazly, M.; Singab, A.N.B. Probing the Antiallergic and Anti-inflammatory Activity of Biflavonoids and Dihydroflavonols from *Dietes bicolor. J. Nat. Prod.*, **2018**, *81*(2), 243-253.
[http://dx.doi.org/10.1021/acs.jnatprod.7b00476] [PMID: 29381070]

[76]   Ito, T.; Yokota, R.; Watarai, T.; Mori, K.; Oyama, M.; Nagasawa, H.; Matsuda, H.; Iinuma, M. Isolation of six isoprenylated biflavonoids from the leaves of Garcinia subelliptica. *Chem. Pharm. Bull. (Tokyo)*, **2013**, *61*(5), 551-558.
[http://dx.doi.org/10.1248/cpb.c12-01057] [PMID: 23649198]

[77]   Fritz, D.; Venturi, C.R.; Cargnin, S.; Schripsema, J.; Roehe, P.M.; Montanha, J.A.; von Poser, G.L. Herpes virus inhibitory substances from *Hypericum connatum* Lam., a plant used in southern Brazil to treat oral lesions. *J. Ethnopharmacol.*, **2007**, *113*(3), 517-520.
[http://dx.doi.org/10.1016/j.jep.2007.07.013] [PMID: 17719731]

[78]   Cao, Y.; Tan, N.H.; Chen, J.J.; Zeng, G.Z.; Ma, Y.B.; Wu, Y.P.; Yan, H.; Yang, J.; Lu, L.F.; Wang, Q. Bioactive flavones and biflavones from Selaginella moellendorffii Hieron. *Fitoterapia*, **2010**, *81*(4), 253-258.
[http://dx.doi.org/10.1016/j.fitote.2009.09.007] [PMID: 19775597]

[79]   Jung, H.J.; Sung, W.S.; Yeo, S.H.; Kim, H.S.; Lee, I.S.; Woo, E.R.; Lee, D.G. Antifungal effect of amentoflavone derived from *Selaginella tamariscina. Arch. Pharm. Res.*, **2006**, *29*(9), 746-751.
[http://dx.doi.org/10.1007/BF02974074] [PMID: 17024847]

[80]   Park, S-Y.; Nguyen, P-H.; Kim, G.; Jang, S-N.; Lee, G-H.; Phuc, N.M.; Wu, Z.; Liu, K-H. Strong and Selective Inhibitory Effects of the Biflavonoid Selamariscina A against CYP2C8 and CYP2C9 Enzyme Activities in Human Liver Microsomes. *Pharmaceutics*, **2020**, *12*(4), 343.
[http://dx.doi.org/10.3390/pharmaceutics12040343] [PMID: 32290339]

[81]   Li, Y.-Y.; Lu, X.-Y.; Sun, J.-L.; Wang, Q.-Q.; Zhang, Y.-D.; Zhang, J.-B.; Fan, X.-H. Potential hepatic and renal toxicity induced by the biflavonoids from Ginkgo biloba. *Chin. J. Nat. Med.*, **2019**, *17*(9), 0672-0681.

[82]   Ogunwa, T.H. Insights into interaction profile and inhibitory potential of amentoflavone with α-glucosidase, tyrosinase and 15-lipoxygenase as validated therapeutic targets. *J. Syst. Biol. Proteome. Res.*, **2018**, *2*(1), 10-20.

[83]   Kim, A.R.; Jin, Q.; Jin, H.G.; Ko, H.J.; Woo, E.R. Phenolic compounds with IL-6 inhibitory activity from *Aster yomena. Arch. Pharm. Res.*, **2014**, *37*(7), 845-851.
[http://dx.doi.org/10.1007/s12272-013-0236-x] [PMID: 24014305]

[84]   Jia, B.X.; Zhou, Y.X.; Chen, X.Q.; Wang, X.B.; Yang, J.; Lai, M.X.; Wang, Q. Structure determination of baeckeins C and D from the roots of *Baeckea frutescens. Magn. Reson. Chem.*, **2011**, *49*(11), 757-761.
[http://dx.doi.org/10.1002/mrc.2803] [PMID: 22002464]

[85]   Jia, B.X.; Ren, F.X.; Jia, L.; Chen, X.Q.; Yang, J.; Wang, Q. Baeckein E, a new bioactive C-methylated biflavonoid from the roots of *Baeckea frutescens. Nat. Prod. Res.*, **2013**, *27*(22), 2069-2075.
[http://dx.doi.org/10.1080/14786419.2013.778852] [PMID: 23521216]

[86]   Lenta, B.N.; Tantangmo, F.; Devkota, K.P.; Wansi, J.D.; Chouna, J.R.; Soh, R.C.; Neumann, B.; Stammler, H-G.; Tsamo, E.; Sewald, N. Bioactive constituents of the stem bark of *Beilschmiedia zenkeri. J. Nat. Prod.*, **2009**, *72*(12), 2130-2134.
[http://dx.doi.org/10.1021/np900341f] [PMID: 19904919]

[87]   Freitas, A.M.; Almeida, M.T.R.; Andrighetti-Fröhner, C.R.; Cardozo, F.T.G.S.; Barardi, C.R.M.; Farias, M.R.; Simões, C.M.O. Antiviral activity-guided fractionation from Araucaria angustifolia leaves extract. *J. Ethnopharmacol.,* **2009**, *126*(3), 512-517.
[http://dx.doi.org/10.1016/j.jep.2009.09.005] [PMID: 19761825]

[88]   Kang, S.S.; Lee, J.Y.; Choi, Y.K.; Song, S.S.; Kim, J.S.; Jeon, S.J.; Han, Y.N.; Son, K.H.; Han, B.H. Neuroprotective effects of naturally occurring biflavonoids. *Bioorg. Med. Chem. Lett.,* **2005**, *15*(15), 3588-3591.
[http://dx.doi.org/10.1016/j.bmcl.2005.05.078] [PMID: 15978805]

[89]   Ryu, Y.B.; Jeong, H.J.; Kim, J.H.; Kim, Y.M. Park, Ji-Y.; Kim, D.; Naguyen, T.T. H.; Park, Su-Jin.; Chang, J.S.; Park, K.H.; Rho, Mun-Chual.; Lee, W.S. Biflavonoids from Torreya nucifera displaying SARS-CoV 3CL[pro] inhibition. *Bioorg. Med. Chem.,* **2010**, *18*, 7940-7947.
[http://dx.doi.org/10.1016/j.bmc.2010.09.035] [PMID: 20934345]

[90]   Ali, A.F.; Sangyong, K.; Shinichiro, K.; Hisako, S.; Hirofumi, S.; Yoshiki, K.; Yoshihisa, T. Biflavonoids from flowers of *Butea monosperma* (Lam.) TAUB. *Heterocycles,* **2011**, *83*(9), 2079-2089.
[http://dx.doi.org/10.3987/COM-11-12275]

[91]   Oliveira, R.F.; Camara, C.A.; de Agra, M.F.; Silva, T.M. Biflavonoids from the unripe fruits of *Clusia paralicola* and their antioxidant activity. *Nat. Prod. Commun.,* **2012**, *7*(12), 1597-1600.
[http://dx.doi.org/10.1177/1934578X1200701215] [PMID: 23413562]

[92]   Negi, N.; Ochi, A.; Kurosawa, M.; Ushijima, K.; Kitaguchi, Y.; Kusakabe, E.; Okasho, F.; Kimachi, T.; Teshima, N.; Ju-Ichi, M.; Abou-Douh, A.M.; Ito, C.; Furukawa, H. Two new dimeric coumarins isolated from Murraya exotica. *Chem. Pharm. Bull. (Tokyo),* **2005**, *53*(9), 1180-1182.
[http://dx.doi.org/10.1248/cpb.53.1180] [PMID: 16141593]

[93]   Stark, T.D.; Germann, D.; Balemba, O.B.; Wakamatsu, J.; Hofmann, T. New highly *in vitro* antioxidative 3,8″-linked biflav(an)ones and flavanone-C-glycosides from *Garcinia buchananii* stem bark. *J. Agric. Food Chem.,* **2013**, *61*, 12572-12581. [94] Stark, T.D.; Matsutomo, T.; Lösch, S.; Boakye, P.A.; Balemba, O.B.; Pasilis, S.P.; Hofmann, T. Isolation and structure elucidation of highly antioxidative 3,8″-linked biflavanones and flavanon-C glycosides from *Garcinia buchananii* bark. *J. Agric. Food Chem.,* **2012**, *60*, 2053-2062.
[http://dx.doi.org/10.1021/jf205175b] [PMID: 22250972]

[95]   Bahia, M.V.; dos Santos, J.B.; David, J.P.; David, J.M. Biflavonoids and other Phenolics from *Caesalpinia pyramidalis* (Fabaceae). *J. Braz. Chem. Soc.,* **2005**, *16*(6B), 1402-1405.
[http://dx.doi.org/10.1590/S0103-50532005000800017]

[96]   Manga, S.S.E.; Tih, A.E.; Ghogomu, R.T.; Blond, A.; Bodo, B. Biflavonoid constituents of *Campylospermum mannii. Biochem. Syst. Ecol.,* **2009**, *37*, 402-404.
[http://dx.doi.org/10.1016/j.bse.2009.04.002]

[97]   Zhang, R-R.; Lin, Z-X.; Lu, X-Y.; Xia, X.; Jiang, R-W.; Chen, Q-B. CGY-1, a biflavonoid isolated from *cardiocrinum giganteum* seeds, improves memory deficits by modulating the cholinergic system in scopolamine-treated mice. *Biomed. Pharmacother.,* **2019**, *111*, 496-502.
[http://dx.doi.org/10.1016/j.biopha.2018.12.100] [PMID: 30594789]

[98]   Asada, Y.; Sukemori, A.; Watanabe, T.; Malla, K.J.; Yoshikawa, T.; Li, W.; Kuang, X.; Koike, K.; Chen, C-H.; Akiyama, T.; Qian, K.; Nakagawa-Goto, K.; Morris-Natschke, S.L.; Lu, Y.; Lee, K-H. Isolation, structure determination, and anti-HIV evaluation of tigliane-type diterpenes and biflavonoid from *Stellera chamaejasme. J. Nat. Prod.,* **2013**, *76*(5), 852-857.
[http://dx.doi.org/10.1021/np300815t] [PMID: 23611151]

[99]   Zhang, C.; Zhou, S-S.; Feng, L-Y.; Zhang, D-Y.; Lin, N-M.; Zhang, L-H.; Pan, J-P.; Wang, J.B.; Li, J. *In vitro* anti-cancer activity of chamaejasmenin B and neochamaejasmin C isolated from the root of *Stellera chamaejasme* L. *Acta Pharmacol. Sin.,* **2013**, *34*(2), 262-270.
[http://dx.doi.org/10.1038/aps.2012.158] [PMID: 23222270]

[100]   Wang, Z.-X.; Cheng, M-C.; Zhang, X.-Z.; Hong, Z.-L.; Gao, M-Z.; Kan, X-X.; Li, Q.; Wang, Y-J.; Zhu, X.-X.; Xiao, H-B. Cytotoxic biflavones from *Stellera chamaejasme. Fitoterapia*, **2014**, *99*, 334-340.
        [http://dx.doi.org/10.1016/j.fitote.2014.10.002] [PMID: 25313014]

[101]   Zhao, Y.; Wu, F.; Wang, Y.; Chen, S.; Han, G.; Liu, M.; Jin, D. Inhibitory action of chamaejasmin A against human HEP-2 epithelial cells: effect on tubulin protein. *Mol. Biol. Rep.*, **2012**, *39*(12), 11105-11112.
        [http://dx.doi.org/10.1007/s11033-012-2016-y] [PMID: 23053997]

[102]   Zhou, G.X.; Jiang, R.W.; Cheng, Y.; Ye, W.C.; Shi, J.G.; Gong, N.B.; Lu, Y. Daphnogirins A and B, two biflavones from *Daphne giraldii. Chem. Pharm. Bull. (Tokyo)*, **2007**, *55*(9), 1287-1290.
        [http://dx.doi.org/10.1248/cpb.55.1287] [PMID: 17827749]

[103]   Awadh, M.M.; Tarus, P.K.; Onani, M.O.; Machocho, A.K.; Hassanali, A. Biflavonoids from an Ethno-Medicinal Plant Ochna holtzii Gilg. *Nat. Prod. Chem. Res.*, **2014**, *2*, 6.

[104]   Chatsumpun, N.; Sritularak, B.; Likhitwitayawuid, K. New Biflavonoids with α-Glucosidase and Pancreatic Lipase Inhibitory Activities from *Boesenbergia rotunda. Molecules*, **2017**, *22*(11), 1862.
        [http://dx.doi.org/10.3390/molecules22111862] [PMID: 29084164]

[105]   Mbwambo, Z.H.; Kapingu, M.C.; Moshi, M.J.; Machumi, F.; Apers, S.; Cos, P.; Ferreira, D.; Marais, J.P.J.; Vanden Berghe, D.; Maes, L.; Vlietinck, A.; Pieters, L. Antiparasitic activity of some xanthones and biflavonoids from the root bark of Garcinia livingstonei. *J. Nat. Prod.*, **2006**, *69*(3), 369-372.
        [http://dx.doi.org/10.1021/np050406v] [PMID: 16562837]

[106]   Castardo, J.C.; Prudente, A.S.; Ferreira, J.; Guimarães, C.L.; Monache, F.D.; Filho, V.C.; Otuki, M.F.; Cabrini, D.A. Anti-inflammatory effects of hydroalcoholic extract and two biflavonoids from *Garcinia gardneriana* leaves in mouse paw oedema. *J. Ethnopharmacol.*, **2008**, *118*(3), 405-411.
        [http://dx.doi.org/10.1016/j.jep.2008.05.002] [PMID: 18555627]

[107]   Messi, B.B.; Ndjoko-Ioset, K.; Hertlein-Amslinger, B.; Lannang, A.M.; Nkengfack, A.E.; Wolfender, J.L.; Hostettmann, K.; Bringmann, G. Preussianone, a new flavanone-chromone biflavonoid from *Garcinia preussii* Engl. *Molecules*, **2012**, *17*(5), 6114-6125.
        [http://dx.doi.org/10.3390/molecules17056114] [PMID: 22614864]

[108]   Okunji, C.; Komarnytsky, S.; Fear, G.; Poulev, A.; Ribnicky, D.M.; Awachie, P.I.; Ito, Y.; Raskin, I. Preparative isolation and identification of tyrosinase inhibitors from the seeds of Garcinia kola by high-speed counter-current chromatography. *J. Chromatogr. A*, **2007**, *1151*(1-2), 45-50.
        [http://dx.doi.org/10.1016/j.chroma.2007.02.085] [PMID: 17367799]

[109]   Campos, P.M.; Prudente, A.S.; Horinouchi, C.D.S.; Cechinel-Filho, V.; Fávero, G.M.; Cabrini, D.A.; Otuki, M.F. Inhibitory effect of GB-2a (I3-naringenin-II8-eriodictyol) on melanogenesis. *J. Ethnoph.*, **2015**, *174*, 224-229.
        [http://dx.doi.org/10.1016/j.jep.2015.08.015] [PMID: 26297636]

[110]   Recalde-Gil, A.M.; Klein-Júnior, L.; Salton, J.; Bordignon, S.; Cechinel-Filho, V.; Matté, C.; Henriques, A. Aromatase (CYP19) inhibition by biflavonoids obtained from the branches of *Garcinia gardneriana* (Clusiaceae). *Z. Naturforsch. C J. Biosci.*, **2019**, *74*(9-10), 279-282, 279-282.
        [http://dx.doi.org/10.1515/znc-2019-0036] [PMID: 31393836]

[111]   Stark, T.D.; Lösch, S.; Salger, M.; Balemba, O.B.; Wakamatsu, J.; Frank, O.; Hofmann, T. A new NMR approach for structure determination of thermally unstable biflavanones and application to phytochemicals from *Garcinia buchananii. Magn. Reson. Chem.*, **2015**, *53*(10), 813-820.
        [http://dx.doi.org/10.1002/mrc.4269] [PMID: 26195084]

[112]   Stark, T.D.; Lösch, S.; Frank, O.; Balemba, O.B.; Hofmann, T. Purification procedure for (2R,3S,2"R,3"R)-manniflavanone and its minor (2R,3S,2"S,3"S)- isomer from *Garcinia buchananii* stem bark extract. *Eur. Food Res. Technol.*, **2015**, *240*, 1075-1080.
        [http://dx.doi.org/10.1007/s00217-014-2411-9]

[113]   Huang, W.; Zhang, X.; Wang, Y.; Ye, W.; Ooi, V.E.; Chung, H.Y.; Li, Y. Antiviral biflavonoids from

Radix Wikstroemiae (Liaogewanggen). *Chin. Med.,* **2010**, *5*, 23.
[http://dx.doi.org/10.1186/1749-8546-5-23] [PMID: 20565950]

[114] Pawellek, A.; Ryder, U.; Tammsalu, T.; King, L.J.; Kreinin, H.; Ly, T.; Hay, R.T.; Hartley, R.C.; Lamond, A.I. Characterisation of the biflavonoid hinokiflavone as a pre-mRNA splicing modulator that inhibits SENP. *eLife,* **2017**, *6*, e27402.
[http://dx.doi.org/10.7554/eLife.27402] [PMID: 28884683]

[115] Yeh, P.H.; Shieh, Y.D.; Hsu, L.C.; Kuo, L.M.; Lin, J.H.; Liaw, C.C.; Kuo, Y.H. Naturally occurring cytotoxic [3′→8″]-biflavonoids from *Podocarpus nakaii. J. Tradit. Complement. Med.,* **2012**, *2*(3), 220-226.
[http://dx.doi.org/10.1016/S2225-4110(16)30103-1] [PMID: 24716136]

[116] Jalil, J.; Jantan, I.; Ghani, A.A.; Murad, S. Platelet-activating factor (PAF) antagonistic activity of a new biflavonoid from *Garcinia nervosa* var. pubescens King. *Molecules,* **2012**, *17*(9), 10893-10901.
[http://dx.doi.org/10.3390/molecules170910893] [PMID: 22964504]

[117] Sasaki, H.; Miki, K.; Kinoshita, K.; Koyama, K.; Juliawaty, L.D.; Achmad, S.A.; Hakim, E.H.; Kaneda, M.; Takahashi, K. β-Secretase (BACE-1) inhibitory effect of biflavonoids. *Bioorg. Med. Chem. Lett.,* **2010**, *20*(15), 4558-4560.
[http://dx.doi.org/10.1016/j.bmcl.2010.06.021] [PMID: 20598535]

[118] Tsalikis, J.; Abdel-Nour, M.; Farahvash, A.; Sorbara, M.T.; Poon, S.; Philpott, D.J.; Girardin, S.E. Isoginkgetin, a natural biflavonoid proteasome inhibitor, sensitizes cancer cells to apoptosis *via* disruption of lysosomal homeostasis and impaired protein clearance. *Mol. Cell. Biol.,* **2019**, *39*(10), e00489-e18.
[http://dx.doi.org/10.1128/MCB.00489-18] [PMID: 30910794]

[119] Shen, G.; Van Kiem, P.; Cai, X.F.; Li, G.; Dat, N.T.; Choi, Y.A.; Lee, Y.M.; Park, Y.K.; Kim, Y.H. Solanoflavone, a new biflavonol glycoside from *Solanum melongena*: seeking for anti-inflammatory components. *Arch. Pharm. Res.,* **2005**, *28*(6), 657-659.
[http://dx.doi.org/10.1007/BF02969354] [PMID: 16042073]

[120] Yang, G.; Chen, D. Biflavanones, flavonoids, and coumarins from the roots of Stellera chamaejasme and their antiviral effect on hepatitis B virus. *Chem. Biodivers.,* **2008**, *5*(7), 1419-1424.
[http://dx.doi.org/10.1002/cbdv.200890130] [PMID: 18649308]

[121] Adaramoye, O.A.; Awogbindin, I.; Okusaga, J.O. Effect of kolaviron, a biflavonoid complex from Garcinia kola seeds, on ethanol-induced oxidative stress in liver of adult wistar rats. *J. Med. Food,* **2009**, *12*(3), 584-590.
[http://dx.doi.org/10.1089/jmf.2008.0138] [PMID: 19627207]

[122] Farombi, E.O.; Abarikwu, S.O.; Adedara, I.A.; Oyeyemi, M.O. Curcumin and kolaviron ameliorate di-n-butylphthalate-induced testicular damage in rats. *Basic Clin. Pharmacol. Toxicol.,* **2007**, *100*(1), 43-48.
[http://dx.doi.org/10.1111/j.1742-7843.2007.00005.x] [PMID: 17214610]

[123] Oluwatosin, A.; Tolulope, A.; Ayokulehin, K.; Patricia, O.; Aderemi, K.; Catherine, F.; Olusegun, A. Antimalarial potential of kolaviron, a biflavonoid from Garcinia kola seeds, against Plasmodium berghei infection in Swiss albino mice. *Asian Pac. J. Trop. Med.,* **2014**, *7*(2), 97-104.
[http://dx.doi.org/10.1016/S1995-7645(14)60003-1] [PMID: 24461521]

[124] Sisein, E.A.; Ayibaene, F-O.; Ayakeme, T.; Ebizimor, W.; Diepreye, E.; Marcellinus, A.E. Inhibitory Effect of a Biflavonoid Antioxidant (Kolaviron) on Benzoyl Peroxide Induced Free Radical Generation in Rat Skin. *Pharm. Chem. J.,* **2016**, *3*(4), 144-149.

[125] Ishola, I.O.; Adamson, F.M.; Adeyemi, O.O. Ameliorative effect of kolaviron, a biflavonoid complex from *Garcinia kola* seeds against scopolamine-induced memory impairment in rats: role of antioxidant defense system. *Metab. Brain Dis.,* **2017**, *32*(1), 235-245.
[http://dx.doi.org/10.1007/s11011-016-9902-2] [PMID: 27631100]

[126] Kehinde, A.; Adefisan, A.; Adebayo, O.; Adaramoye, O. Biflavonoid fraction from *Garcinia kola* seed

ameliorates hormonal imbalance and testicular oxidative damage by anti-tuberculosis drugs in Wistar rats. *J. Basic Clin. Physiol. Pharmacol.,* **2016**, *27*(4), 393-401.
[http://dx.doi.org/10.1515/jbcpp-2015-0063] [PMID: 27089414]

[127] Ren, Y.; Lantvit, D.D.; Carcache de Blanco, E.J.; Kardono, L.B.S.; Riswan, S. Chai, Heebyung.; Cottrell, Charles, E.; Farnsworth, N.R.; Swanson, S. M.; Ding, Yuanqing.; Li, Xing-Cong.; Marais, J.P.J.; Ferreira, Daneel.; Kinghorn, A.D. Proteasomeinhibitory and cytotoxic constituents of *Garcinia lateriflora*: Absolute configuration of caged xanthones. *Tetrahedron,* **2010**, *66*(29), 5311-5320.
[http://dx.doi.org/10.1016/j.tet.2010.05.010] [PMID: 20730041]

[128] Navarat, T.; Pyne, S.G.; Prawat, U.; Tuntiwachwuttikul, P. Isolation of linobiflavonoid, a novel biflavonoid from *Linostoma pauciflorum* Griff. *Phytochem. Lett.,* **2011**, *4*, 383-385.
[http://dx.doi.org/10.1016/j.phytol.2011.08.009]

[129] Tih, A.E.; Ghogomu, R.T.; Sondengam, B.L.; Caux, C.; Bodo, B. Minor biflavonoids from Lophira alata leaves. *J. Nat. Prod.,* **2006**, *69*(8), 1206-1208.
[http://dx.doi.org/10.1021/np050169w] [PMID: 16933877]

[130] Cane, H.P.C.A.; Saidi, N.; Yahya, M.; Darusman, D.; Erlidawati, E.; Safrida, S.; Musman, M. Macrophylloflavone: A New Biflavonoid from *Garcinia macrophylla* Mart. (Clusiaceae) for Antibacterial, Antioxidant, and Anti-Type 2 Diabetes Mellitus Activities. *ScientificWorldJournal,* **2020**, *2020*, 2983129.
[http://dx.doi.org/10.1155/2020/2983129] [PMID: 32454801]

[131] Fossen, T.; Rayyan, S.; Holmberg, M.H.; Nimtz, M.; Andersen, O.M. Covalent anthocyanin-flavone dimer from leaves of *Oxalis triangularis. Phytochemistry,* **2007**, *68*(5), 652-662.
[http://dx.doi.org/10.1016/j.phytochem.2006.10.030] [PMID: 17182069]

[132] Balemba, O.B.; Stark, T.D.; Lösch, S.; Patterson, S.; McMillan, J.S.; Mawe, G.M.; Hofmann, T. (2R,3S,2″ R,3″R)-manniflavanone, a new gastrointestinal smooth muscle L-type calcium channel inhibitor, which underlies the spasmolytic properties of *Garcinia buchananii* stem bark extract. *J. Smooth Muscle Res.,* **2014**, *50*, 48-65.
[http://dx.doi.org/10.1540/jsmr.50.48] [PMID: 26081368]

[133] Gontijo, V.S.; de Souza, T.C.; Rosa, I.A.; Soares, M.G.; da Silva, M.A.; Vilegas, W.; Viegas, C.; Dos Santos, M.H. Isolation and evaluation of the antioxidant activity of phenolic constituents of the *Garcinia brasiliensis* epicarp. *Food Chem.,* **2012**, *132*(3), 1230-1235.
[http://dx.doi.org/10.1016/j.foodchem.2011.10.110] [PMID: 29243605]

[134] Stark, T.D.; Lösch, S.; Wakamatsu, J.; Balemba, O.B.; Frank, O.; Hofmann, T. UPLC-ESI-TOF MS-based metabolite profiling of the antioxidative food supplement *Garcinia buchananii. J. Agric. Food Chem.,* **2015**, *63*(32), 7169-7179.
[http://dx.doi.org/10.1021/acs.jafc.5b02544] [PMID: 26226176]

[135] Hu, X.; Wu, J-W.; Wang, M.; Yu, M-H.; Zhao, Q-S.; Wang, H-Y.; Hou, A-J. 2-Arylbenzofuran, flavonoid, and tyrosinase inhibitory constituents of *Morus yunnanensis. J. Nat. Prod.,* **2012**, *75*(1), 82-87.
[http://dx.doi.org/10.1021/np2007318] [PMID: 22165973]

[136] Saied, S.; Nizami, S.S.; Anis, I. Two new coumarins from *Murraya paniculata. J. Asian Nat. Prod. Res.,* **2008**, *10*(5-6), 515-519.
[http://dx.doi.org/10.1080/10286020801967292] [PMID: 18470803]

[137] Pan, L.; Hu, H.; Wang, X.; Yu, L.; Jiang, H.; Chen, J.; Lou, Y.; Zeng, S. Inhibitory effects of neochamaejasmin B on P-glycoprotein in MDCK-hMDR1 cells and molecular docking of NCB binding in P-glycoprotein. *Molecules,* **2015**, *20*(2), 2931-2948.
[http://dx.doi.org/10.3390/molecules20022931] [PMID: 25679052]

[138] Moon, T.C.; Hwang, H.S.; Quan, Z.; Son, K.H.; Kim, C.H.; Kim, H.P.; Kang, S.S.; Son, J.K.; Chang, H.W. Ochnaflavone, naturally occurring biflavonoid, inhibits phospholipase A_2 dependent phosphatidylethanolamine degradation in a CCl_4-induced rat liver microsome. *Biol. Pharm. Bull.,*

2006, *29*(12), 2359-2361.
[http://dx.doi.org/10.1248/bpb.29.2359] [PMID: 17142963]

[139] Son, M.J.; Moon, T.C.; Lee, E.K.; Son, K.H.; Kim, H.P.; Kang, S.S.; Son, J.K.; Lee, S.H.; Chang, H.W. Naturally occurring biflavonoid, ochnaflavone, inhibits cyclooxygenases-2 and 5-lipoxygenase in mouse bone marrow-derived mast cells. *Arch. Pharm. Res.*, **2006**, *29*(4), 282-286.
[http://dx.doi.org/10.1007/BF02968571] [PMID: 16681032]

[140] Kang, Y-J.; Min, H-Y.; Hong, J-Y.; Kim, Y.S.; Kang, S.S.; Lee, S.K. Ochnaflavone, a Natural Biflavonoid, Induces Cell Cycle Arrest and Apoptosis in HCT-15 Human Colon Cancer Cells. *Biomol. Ther. (Seoul)*, **2009**, *17*(3), 282-287.
[http://dx.doi.org/10.4062/biomolther.2009.17.3.282]

[141] Lee, J.H. Involvement of T-cell immunoregulation by ochnaflavone in therapeutic effect on fungal arthritis due to *Candida albicans. Arch. Pharm. Res.*, **2011**, *34*(7), 1209-1217.
[http://dx.doi.org/10.1007/s12272-011-0720-0] [PMID: 21811929]

[142] Makhafola, T.J.; Samuel, B.B.; Elgorashi, E.E.; Eloff, J.N. Ochnaflavone and ochnaflavone 7--methyl ether two antibacterial biflavonoids from *Ochna pretoriensis* (Ochnaceae). *Nat. Prod. Commun.*, **2012**, *7*(12), 1601-1604.
[http://dx.doi.org/10.1177/1934578X1200701216] [PMID: 23413563]

[143] Xiao, S.; Mu, Z-Q.; Cheng, C-R.; Ding, J. Three new biflavonoids from the branches and leaves of *Cephalotaxus oliveri* and their antioxidant activity. *Nat. Prod. Res.*, **2018**, •••, 1-7.
[PMID: 29544363]

[144] Ngo Mbing, J.; Enguehard-Gueiffier, C.; Atchadé, Ade.T.; Allouchi, H.; Gangoué-Piéboji, J.; Mbafor, J.T.; Tih, R.G.; Pothier, J.; Pegnyemb, D.E.; Gueiffier, A. Two biflavonoids from *Ouratea nigroviolacea. Phytochemistry*, **2006**, *67*(24), 2666-2670.
[http://dx.doi.org/10.1016/j.phytochem.2006.07.027] [PMID: 16950483]

[145] Liu, Y.; Kelsang, N.; Lu, J.; Zhang, Y.; Liang, H.; Tu, P.; Kong, D.; Zhang, Q.; Oxytrodiflavanone, A.; Oxytrochalcoflavanones, A. Oxytrodiflavanone A and Oxytrochalcoflavanones A,B: New Biflavonoids from *Oxytropis chiliophylla. Molecules*, **2019**, *24*(8), 1468.
[http://dx.doi.org/10.3390/molecules24081468] [PMID: 31013944]

[146] Jia, C.; Han, T.; Xu, J.; Li, S.; Sun, Y.; Li, D.; Li, Z.; Hua, H. A new biflavonoid and a new triterpene from the leaves of *Garcinia paucinervis* and their biological activities. *J. Nat. Med.*, **2017**, *71*(4), 642-649.
[http://dx.doi.org/10.1007/s11418-017-1092-7] [PMID: 28550652]

[147] Yao, G.M.; Ding, Y.; Zuo, J.P.; Wang, H.B.; Wang, Y.B.; Ding, B.Y.; Chiu, P.; Qin, G.W. Dihydrochalcones from the leaves of *Pieris japonica. J. Nat. Prod.*, **2005**, *68*(3), 392-396.
[http://dx.doi.org/10.1021/np049698a] [PMID: 15787442]

[148] Jaitak, V.; Sharma, K.; Kalia, K.; Kumar, N.; Singh, H.P.; Kaul, V.K.; Singh, B. Antioxidant activity of Potentilla fulgens: An alpine plant of western Himalaya. *J. Food Compos. Anal.*, **2010**, *23*, 142-147.
[http://dx.doi.org/10.1016/j.jfca.2009.02.013]

[149] Stark, T.D.; Salger, M.; Frank, O.; Balemba, O.B.; Wakamatsu, J.; Hofmann, T. Antioxidative compounds from *Garcinia buchananii* stem bark. *J. Nat. Prod.*, **2015**, *78*(2), 234-240.
[http://dx.doi.org/10.1021/np5007873] [PMID: 25625705]

[150] Mohammadi, M.; Yousefi, M.; Habibi, Z.; Shafiee, A. Two new coumarins from the chloroform extract of *Angelica urumiensis* from Iran. *Chem. Pharm. Bull. (Tokyo)*, **2010**, *58*(4), 546-548.
[http://dx.doi.org/10.1248/cpb.58.546] [PMID: 20410639]

[151] Kamara, B.I.; Manong, D.T.L.; Brandt, E.V. Isolation and synthesis of a dimeric dihydrochalcone from *Agapanthus africanus. Phytochemistry*, **2005**, *66*(10), 1126-1132.
[http://dx.doi.org/10.1016/j.phytochem.2005.04.007] [PMID: 15907963]

[152] Machado, M.B.; Lopes, L.M.X. Chalcone-flavone tetramer and biflavones from *Aristolochia ridicula*.

Phytochemistry, **2005**, *66*(6), 669-674.
[http://dx.doi.org/10.1016/j.phytochem.2005.01.016] [PMID: 15771888]

[153] Machado, M.B.; Lopes, L.M.X. Tetraflavonoid and biflavonoids from *Aristolochia ridicula.* *Phytochemistry,* **2008**, *69*(18), 3095-3102.
[http://dx.doi.org/10.1016/j.phytochem.2008.04.025] [PMID: 18561961]

[154] Wang, L.Y.; Unehara, T.; Kitanaka, S. Anti-inflammatory activity of new guaiane type sesquiterpene from *Wikstroemia indica. Chem. Pharm. Bull. (Tokyo),* **2005**, *53*(1), 137-139.
[http://dx.doi.org/10.1248/cpb.53.137] [PMID: 15635251]

[155] Li, J.; Lu, L.Y.; Zeng, L.H.; Zhang, C.; Hu, J.L.; Li, X.R.; Sikokianin, D. Sikokianin D, a new C-3/- -3"-biflavanone from the roots of Wikstroemia indica. *Molecules,* **2012**, *17*(7), 7792-7797.
[http://dx.doi.org/10.3390/molecules17077792] [PMID: 22735781]

[156] Yan, H.W.; Zhu, H.; Yuan, X.; Yang, Y.N.; Feng, Z.M.; Jiang, J.S.; Zhang, P.C. Eight new biflavonoids with lavandulyl units from the roots of *Sophora flavescens* and their inhibitory effect on PTP1B. *Bioorg. Chem.,* **2019**, *86*, 679-685.
[http://dx.doi.org/10.1016/j.bioorg.2019.01.058] [PMID: 30831529]

[157] Adjapmoh, M.F.E.; Toze, F.A.A.; Songue, J.L.; Langat, M.K.; Kapche, G.D.W.F.; Hameed, A.; Lateef, M.; Shaiq, M.A.; Mbaze, L.M.; Wansi, J.D.; Kamdem, A.F.W. A New Ceramide and Biflavonoid from the Leaves of *Parinari hypochrysea* (Chrysobalanaceae). *Nat. Prod. Commun.,* **2016**, *11*(5), 615-620.
[http://dx.doi.org/10.1177/1934578X1601100515] [PMID: 27319132]

[158] Arimboor, R.; Rangan, M.; Aravind, S.G.; Arumughan, C. Tetrahydroamentoflavone (THA) from *Semecarpus anacardium* as apotent inhibitor of xanthine oxidase. *J. Ethnoph.,* **2011**, *133*, 117-112.
[http://dx.doi.org/10.1016/j.jep.2010.10.027]

[159] Zheng, J.X.; Wang, N.L.; Liu, H.W.; Chen, H.F.; Li, M.M.; Wu, L.Y.; Fan, M.; Yao, X.S. Four new biflavonoids from *Selaginella uncinata* and their anti-anoxic effect. *J. Asian Nat. Prod. Res.,* **2008**, *10*(9-10), 945-952.
[http://dx.doi.org/10.1080/10286020802181166] [PMID: 19003613]

[160] Chen, L-Y.; Chen, I-S.; Peng, C-F. Structural elucidation and bioactivity of biflavonoids from the stems of *Wikstroemia taiwanensis. Int. J. Mol. Sci.,* **2012**, *13*(1), 1029-1038.
[http://dx.doi.org/10.3390/ijms13011029] [PMID: 22312302]

[161] Alimova, D.F.; Kuliev, Z.A.; Nishanbaev, S.Z.; Vdovin, A.D.; Abdullaev, N.D.; Aripova, S.F. New oligomeric proanthocyanidins from *Alhagi pseudalhagi. Chem. Nat. Compd.,* **2010**, *46*, 352-356.
[http://dx.doi.org/10.1007/s10600-010-9615-4]

[162] Lin, H-C.; Lee, S-S. Proanthocyanidins from the leaves of *Machilus philippinensis. J. Nat. Prod.,* **2010**, *73*(8), 1375-1380.
[http://dx.doi.org/10.1021/np1002274] [PMID: 20568785]

[163] Ndoile, M.M.; van Heerden, F.R. Total synthesis of ochnaflavone. *Beilstein J. Org. Chem.,* **2013**, *9*, 1346-1351.
[http://dx.doi.org/10.3762/bjoc.9.152] [PMID: 23946830]

[164] Sum, T.J.; Sum, T.H.; Galloway, W.R.J.D.; Twigg, D.G.; Ciardiello, J.J.; Spring, D.R. Synthesis of structurally diverse bioflavonoids. *Tetrahedron,* **2018**, *74*, 5089-5101.
[http://dx.doi.org/10.1016/j.tet.2018.05.003]

[165] Sum, T.H.; Sum, T.J.; Collins, S.; Galloway, W.R.J.D.; Twigg, D.G.; Hollfelder, F.; Spring, D.R. Divergent synthesis of biflavonoids yields novel inhibitors of the aggregation of amyloid β (1-42). *Org. Biomol. Chem.,* **2017**, *15*(21), 4554-4570.
[http://dx.doi.org/10.1039/C7OB00804J] [PMID: 28513756]

[166] Mathai, K.P.; Sethna, S. Chromones and Flavones, Part 5. Synthesis of Some 3',3'-and 6,6'- Biflavonyls. *J. Indian Chem. Soc.,* **1964**, *41*, 347-351.

[167] Lin, G-Q.; Zhong, M. The first enantioselec tive synthesis of optically pure (*R*)- and (*S*)-5,5-
-dihydroxy-4′,4‴,7,7″-tetramethoxy-8,8″-biflavone and the reconfirmation of their absolute
configuration. *Tetrahedron Lett.,* **1997**, *38*, 1087-1090.
[http://dx.doi.org/10.1016/S0040-4039(96)02475-6]

[168] Chen, F.C.; Lin, Y-M.; Huang, S-K.; Ueng, T. Synthesis of Hexa-*O*-methyl-6,8″-binaringenin.
Heterocycles, **1976**, *4*, 1913-1915.
[http://dx.doi.org/10.3987/R-1976-12-1913]

[169] Echavarren, A.M.; Stille, J.K. Palladium-catalyzed coupling of aryl triflates with organostannanes. *J.
Am. Chem. Soc.,* **1987**, *109*, 5478-5486.
[http://dx.doi.org/10.1021/ja00252a029]

[170] Muller, D.; Fleury, J.P. A new strategy for the synthesis of biflavonoids *via* arylboronic acids.
Tetrahedron Lett., **1991**, *32*, 2229-2232.
[http://dx.doi.org/10.1016/S0040-4039(00)79688-2]

[171] Okigawa, M.K.; Nobusuke, ; Aqil, M.; Rahman, W. Ochnaflavone and its derivatives: a new series of
diflavonyl ethers from Ochna squarrosa Linn. *J. Chem. Soc., Perk. Trans. 1,* **1976**, *5*, 580-583.

[172] Zembower, D.E.; Zhang, H. Total Synthesis of Robustaflavone, a Potential Anti-Hepatitis B Agent. *J.
Org. Chem.,* **1998**, *63*, 9300-9305.
[http://dx.doi.org/10.1021/jo981186b]

[173] Molyneux, R.J.; Waiss, A.C., Jr; Haddon, W.F. Oxidative coupling of apigenin. *Tetrahedron,* **1970**,
26, 1409-1416.
[http://dx.doi.org/10.1016/S0040-4020(01)92970-9]

[174] Nakazawa, K. Syntheses of Ring-substituted Flavonoids and Allied Compounds. XI. Synthesis of
Hinokiflavone. *Chem. Pharm. Bull. (Tokyo),* **1968**, *16*, 2503-2511.
[http://dx.doi.org/10.1248/cpb.16.2503]

[175] Chen, A-H.; Cheng, C-Y.; Chen, C-W. Synthesis of 2,2′-Biflavanones from Flavone *via* Electrolytic
Reductive Coupling. *J. Chin. Chem. Soc. (Taipei),* **2002**, *49*, 1105-1109.
[http://dx.doi.org/10.1002/jccs.200200159]

[176] Wang, Q.; Zhu, J.; Li, Y. Study on the synthesis of some new Biflavonoids (VI) -- the catalytic hydro
genation of 3,3″-biflavones. *Chin. Sci. Bull.,* **1990**, *35*, 744-746.

CHAPTER 4

Plant Metabolites may Protect Human Cells against Radiation-associated Damage: An Integrative Review

Cristiane Pimentel Victório[1], Fernanda Marques Peixoto[1], Edmilson Monteiro de Souza[1], João Bosco de Salles[1], Alexander Machado Cardoso[1] and Maria Cristina de Assis[1,*]

[1] *Western Rio Janeiro State University - UEZO, Avenida Manuel Caldeira de Alvarenga, 1203, Rio de Janeiro - RJ, 23070200, Brazil*

Abstract: The human body is exposed to natural sources of ionizing radiation including cosmic rays, radionuclides disposed on the Earth's crust, air, water, and food. In addition, man-made radiation sources for military and civil purposes such as the use of radiation in health care, medical procedures in the diagnosis and treatment of diseases, scientific researches, and energy production can contribute to the increased exposure and may affect the human cells. Many derivatives of plant extracts or genetically modified plants have been employed as radiomodifiers as they are compounds that can modify the biological response to the damage induced by the radiation. On the other hand, radiomodulators can be used for varied medical applications such as radioprotection and radiosensitization of tumor cells. This chapter aims to identify, analyze, and synthesize results of independent studies through an integrative review, which evaluated the protective effects of plant metabolites on cell injury caused by radiation therapy against cancer and high doses of radiation exposure.

Keywords: DNA damage, Ionizing radiation, Lipid peroxidation, Natural products, Plant extracts, Plant families, Radiomodifiers, Radioprotection, Secondary metabolite.

INTRODUCTION

Ionizing Radiation and Human Health

"Don't talk to me about X-rays", he said. *"I am afraid of them. I stopped experimenting with them two years ago, when I came near to losing my eyesight*

* **Corresponding author Maria Cristina de Assis:** Western Rio Janeiro State University - UEZO, Avenida Manuel Caldeira de Alvarenga, 1203, Rio de Janeiro - RJ, 23070200, Brazil; Tel: +55(21)23327535; E-mail: mariacristina@uezo.edu.br and cristinauezo@gmail.com

Atta-ur-Rahman (Ed.)

and Dally, my assistant practically lost the use of both of his arms. I am afraid of radium and polonium too, and I don't want to monkey with them". With this quick sentence spoken to a reporter from the New York World Journal in 1903, the famous inventor Thomas Edison expressed worry about the risks associated with the use of ionizing radiation [1]. Nevertheless, in 1928, during the *Second International Congress of Radiology*, the ICRP (*International Commission on Radiological Protection*) was created in response to the growing concerns of the medical community and population about the undesirable effects of ionizing radiation [2].

Ionizing radiation is any radiation that can remove electrons from atoms and molecules with or without resting mass. It is divided into two categories, according to how they transfer their energy to matter: directly ionizing radiation and indirectly ionizing radiation. Directly ionizing radiation acts primarily through its electric field and transfers its energy to many atoms at the same time. These are radiations with an electrical charge, such as electrons, protons, alpha particles, beta, and fission fragments. Indirectly ionizing radiation interacts individually, transferring its energy to electrons, which will cause new ionizations. Indirectly ionizing radiations are those that do not have charges, such as electromagnetic radiation X and gamma and neutrons [3].

Radiation has existed on our planet long before life appeared on it. However, they were only formally revealed to humanity with the discovery of X-rays by the German physicist Wilhelm Conrad Röntgen in 1895, and later with the discovery of Gamma-rays through the experiments developed by Henri Becquerel in 1896 and by the couple Pierre and Marie Curie in 1898 [4 - 6]. Since then, there has been a growing interest in research involving the use of ionizing radiation in health, industry, agriculture, and energy generation [7].

However, the unrestrained use of ionizing radiation, the disrespect for good radiological protection practices, and the use for war purposes show to the world the possible deleterious consequences of the misuse of ionizing radiation. Adverse effects, which can cause from superficial tissue damage (radiation dermatitis) to severe damage such as the induction of mutations caused by the breakdown of the DNA molecules in cells, are the main concerns of different institutions, such as the *International Atomic Energy Agency* (IAEA), the *United Nations Scientific Committee on the Effects of Atomic Radiation* (UNSCEAR/ONU), and the *National Nuclear Energy Commission* – CNEN, whose mission is to evaluate the doses, effects, and risks of radiation, and establish new processes and products to minimize the undesirable effects of radiation on humans, such as the development of novel radiomodifiers.

BIOLOGICAL EFFECTS OF IONIZING RADIATION

Deleterious Effects of Ionizing Radiation and Oxidative Stress

Ionizing radiation has enough energy to remove electrons from biomolecules, which can cause direct or indirect damage to their cellular structures [8, 9]. Among the main direct effects of the interaction of radiation with biomolecules, those caused in the DNA molecules stand out, such as the formation of mutations, insertions, and deletions [10, 11]. Ionizing radiation can also compromise the heterozygosis process, stimulating carcinogenesis [11].

In addition to the direct effects of ionizing radiation, DNA and other important macromolecules, including proteins and lipids, along with cellular structures such as the cell membrane, can suffer indirect effects of this radiation through the Reactive Oxygen Species (ROS) generated by water radiolysis (Fig. 1) [12, 13] and Reactive Nitrogen Species (RNS) generated by the induction of transient mitochondrial permeability stimulated by radiation [14, 15].

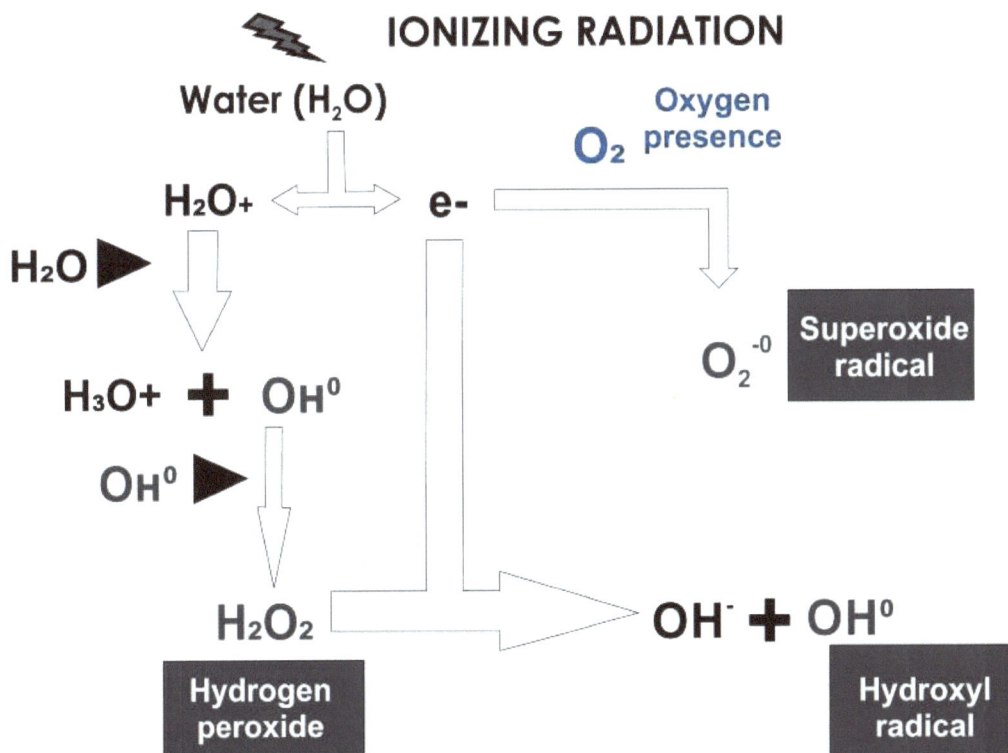

Fig. (1). Simplified scheme for the formation of the main Reactive Oxygen Species (ROS) as a result of water radiation induced by ionizing radiation.

Membrane lipid peroxidation is one of the major cellular damage caused by ionizing radiation. This peroxidation results in the structural and functional loss of cellular machinery, leading to cross-linking between lipids that promote the increase of the dielectric constant inside the membrane, with a consequent alteration in its microviscosity and permeability in ionic transport [16].

Cellular proteins can also suffer direct or indirect effects of ionizing radiation, the most common being cross-linking, oxidation, carbonylation, and cleavages [11, 17, 18]. Oxidation of the lateral chain of cysteine can lead to the formation of mixed disulfides between the thiol group of proteins and low-weight molecules such as reduced glutathione (GSH) [19].

Among the main ROS are the radicals: hydroxyl (OH), superoxide (O_2^-), peroxyl (ROO^-), and alkoxide (RO); and non-radical: oxygen, hydrogen peroxide, and hypochlorous acid. While RNS are represented by nitric oxide (NO), nitrous oxide (N_2O_3), nitrous acid (HNO_2), nitrites (NO_2^-), nitrates (NO_3^-), and peroxynitrites ($ONOO^-$) [20 - 23].

Hydroxyl is the most deleterious free radical to the cells because it reacts promptly with several macromolecules before being kidnapped by the antioxidants present. Its action occurs through oxidation [24]. Although hydroxyl is easily sequestered *in vitro* by numerous antioxidant agents, these molecules are not very effective *in vivo* since administration in high doses is necessary to reach sufficient concentration inside cells for the suppression of this free radical. Therefore, to control the harmful effects of the hydroxyl radical, it is necessary to prevent its formation or repair the damage caused [24].

Hydroxyl damages DNA, RNA, proteins, and cell membranes. The attack on DNA occurs through nitrogenous bases and deoxyribose. The attack on deoxyribose promotes the removal of one of the hydrogen atoms, usually leading to the breaking of the DNA chain [20 - 23]. Hydroxyl attacks protein side chains and can cause damage such as cleavages, resulting in loss of enzymatic activity, difficulties in active transport across cell membranes, cytolysis, and cell death [25]. Lipids, especially polyunsaturated ones, are also very susceptible to hydroxyl attacks. When this attack occurs, lipid-free radicals are formed that can attack membrane proteins, damaging cells. Furthermore, genotoxic products are generated by the peroxidation of lipids, including α,β-unsaturated aldehydes 4-hydroperoxy-2-nonenal, 4-hydroxy-2-nonenal, 4-oxo-2-nonenal, and 4,5-epoxy - 2(E)-decennial [24, 26].

Under normal conditions, enzymes and endogenous antioxidant agents maintain the balance between the production and removal of ROS and RNS. These include glutathione reduced (GSH), histidine peptides, iron-binding proteins (transferrin and ferritin), dihydrolipoic acid and dihydroquinone (CoQH2), and dietary antioxidants such as a-tocopherol (vitamin-E), β- carotene (pro-vitamin-A), ascorbic acid (vitamin-C), phenolic compounds, flavonoids, and polyflavonoids [27, 28]. The main antioxidant enzymes are Glutathione peroxidase (GPx), catalase (CAT), and superoxide dismutase (SOD) [29].

ROS and RNS have several cellular functions. They are involved in phagocytosis, regulation of cellular and intercellular signaling, anabolic and catabolic reactions [24]. However, when in excess, ROS and RNS can have harmful effects such as the injury of DNA, proteins, carbohydrates, and membrane lipids [30].

STOCHASTIC AND DETERMINISTIC BIOLOGICAL EFFECTS OF RADIATION EXPOSURE

Depending on the dose of radiation, the effects on a tissue can be divided into two types: deterministic and stochastic. Stochastic effects are those that do not have a dose threshold, having a probabilistic character of occurrence [31]. Stochastic effects are generally delayed and caused by exposure to low doses of radiation. They can be generated even by naturally-occurring background radiation. The probability of occurrence is proportional to the absorbed dose. However, the severity of the effects is independent of the dose. Examples of stochastic effects of ionizing radiation on human health are radio-induced cancers [32].

On the other hand, high doses of ionizing radiation can cause very expected effects, which can be easily associated with certain exposure. These effects are known as deterministic, ranging from blood and chromosomal aberrations to death. They depend on factors such as immune resistance, dose received, exposure time, and type of radiation [32]. The higher the doses received, the more severe these effects are [31].

Exposure to high doses promotes acute radiation syndrome (ARS) characterized by gastrointestinal and hematopoietic disorders, lesions in the skin, and neurovascular system [33]. In contrast, due to the radiosensitivity of the hematopoietic system, the hematopoietic syndrome may also occur in exposures doses much lower than those necessary for the occurrence of other manifestations [33]. High doses of ionizing radiation, around 10 Gy, can be fatal, as they promote, just in a few days, the complete loss of the mucosa from the digestive tract, as well as the breakdown of neurological and cardiovascular systems [34, 35].

RADIOMODULATORS

Radiomodulators are synthetic or natural substances capable of modifying the biological effects generated by radiation. There are two distinct types of radio-modulators: radioprotectors and radiosensitizers.

Radioprotectors

Radioprotectors are substances that prevent or reduce the damage caused to the living organism due to exposure to radiation [36 - 38]. Substances are considered radio-protective only when they are administered before irradiation [39]. If they are administered during or immediately after irradiation, before the appearance of clinical manifestations, they are considered mitigators, and if administered after the appearance of clinical manifestations, they are considered therapeutics [39].

Several constituents of natural and artificial sources have been evaluated to identify novel, safe, and effective radioprotective agents. Ideal radioprotectors should have the following skills [40]:

a. Repair DNA and cellular damage;
b. Assist in repopulation of damaged organs;
c. Immunomodulation;
d. Free radical scavenging;
e. Decrease oxidative stress.

Radiosensitizers

Radiosensitizers are substances used in radiotherapy to increase their efficiency in killing cancer cells and shrinking tumors. Different definitions have been applied to radiosensitizers such as:

- *"Radiosensitizers are compounds that when combined with radiation will achieve greater tumor inactivation than would have been expected from the additive effect of each modality"* [41].
- *"Radiosensitizers are agents that do not have a therapeutic effect of their own but act to enhance the therapeutic effect of radiation"* [42].
- *"Radiosensitizers are chemicals or pharmaceutical agents that can enhance the killing effect on tumor cells by accelerating DNA damage and producing free radicals indirectly"* [43].

The most-reported mechanisms involved in radiosensitization are 1) enhanced generation of ROS/RNS; 2) selective depletion of tumor cells by antioxidants and antioxidant enzymes; 3) increased lipid peroxidation and depletion of glutathione; 4) elevated levels of lipid peroxidation and DNA damage of tumor cells; 5) formation of DNA adducts (a segment of DNA bound to a cancer-causing chemical); 6) inhibition of DNA repair; 7) inhibition of DNA synthesis; 8) induction of cell cycle arrest; 9) induction of apoptosis; 10) depletion of protein kinase C [44, 45].

DEVELOPMENT OF RADIO-PROTECTIVE DRUGS

Considering that exposure to ionizing radiation can occur in different circumstances such as radiotherapy, space travel, nuclear accidents, and war, it is crucial to develop radio-protective agents that can prevent and mitigate the effects of this radiation [46, 47]. Research for the development of radio-protective drugs began in the middle of the last century when the protective effect of cysteine against X-radiation was reported [48]. Many countries, including the United States, the USSR, Germany, and China, disputed especially during the Cold War period, the development of novel synthetic radio-protective drugs [44, 49 - 52], the most promising being compounds based on sulfhydryls. Only the Walter Reed Army Institute of Research (USA) synthesized and tested over 5,000 compounds in the 1980s [53 - 55].

Several drugs such as amifostine (WR-2721 or Ethiophos), glucocorticoids, phosphorothioates, and thiosulfonates (WR-159243, WR-3302, WR-1551, and WR-2926) have achieved a good radio-protective effect [56 - 58]; however, their effectiveness was unfavorable in oral administration due to the low availability through this route. In addition, these drugs were not successful because of their narrow therapeutic windows, important side effects, and toxicity [56].

More recently, new synthetic drugs such as cerium oxide [59] and fullerenol [60] have been administered in the form of nanoparticles with excellent radio-protective effects *in vivo*. In addition to nanoparticles having low solubility, short half-life, fast metabolism, and high synthesis cost [61], several studies have shown that they have some side effects such as pro-oxidant activities resulting in ROS production and cytotoxicity, inflammation, necrosis, fibrosis, and apoptosis [62, 63]. It has been suggested that the use of nanoparticles for radioprotection is inadvisable, considering their toxicity, limited routes of administration, limited protection of the central nervous system, and their high cost. To overcome these limitations, many researchers have been looking for novel compounds that are effective and non-toxic [64].

Plant-derived Compounds and Radioprotection

About 80% of the world's population uses traditional methods to treat their illnesses [65, 66]. In recent decades, many studies with plants, especially those for medicinal use, have grown a lot. Consequently, many researchers have demonstrated the diverse medicinal properties of plants such as antioxidant, anti-inflammatory, anticancer, antimicrobial, analgesic, and antibiotic agents [67].

Considering that synthetic radioprotectors available are generally toxic in their effective doses, the search for plant extracts and their respective metabolites with efficient radio-protective effects to replace synthetic drugs has increased [40]. Some plants (their extracts or their respective phytochemicals) have already been successfully used to mitigate the harmful effects of ionizing radiation in cases of accidents and nuclear conflicts. For example, *Gingko biloba* extracts and plant phenols have suppressed clastogenic factors in the plasma of workers from the worst nuclear accident in history at Chernobyl [68, 69], and the consumption of fruits and green-yellow vegetables by survivors of the atomic bomb in Japan resulted in protection against bladder cancer [70].

Throughout history, accidents involving radiation have been recorded in a few events. However, the severity of the damage and the magnitude of related accidents justify studies aimed at developing novel radio-protective substances. Studies on the search for effective radio-protective agents from plants to replace limited synthetic radio-protective drugs permeate the scientific literature. However, for a natural radio-protective to replace a synthetic chemical drug, its efficiency needs to be evaluated and validated [71]. Many *in vitro* and *in vivo* studies have shown promising radio-protective effects by total extracts, fractions, and compounds isolated from plants, such as curcumin, extracted from the rhizome of *Curcuma longa* (*Zingiberaceae*) [72], *Diospyros kaki* (*Ebenaceae*) [73], *Panax ginseng* (*Araliaceae*) [74], *Gymnema sylvestre* (*Asclepiadaceae*) [75], *Chrysophyllum cainito* (*Sapotaceae*) [76], and *Nigella sativa* (*Ranunculaceae*) [77].

INTEGRATIVE REVIEW OF THE USE OF PLANTS AND PHYTOSUBSTANCES TO PROTECT AGAINST IONIZING RADIATION

This research was carried out on the basis of an integrative review including theoretical and empirical literature, as well as studies with different methodologies. For the preparation of this study, the following steps were taken: establishment of the hypothesis and objective of the integrative review; definition of inclusion and exclusion criteria for sample selection, the definition of information to be extracted from the articles, analysis of results, and presentation of possible mechanisms involved in the protection against ionizing radiation from phytosubstances.

The following question guided this study: what are the plant families and plant metabolites most frequently used in radioprotection studies against ionizing radiation? Searches were performed in electronic journals such as the Latin American and Caribbean Center for Health Sciences (LILACS), the Medical Literature Online (MEDLINE) databases, the Scientific Electronic Library Online (SciELO), and Science Direct electronic support. The criteria for selecting the articles were: i) Articles available online in full in Portuguese and English, published in the last 10 years (2011 to 2021); ii) Contents related to the focus of this study. The following descriptors were used: *"ionizing radiation and phytochemical"*, *"radioprotection and plant extracts"*, and *"phytochemical and radioprotection"*.

After searching the descriptors in the databases, 287 articles were found, initially selected based on the title, abstract, study approach, adequacy to the guiding question, and inclusion criteria. After a critical analysis, the final sample consisted of 73 articles, of which 13 were outside the focus of the study, leaving 60 articles for final analysis. For data analysis, a script was established with the following information: plant species; the popular name of the plant species, type of extract, part of the plant used in the preparation of the extract, chemical class, phytosubstance, biological effect, the experimental model used, study title, authors, journal, and year of publication. 60 articles were grouped into two categories: 41 reviews and 19 experimental articles. The review papers were considered to survey the most frequently botanical families associated with radiation protection. Experimental articles were also analyzed to verify the data of isolated phytosubstances. Data analyses were presented as tables (Tables **1** and **2**) and graph (Fig. **2**) for a better understanding.

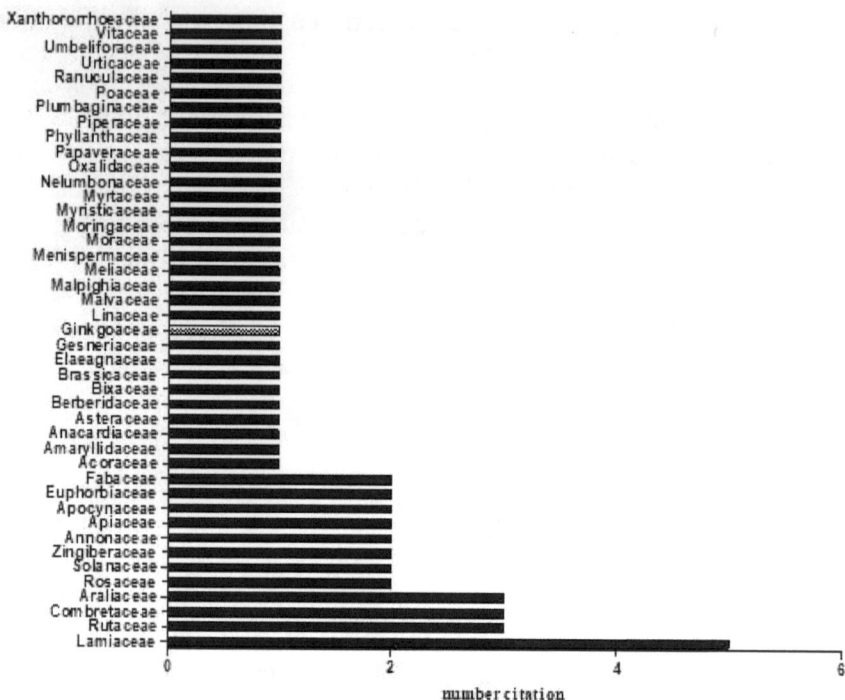

Fig. (2). Number of citations of Plant families in scientific articles involving studies about radioprotection. Except for the family Ginkgoaceae (Gimnospermae), the other families are of the Angiospermae group.

Table 1. Natural products that exhibited radioprotective property in different models of ionizing radiation injury.

Plant* and Metabolites	Concentration*	Radiation Type /Dose	Model	Route Administration/ before (BI) or after irradiation (AI)	Radioprotective mechanisms	References
Morus nigra	200 mg/Kg	γ ray (3 and 6 Gy) whole body	Rat (bone marrow cells and liver)	Intraperitoneal 3 days BI and 3 days AI	Decreased the level of malondialdehyde (MDA) and superoxide dismutase (SOD), as well as enhanced the total thiol content and catalase activity; Antioxidant activity reduced the genotoxicity and cytotoxicity induced by gamma irradiation in bone marrow cells and liver in the rat.	Ghasemnezhad *et al.* (2017)

(Table 1) cont.....

Tinospora cordifolia	75 mg/Kg	γ ray (2,5Gy)	Rat (testes)	Oral Gavage 5 days half an hour (BI)	Effectively prevented radiation-induced alterations in body weight, tissue weight, weight index, tubular diameters and reduced of lipid peroxidation levels, increased glutathione and catalase activity in testes and restored almost a normal structure of testes.	Sharma *et al.* (2015)
Sanguisorba officinalis, Erigeron canadenses, Fragaria vesca, Rubus plicatus	1 a 30µg/mL	γ ray (15, 100 and 200 Gy)	The peripheral blood human mononuclear cells (lymphocyte)	1 hour (BI)	Reduced lipid peroxidation and DNA damage Antioxidant activity.	Szejk *et al.* (2017)
Pilea microphylla	12.5, 25, 50 g/mL	γ ray (2, 4, 6, 8 and 10 Gy)	Chinese hamster normal lung fibroblasts (V79 cells) (NCCS)	30 min (BI)	Decreased lipid peroxidation; Inhibited radiation-induced DNA breaks in micronuclei assay; Protection against oxidative damage.	Paul *et al* (2012)
Acorus calamus	250 mg/kg	γ ray (2, 6 and 10 Gy) whole body	Mice (peripheral blood ,brain, liver, and kidney)	Oral Gavage 1 hour (BI)	Decreased lipid peroxidation Increased the activities of major enzymes of the antioxidant defense system specially SOD, catalase and GPx and levels of GSH. Protected the cellular DNA in peripheral blood leucocytes, bone marrow cells, and spleenocytes from radiation induced damages.	Sandeep *et al.* (2012)
Terminalia Chebula	80 mg/kg	γ ray (6, 8 and 10 Gy) whole body	Rats (peripheral blood and intestinal histopathological studies)	Oral (ad libitum.) 5 days (BI)	Reduced radiation-induced cellular DNA damage and gastrointestinal cell death.	Dixit *et al.* (2013)

(Table 1) cont.....

Xylopia aethiopica	250 mg/Kg	γ ray (5 Gy) whole body	Rats (Liver and kidney)	Oral (ad libitum.) 6 weeks (BI) and 8 weeks (AI)	Increased the activities of enzymes of the antioxidant defense system specially SOD, catalase and levels of GSH.	Oluwatosin *et al.* (2011)
Aloe vera	50 mg/ kg	γ ray (2 Gy) whole body	Mice (Liver and kidney tissues)	Oral Alternate days for 30 days BI (15 times)	Reduction in ROS/lipid peroxidation and levels, LDH activity and anti-genotoxic effects	Bala *et al.* (2018)
Lycopene and curcumin**	20 mg/Kg- Lycopene, 50 mg/Kg - Curcumin	γ ray (20 Gy) Parotid glands	Rats (Parotid glands of 40 female)	Intraperitoneal 24 hours (BI)	Reduced the structural damage to the salivary glands	Lopez-Jorne *et al.* (20160
Polyalthia longifólia	250, 500mg/Kg	X ray (10Gy) whole body	Mice (Peripheral blood, small intestine, spleen and liver)	Oral 15 days (BI)	Inhibited the decline in the intracellular antioxidant enzymes in the liver and intestine	Jothy *et al.* (2015)
Umbelliferone**	31, 62, 124, 186, 248 and 310 μM	γ ray (1, 2, 3 4 and 5 Gy)	Lymphocytes collected peripheral blood samples from non-smoking healthy individuals (22–25 years old	30 min (BI)	Inhibited reactive oxygen species generation and its subsequent toxicity. decreased % of apoptotic cells and prevented radiation induced mitochondrial depolarization in lymphocytes	Kanimozhi *et al.* (2011)
Curcumin**	1,5 and 10 μg/mL	γ ray (1, 2, and 4 Gy)	Lymphocytes collected peripheral blood samples from non-smoking healthy individuals (22–25 years old)	30 min (BI)	Decreased the frequency of micronucleus and dicentric aberration; activities of SOD, CAT and GPx significantly increased levels; Decreased lipid peroxidation; Improved antioxidant status conferring protection against oxidative damage.	Srinivasan *et al.* (2006)
Malpighia gabra	1 mL/100 g of body weight	Iodine - 131 (25μCi or 0.925 MBq/100g body weight	Rats (Bone marrow cells)	Oral (Gavage) 5 days (BI), 5 days (AI) and simultaneous	Effects antimutagenic in acute and subchronic tretaments, attributed to its ability to scavenge free radicals	Düsman *et al.* (20140

(Table 1) cont.....

Lycium barbarum	50, 100, 200 mg/Kg	X ray (4Gy) whole body	Mice (Bone marrow mononuclear cells)	Intraperitoneal 2 h (AI) by 14 days (AI)	Effects antiapoptotic and antioxidante on bone marrowmononuclear cells (BMNC) Enabled the maintenance of the redox balance and protected cells against radiation damage)	Zhou *et al.*, 2016
Vitis vinifera	Grape juice (diluted 1:3 with water along seven days of treatmnt	X ray (6Gy) whole body	Mice	Oral 7 days (AI)	Improving anxiety and locomotion within 24 to 72 hours after sub-lethal X-irradiation.	Soares *et al.* (2014)
Vitis labrusca	Ingest a maximum of 10 ml of test compound (grape juice)	X ray (6Gy) whole body	Rats (Liver tissue)	Oral (ad libitum.) 6 days (BI) and 15 days (AI)	Decrease in liver lipid peroxidation and the increase in Cu/ZnSOD and GPx antioxidant enzyme activities	Andrade *et al.*(2011)
Resveratrol**	50, 100 mg/kg	γ ray (2 Gy) whole body	Mice (Peripheral blood lymphocyte)	Intraperitoneal 2 h (BI)	Decreased the Total Comet Score and the % Damaged Cell radiation induced	Koohian *et al.* (2017)
Quercetin**	50 mg/Kg	N/A (20 Gy) (Cranium region)	Rats (Brain tissue and blood)	Oral 15 days (BI)	Reduced by lipid peroxidation and its positive effects on the antioxidant system. Histopathological evaluation of the tissues also demonstrated a significant decrease in cellular degeneration and infiltration parameters	Kale *et al.* 2018
Purified Baicalein	1 or 10 mM (Neural progenitor cells-NPCs) 10 mg/kg (Mice)	γ ray (5 Gy) - NPCs γ ray (16 Gy) - mice	Neural progenitor cell (NPCs) from a neonatal mouse cerebellum mice	7 days (BI)	Protected NPCs from irradiation-induced cell death via a mechanism other than an antioxidative mechanism.	Bi Oh *et al.* (2012)

Botanical Families Associated with Radiation Protection

Plants are at the base of the ecosystem, essential to human life, in the abiotic dynamics, and support the survival of living beings on the planet. Also, they are used in food preparation, religious rituals, and also as therapeutics in the treatment of illnesses [78]. The cultural use is perpetuated in traditional communities as riverside dwellers, quilombolas, indigenous people and is inherited from the empirical knowledge of ancestors. In many cases, the traditional use of plants prevails over-commercialized drugs, as it is the only medicine resource, easy to access, and at a low cost. In addition, the dynamic relationships between man and plants like ethnobotany, ethnopharmacology, which encourages phytochemical studies, prospecting for novel plant drugs, and their biological evaluation have been demonstrated [79].

After discovering their chemical structure, many of these substances are synthesized by man for the production of drugs. The use of plants in their raw state is easy and cheap, often reveals the relevance of that species as medicinal and therapeutic; it is a valuable empirical way where popular knowledge anticipates scientific evidence. It is worth noting the importance of chemosystematics in directing studies on the biological activity of plants, since only the cultural use, although very relevant in the discovery of therapeutic and pharmacological substances, presents a much smaller scale compared to the latent phytochemical diversity [80].

In the current perspective of novel molecular development, chemophenetics studies give insights into chemosystematics by addressing the variety of specialized natural products that corroborate the phylogenetic relationships [81]. The chemodiversity is high and expands the achievement of new alternatives for drugs considering the phylogenetic component. Given the plant diversity, many substances produced by plants have not yet been studied or identified, which makes scientific studies with the flora essential. Considering the flora of tropical countries, especially in Brazil, which is a megadiverse area, distributed in many biomes such as the Amazon Forest, Atlantic Forest Cerrado, Chaco, Pantanal Caatinga, and Pampa. It is estimated that more than 200 species are discovered and described each year and that there is a high degree of endemism [82].

Considering the last 10 years, there is a predominance of review articles related to the use of plants, plant extracts and/or their metabolites to mitigate the harmful effects of radiation. Among the articles, it was possible to observe a diversity of botanical families used to prevent and treat exposure to ionizing radiation. There were 8.19% of citations for the *Lamiaceae* family, for example, and 4.92% for each of these families *Araliaceae, Combretaceae, and Rutaceae*, the most cited (n= 61 citations in articles) in the last 10 years. Fig. (**3**) Many of these plants come from the Asian and European continents. The articles evaluated have no record for using these plants in Brazil as radioprotectors, radiation mitigators, and therapeutic agents. Among the plants mentioned in the studies, there is a wide diversity of plant species distributed in 44 botanical families, one species representing the group of Gymnosperms, division *Ginkgophyta*, family *Ginkgoaceae* (*Ginkgo biloba* L.) [83, 84].

The species *G. biloba*, a plant of the Chinese flora, is the only living representative of the Ginkgo lineage and the oldest record of medicinal use, described in the Chinese Pharmacopoeia. It presents extensive interaction in aspects of Eastern human culture from food and medicinal use to artistic and religious expressions, being rich in flavonoid glycosides, terpene lactones, biflavones, and proanthocyanidins responsible for biological activities [83, 84]. It has been widely used orally to treat diseases and alterations associated with the central nervous system [84]. Studies have shown that the high antioxidant activity of *G. biloba* is extremely relevant in protecting against gamma radiation and reducing oxidative stress [85].

The most cited family was *Lamiaceae*, with representatives from Europe such as the aromatic genera *Coleus, Mentha,* and *Ocimum* [86 - 88]. This family is popularly used in the preparation of infusions as medicine, condiment, and flavoring. The chemical identity of *Lamiaceae* is marked by the presence of volatile substances, rich in mono and sesquiterpenes, produced and accumulated in glandular trichomes [89, 90]. Other families, cited about two to three times, are *Zingiberaceae, Rutaceae, Rosaceae, Araliaceae, Annonaceae, Poaceae,* and *Combretaceae*. The tropical family *Zingiberaceae* has species of the genus *Curcuma* and *Zingiber* [91], rich in volatile substances (essential oils) responsible for the use as a condiment, mainly in Asia, and with high therapeutic relevance [92, 93]. In addition to phenolic substances such as curcumin addressed in radioprotection studies, all plant organs produce volatile substances. The use of rhizomes for therapeutic purposes is quite common.

The *Poaceae* and *Rutaceae* families are present on all continents and are quite representative in the world's diet, with the genera *Oryza* and *Citrus*, respectively, among the most used plants as radioprotectors [94, 95]. Rice (*Oryza* sp.), mostly used in food, has very old records of medicinal use dating back to 2,800 BC. Recent studies indicate rice as an immunostimulant and therapeutic, associated with polysaccharides and lipopolysaccharides [96] and the presence of phenolic substances, carotenoids, and vitamins [97].

The *Rutaceae* species, mentioned in more than two works, were *Aegle marmelos* (L.) Corr. Serr., popularly known as Bael and considered sacred by Hindus, native to the Asian continent in the region of India and nearby and with many studies and applications in the Indian Ayurvedic health system (Kma 2014). The fruits and leaves of this species have therapeutic effects. This plant is rich in monoterpenes (cineol, eugenol, limonene), triterpenes (lupeol), marmelin, and flavonoids such as rutin [97].

Plant organs (leaves, flowers, stems, roots, and fruits) can be used in the preparation of extracts and fractions to obtain phytosubstances isolated from the extracts (secondary metabolites) and also substances from metabolism primary as the polysaccharides that have been used in experimental models *in vitro* and *in vivo* to assess the radio-protective effect [73]. Many plants indicated in the articles are relevant for human consumption as food, condiment, or medicinal through infusions or other domestic preparations. And there is mention of plants used in traditional medicine in India, one of the oldest in mankind – Ayurvedic, as an example Triphala, the name given to a group of medicinal plants – fruits of the species *Emblica officinalis* (*Euphorbiaceae*), *Terminalia bellerica*, and *Terminalia chebula* (*Combretaceae*); and plants from ancient Chinese medicine that reveal the historical and cultural importance of human-plant relationships [98].

The indication of botanical families guides studies of natural products because the kinship of plant species in each family is already known and presents genetic proximity that affects the metabolome (production of chemical classes and/or primary and secondary metabolites of plants) [99]. It is possible to invest in other species of the same family that have already been studied for a specific purpose, as there is a micromolecular evolution that allows predicting a chemical profile for the taxon [80]. Both ethnopharmacological knowledge and chemosystematics/chemophenetics are important scientific tools in the study of plants and the discovery of novel substances that will be applied.

Plant Metabolites Modify the Harmful Effects of Ionizing Radiation on Living Tissues

Organisms exposed to harmful radiation suffer their effects progressively. In response to injuries, repair mechanisms are activated in cells; many changes may occur that lead to cancer, genetic disorders, and morbidity. There are different mechanisms of action from radio-protective agents, depending on the type of damage and the extent of the damage caused by it. It has shown that the radio-protective effects of plants are expressed through various mechanisms such as repair the DNA damage, antioxidant, and anti-inflammatory action, as well as interfering with intracellular signaling preventing cell death, and promoting cell regeneration [100].

Biological Effects of Ionizing Radiation Observed in Experimental Studies

From the analysis of the 19 experimental articles (Table **1**), it was observed that

68.42% used Gamma-rays as a radiation source; 26.31% X-rays and 5.26% used other types of radiation. Radiation doses varied due to the experimental models, most papers used doses equal to or less than 6 Gy (Gray) since the lethal dose of 50% in 30 days (LD50/30) in animal models used. Doses equal to or greater than 8 Gy were used when analyzes were performed in *ex vivo* or *in vitro* models. The doses used are related to established effects, associated with the occurrence of deterministic effects [100].

The route of administration of crude extracts or purified phytosubstances was predominantly oral in the experimental models (Table **1**). This route has been characterized as preferred, due to the ease of administration, besides being a preferential route for drug administration in case of possible mass radiation exposure [87]. Regarding the time of administration of doses, it was observed that 5.26% of the experimental models used only the treatment before radiation exposure, 26.31% opted for previous and subsequent treatment, while 68.42% only administered the phytosubstances after exposure to ionizing radiation. These data suggest that most authors were concerned with evaluating the efficacy of plant-derived extracts/compounds after radiation exposure as a potential clinical use for radiation effects, especially in difficult-to-predict scenarios as exposures result from accidents with nuclear installations.

The main effects of ionizing radiation observed in all experimental models analyzed were the production of ROS and lipid peroxidation, generating cellular damage, mutagenic action, and cell death. Therefore, antioxidant agents present within the cell neutralize the effects of these radicals play an important role in protecting against the effects of ionizing radiation, acting as protectors and repairers of radiation damage [40].

Antioxidants act in different ways in controlling ROS. First, compounds such as aminothiols (thiols) can promote hypoxia and consequent mitigation of ROS generation, reducing the amount of oxygen in the cell through its conversion into disulfide and hydrogen peroxide [101]. On the other hand, radioprotector amifostine (thiophosphate) promotes ROS scavenging mediated by oxygen and hydroxyl radical [102]. In addition, enzymatic antioxidants such as Glucose--phosphate dehydrogenase, glutathione reductase, and glutathione S-transferase (GST) can inactivate ROS into non- or less reactive intermediates [103].

Mammalian cells have a complex antioxidant mechanism, fundamental to neutralize oxidative stress generated by exposure to various environmental aggressions, including ionizing radiation (Fig. **3**).

The radio-protective effects observed in experimental models are associated with protection against oxidative stress, induction of antioxidant enzymes, inhibition of lipid peroxidation, and reduction of genotoxicity and cell death. The radio-protective effects of purified extracts and phytosubstances are summarized in Table **1**.

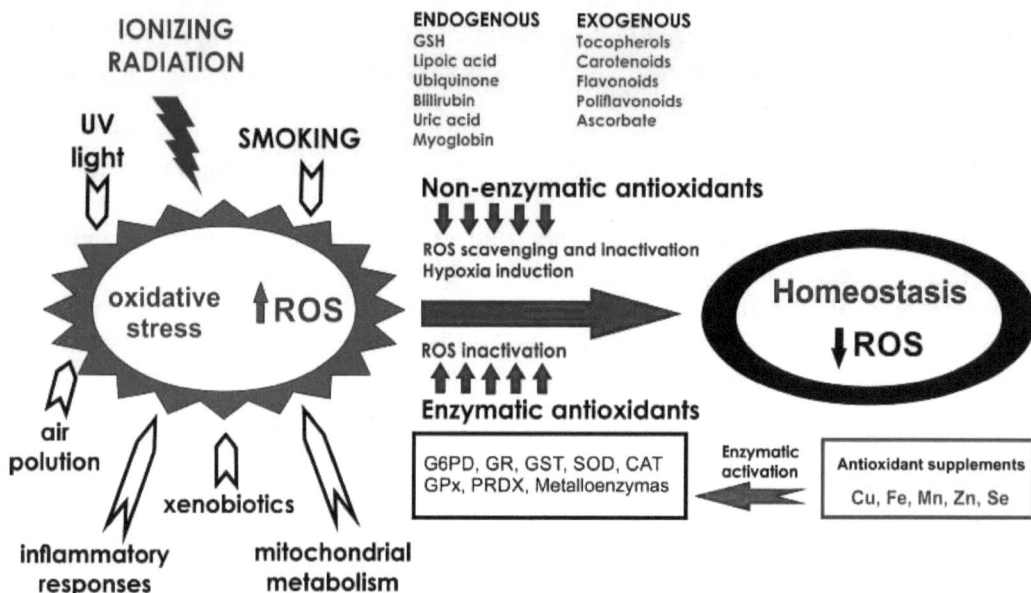

Fig. (3). Antioxidant defense mechanisms in mammals. The cell oxidative stress is generated by reactive oxygen species (ROS) from biotic and abiotic sources. Enzymatic and non-enzymatic antioxidants restore cell homeostasis. Definitions: GSH (Glutathione reduced); G6PD (Glucose-6-phosphate dehydrogenase); GR (Glutathione Reductase); GST (Glutathione S-transferase); SOD (Superoxide Dismutase); CAT (Catalase); GPx (Glutathione peroxidase); PRDX (Peroxiredoxin) [101 - 103].

Main Sources of Phytochemical Compounds Tested

Among the articles analyzed (Table **2**), which reported the description of the type of material tested, a percentage of 15.80% were observed that used aqueous, ethanolic extracts, and fruit juices. For methanol extracts, this percentage stood at 10.53%, in the total of the 19 articles analyzed. In addition, purified/isolated compounds were also tested, representing 42.10% of the total articles. Among the plant extracts tested, a great diversity of compounds was observed, contributing to the diversity of extraction methods. The solubility of phenolic compounds, the polarity of the solvent used, the degree of polymerization of phenolics, the degree of division, their interactions with other constituents of vegetables, time, and temperature directly influence the efficiency of the extraction method. Most phenolic compounds are not found in free form in nature, but in the form of esters or heterosides. They are therefore more soluble in water and polar organic solvents, which is why polar solvents were applied with predominance size [104].

Table 2. Main Sources of Phytochemical Compounds Tested.

Plant (Botany family)	Plant organ	Tested source	Metabolites	Chemical class	Reference
Morus nigra (*Moraceae*)	Fruits	(aqueous extract)	--	Phenolics (anthocyanins, proanthocyanidins, procyanidins)	Ghasemnezhad *et al.* (2017)
Tinospora cordifolia (*Menispermaceae*)	Roots	(aqueous extract)	--	Phenolics (flavonoid)	Sharma *et al.* (2015)
Sanguisorba officinalis (*Rosaceae*) *Erigeron Canadensis* (*Asteraceae*) *Fragaria vesca* (*Rosaceae*) *Rubus plicatus* (*Rosaceae*)	Flowers Flowers Leaves Leaves	Purified*	Glycoconjugated/aglycones (SoA, EcA, FvA and RpA, respectively)	Phenolics	Szejk *et al.* (2017)
Pilea microphylla (*Urticaceae*)	Whole plant	(Etanolic extract)	--	Phenolics	Paul *et al* (2012)
Acorus calamus (*Acoraceae*)	Roots	(Etanolic extract)	--	Phenilpropanoid (asarone)	Sandeep *et al.* (2012)
Terminalia chebula (*Combretaceae*)	--	(Etanolic extract)	--	Phenolics, (flavonoids), triterpenoids	Dixit *et al.* (2013)
Xylopia aethiopica (*Annonaceae*)	Fruits	(metanolic extract)	--	--	Oluwatosin *et al.* (2011)
Aloe vera (*Xanthorrhoeaceae*)	Leaves (mucilage)	(aqueous extract)	--	Carbohydrates and Phenolic (tannins, anthraquinones)	Bala *et al.* (2018)
--	--	Purified*	Lycopene and Curcumin	Tetraterpenoids (lycopene) and Phenolic compounds (curcumin)	Lopez-Jorne *et al.* (20160
Polyalthia longifolia (*Annonaceae*)	Leaves	(metanolic extract)	--	Phenolics (rutin)	Jothy *et al.* (2015)
--	--	Purified*	Umbelliferone	Phenolics (umbelliferone)	Kanimozhi *et al.* (2011)
Curcuma longa (*Zingiberaceae*)	Roots	Purified*	Curcumin	Phenolics (curcumin)	Srinivasan *et al.* (2006)

(Table 2) cont.....

Malpighia gabra (*Malpighiaceae*)	Fruits	(fruit pulp)	--	Phenolics (anthocyanins, flavonoids), tetraterpenoids (carotenes)	Düsman *et al.* (20140
Lycium barbarum (*Solanaceae*)	Fruits	Purified*	Polyssaccharides	--	Zhou *et al.*, 2016
Vitis vinifera (*Vitaceae*)	Fruits	Purple grape juice	---	Phenolics (resveratrol, quercetin, rutin, gallic acid, caffeic acid)	Soares *et al.* (2014)
Vitis labrusca (*Vitaceae*)	Fruits	Black grape juice	--	Phenolics (resveratrol, quercetin, rutin, gallic acid, caffeic acid, total flavonoids).	Andrade *et al.*(2011)
--	--	Purified*	Resveratrol	Phenolics	Koohian *et al.* (2017)
--	--	Purified*	Quercetin	Phenolics (flavonoid)	Kale *et al.* (2018)
Scutellaria baicaiensis (*Lamiaceae*)	Roots	Purified*	Baicalein	Phenolics (flavonoid)	Bi Oh *et al.*(2012)

*Isolated and marketed. (--) Not quoted.

It is worth mentioning that when these components are very complex (with high molecular weight), they are highly water-insoluble [105]. Solvents used to extract these compounds include methanol, ethanol, acetone, water, ethyl acetate, propanol, dimethyl formaldehyde, and its combinations [106]. Ethanol and water are the main solvents used to extract this class of compounds, being water of great relevance because it presents greater abundance and ease of obtaining and handling, besides providing a very efficient extraction [107]. In addition, several studies indicate the ethanic mixture at 70% (w/w) as the ideal solvent system for the extraction of some classes of phenolic compounds [108, 109]. Methanol confers high efficiency in the extraction of phenolic compounds; however, due to its high toxicity, it should be carefully used [110].

About 42% of the articles analyzed (Table **2**), the authors performed their tests from purified/isolated commercial compounds. This approach represents the classic strategy for the discovery of new drugs from natural products, however, the literature reports that the synergistic effects resulting from the combination of substances produce a greater effect than one might expect based on the individual contribution of their components [111].

Regarding the extraction methodologies used, none received prominence, but there are reports in the literature of several methods used in the process of extract extraction and manufacture, among them: macerating, percolation, infusion, decoction, extraction with supercritical CO_2, microwave-assisted extraction, ultrasound-assisted extraction, distillation, among others [109]. It is noteworthy that infusion and decoction are also popular methods used in the home environment and by many traditional communities over time.

Classes of Metabolites Involved in Radioprotection

The high complexity in the composition of plant extracts is known, however, some classes of compounds have been extensively explored. Among the experimental articles, it was possible to verify the identification and quantification of a variety of substances, with phenolic compounds being the most relevant, representing 89.47% of the total compounds selected by the studies (Table **2**). These compounds bring together secondary or special plant metabolites produced by the biosynthetic pathways of shikimic acid and the pentose phosphate pathway [112] and are structurally characterized by the presence of at least one benzene ring linked to one or more hydroxyl groups [113, 114].

Phenolic compounds represent a wide class of compounds, classified according to their chemical nature, belonging to different classes. There are about five thousand phenolic compounds described, such as flavonoids, phenolic acids, simple phenols, coumarins, tannins, lignins, and tocopherols; however the flavonoids, phenolic acids, and coumarins are most widely found in plant species [105, 115]. Among the studies analyzed, the flavonoid compounds represent 63.16%, with rutin, luteolin, quercetin, and baicalein being the most studied, corroborating with previous works, which report results of similar antioxidant activity [116]. In addition, other phenolic compounds were identified and quantified, which include phenolic acids (chlorogenic acid, rosmarinic acid, gallic acid, and ferulic acid), stilbene (resveratrol), in addition to tannins, anthraquinones, and other classes of compounds such as tetraterpenoids (lycopene) [117], curcuminoids (curcumin), and 7-hydroxycoumarin (umbelliferone) also demonstrate relevance as antioxidant agents.

Flavonoid compounds present a structural diversity due to the wide variety of combinations that occur during their biosynthesis. Its common structure shows the pattern of C6-C3-C6, consisting of two aromatic rings, called rings A and B, joined by three carbons that form a heterocyclic ring called ring C (Fig. **4**).

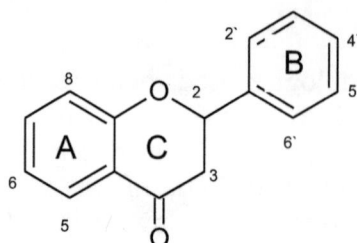

Fig. (4). Representation of the three rings (A, B, and C) characteristic of the basic structure of flavonoids, with their respective positions.

According to the oxidation degree and the C ring substitution pattern, the flavonoid subclasses are classified accordingly to the substitution pattern in the A and B rings [118]. The anthocyanins, flavonols, flavanols, flavanones, flavones, and isoflavones are part of this subcategory. Flavonoids can be found in the form of glycosides and/or methylated and/or acylated derivatives, with the presence or absence of double bonds and carbonyl groups in the C ring being the major differences between the subclasses [119].

Mechanisms of Action of Phytosubstances in Radioprotection

There are two main groups of phytosubstances that act as antioxidant agents, namely, the primary or chain-breaking antioxidants and the secondary or preventive antioxidants [120]. The primary antioxidants act by interrupting the chain reaction by donating hydrogen atoms by promoting the removal or inactivation of free radicals formed during the initiation and propagation stages. Phenolic compounds are good examples of electron donor groups in the ortho positions. The secondary antioxidants act promoting their autooxidation, capturing the oxygen present in the medium through chemical reactions that stabilize the oxidizing agents, making them unavailable to act as propagators, being called secondary agents [121, 122].

As flavonoids are the substances that have been mostly studied, it is relevant to study in detail the mechanisms involved in their chemical interaction with reactive oxygen and nitrogen species generated during tissue exposure to radiation. Several studies indicate that there may be common patterns in the structure-activity relationship of flavonoids and that this activity is positively correlated with the rearrangement of functional groups linked to the main core of the compound [123], more precisely of the hydroxyl groups present [124], which due to their low reduction potential (0.23-0.75 V), are capable of yielding electrons to free radicals [125], resulting in a less reactive and more stable radical [126]. The reaction takes place as follows:

$$FLA\text{-}OH + R* > FLA\text{-}O* + RH$$

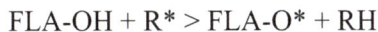

Where: FLA= Flavonoid, R*= free radical and O*= flavonoid free radical.

Furthermore, free radicals must have higher reduction potentials (2.3-1.0 V) than phenolic compounds, as this characteristic will enable the reduction and stabilization of the free radical and the oxidation of flavonoids [127]. Additionally, the flavonoids' ability to reduce free radicals is also generally associated with the number of hydroxyl groups present in their molecule [128].

The presence of hydroxyl groups can occur in the three rings of the flavonoid structure; however, it was observed that the replacement of the A ring has a lesser influence on the antioxidant activity of the flavonoids. The presence of hydroxyl groups in the ortho positions (positions 5 and 6) seems to be responsible for a greater activity than the presence of hydroxyl groups in the meta positions (positions 5 and 7) (Fig. **5**).

The configuration and number of hydroxyl groups present in the B ring are the main factors that impact the antioxidant activity of flavonoids against reactive oxygen and nitrogen species. Compounds with a dihydroxylated structure (catechol) in the B ring, such as the ortho or 3',4'-dihydroxylated, have a superior antioxidant activity due to their favorable reduction potential; when the B-ring flavonoid is monohydroxylated in the 4' position, it has weak antioxidant activity [129].

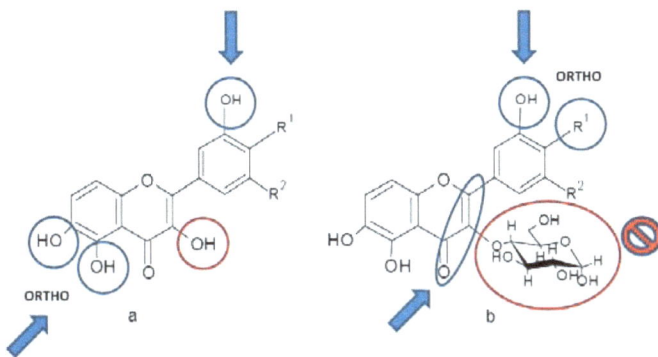

Fig. (5). Basic structures of the aglycone (**A**) and glycosylated (**B**) forms of the flavonoids with an indication of the main sites of antioxidant action. In ring A: Presence of hydroxyls in the ortho positions; Ring B: 1) presence of the free hydroxyl group at position 3; 2) Presence of dihydroxy (catechol) substitutions (preferably) in the ortho position; 3) Hydroxyl in position 3: main binding site with radical species, preferably in ortho position with another hydroxyl; the hydroxyl groups of ring B form hydrogen bonds with the hydroxyl at the 3-position of ring C; Ring C: 1) presence of a free hydroxyl group in free 3-position, allows delocalization of electrons 2) allow conjugation between aromatic rings; 3) presence of unsaturated 2–3 bond in conjunction with function 4-oxo, allows delocalization of electrons; 4) presence of glycosylation at position 3 reduces antioxidant capacity.

The angle of the B ring concerning the rest of the molecule, guided by the presence of the free hydroxyl group in position 3, positively influences the ability to reduce free radicals. Thus, flavonol compounds and flavanols with hydroxyls in position 3 are planar, while flavones and flavanones, without this grouping, have different conformations. This planarity allows for conjugation, and electronic delocalization, providing a corresponding increase in the stability of the flavonoid radical [123, 130]. The hydroxyl groups of ring B form hydrogen bonds with the hydroxyl in position 3 of ring C, aligning the three rings: B, heterocyclic and ring A). When the molecule is unable to form this hydrogen bond, the small twist of the B ring is compromised, compromising the ability to delocalize electrons [123].

The C, heterocyclic ring also contributes to antioxidant activity by the presence of a free hydroxyl group at position 3 and by allowing conjugation with aromatic rings, characteristics that seem to be determinant in flavonoids [130]. The formation of the C ring occurs from the closure of the chalcone structure, but the closure of the ring does not seem to be a determining factor, as chalcones have significant reducing potential. During flavonoid biosynthesis, chalcone isomers (cis and trans), known as 1,3-diphenyl-2-propen1-one, are common intermediates [131] (Fig. **5**).

Furthermore, another structural feature of the C ring, which is associated with the antioxidant activity of flavonoids, is the presence of the unsaturated 2–3 bond in conjunction with the 4-oxo functions. Several studies have sought to determine the importance of 2–3 unsaturation and the 4-carbonyl group [132]. Some works using catechins and anthocyanidins suggest that they may be unnecessary as long as other structural criteria are met. However, the conjugation of these two bonds allows a resonance effect of the aromatic nuclei that stabilizes the resulting flavonoid radical [133].

Aglycones are more potent antioxidants than their corresponding glycosides [134]. It has been demonstrated that the antioxidant activity increases with the increase in the number of hydroxyl groups in the molecule and decreases with the glycosylation of anthocyanidins, belonging to the flavonoid class [135]. Additionally, it has been suggested that the glycosylation of anthocyanins decreased the scavenging capacity of free radicals compared to the respective aglycone since it reduces the ability of the C ring to displace electrons [136]. In addition to the mere presence and total number, sugar position and structure play an important role due to the same steric blockage seen with O-methylations. Like methylation, O-glycosylation also interferes with the coplanarity of the B ring and, therefore, with the rest of the flavonoid, impacting its ability to displace electrons [137].

CONCLUDING REMARKS

The integrative review presents us with a set of information that can guide the continuity of studies of natural substances to treat the effects of radiation. Plants of the Family Lamiaceae were the most cited such as *Ocimum sanctum*, *Mentha piperita*, and *Coleus aromaticus*, considering reviews and experimental articles published. Nevertheless, it is worth mentioning that these plants are globally used, and there are still many unexplored families in tropical ecosystems. Among the plant metabolites, the flavonoid class represented the highest percentage of citations as expected, mainly because of its high antioxidant capacity and indicating the polar solvent extraction as the most promising method.

Studies of plant-based radiomodifiers have shown potential results in radioprotection or mitigation of undesirable effects of ionizing radiation on animal models. However, the radioprotection of these phytosubstances in humans depends on pharmacokinetic and bioavailability analyses. Studies of the pharmacokinetic properties of phytochemicals are limited. In order to increase their bioavailability and therapeutic efficacy the use of nanocrystal and encapsulation technologies has been applied to plant metabolites such as flavonoids. Futhermore, the establishment of an *in vivo* model system that allows proof of the efficacy of radioprotection in physiological tissues during radiotherapy and field application in cases of possible accidents, wars, or nuclear terrorism is mandatory.

CONSENT FOR PUBLICATION

Not applicable.

CONFLICT OF INTEREST

The authors confirm that this chapter's contents have no conflict of interest.

ACKNOWLEDGEMENTS

The authors acknowledge Fundação Carlos Chagas Filho de Amparo à Pesquisa do Estado do Rio de Janeiro (FAPERJ) for financial support and the staff of UEZO for insightful discussions and comments. The funders had no role in study design, data collection and analysis, decision to publish, or preparation of the manuscript.

REFERENCES

[1]   Edison Fears Hidden Perils of the X-rays. *New York World,* **1903**.https://web.archive.org/web/20110816170318/http://home.gwi.net/~dnb/read/edison/edison_xrays.h

[2]   Clarke, R.H.; Valentin, J. *The history of ICRP and the evolution of its policies.*, **2009**.
       [http://dx.doi.org/10.1016/j.icrp.2009.07.009]

[3]   Attix, F.H. *Introduction to radiological physics and radiation dosimetry*; J. Wileyand Son: New York,
       1986.
       [http://dx.doi.org/10.1002/9783527617135]

[4]   Frankel, R.I. Centennial of Röntgen's discovery of x-rays. *West. J. Med.*, **1996**, *164*(6), 497-501.
       [PMID: 8764624]

[5]   Becquerel, H. Emission des radiations nouvelles par l'uranium metallique. *C. R. Acad. Sci. Paris*,
       1896, *122*, 1086.

[6]   Curie, M. Rayonsemis par lescomposes de l'uranium et duthorium. *C. R. Acad. Sci. Paris*, **1896**, *126*,
       1101.

[7]   Walter, A.E. The medical, agricultural, and industrial applications of nuclear technology. *Global 2003:
       Atoms for Prosperity: Updating Eisenhowers Global Vision for Nuclear Energy*, **2003**, 22-33.

[8]   Kuntić, V.S.; Stanković, M.B.; Vujić, Z.B.; Brborić, J.S.; Uskoković-Marković, S.M. Radioprotectors
       - the evergreen topic. *Chem. Biodivers.*, **2013**, *10*(10), 1791-1803.
       [http://dx.doi.org/10.1002/cbdv.201300054] [PMID: 24130023]

[9]   Lachumy, S.J.; Oon, C.E.; Deivanai, S.; Saravanan, D.; Vijayarathna, S.; Choong, Y.S.; Yeng, C.;
       Latha, L.Y.; Sasidharan, S. Herbal remedies for combating irradiation: a green anti-irradiation
       approach. *Asian Pac. J. Cancer Prev.*, **2013**, *14*(10), 5553-5565.
       [http://dx.doi.org/10.7314/APJCP.2013.14.10.5553] [PMID: 24289545]

[10]   Neijenhuis, S.; Verwijs-Janssen, M.; Kasten-Pisula, U.; Rumping, G.; Borgmann, K.; Dikomey, E.;
       Begg, A.C.; Vens, C. Mechanism of cell killing after ionizing radiation by a dominant negative DNA
       polymerase beta. *DNA Repair (Amst.)*, **2009**, *8*(3), 336-346.
       [http://dx.doi.org/10.1016/j.dnarep.2008.11.008] [PMID: 19059500]

[11]   Nambiar, D.; Rajamani, P.; Singh, R.P. Effects of phytochemicals on ionization radiation-mediated
       carcinogenesis and cancer therapy. *Mutat. Res.*, **2011**, *728*(3), 139-157.
       [http://dx.doi.org/10.1016/j.mrrev.2011.07.005] [PMID: 22030216]

[12]   Riley, P.A. Free radicals in biology: oxidative stress and the effects of ionizing radiation. *Int. J.
       Radiat. Biol.*, **1994**, *65*(1), 27-33.
       [http://dx.doi.org/10.1080/09553009414550041] [PMID: 7905906]

[13]   LaVerne, J.A. OH radicals and oxidizing products in the gamma radiolysis of water. *Radiat. Res.*,
       2000, *153*(2), 196-200.
       [http://dx.doi.org/10.1667/0033-7587(2000)153[0196:ORAOPI]2.0.CO;2] [PMID: 10629619]

[14]   Vercesi, A.E.; Kowaltowski, A.J.; Grijalba, M.T.; Meinicke, A.R.; Castilho, R.F. The role of reactive
       oxygen species in mitochondrial permeability transition. *Biosci. Rep.*, **1997**, *17*(1), 43-52.
       [http://dx.doi.org/10.1023/A:1027335217774] [PMID: 9171920]

[15]   Leach, J.K.; Van Tuyle, G.; Lin, P.S.; Schmidt-Ullrich, R.; Mikkelsen, R.B. Ionizing radiation-
       induced, mitochondria-dependent generation of reactive oxygen/nitrogen. *Cancer Res.*, **2001**, *61*(10),
       3894-3901.
       [PMID: 11358802]

[16]   Yonei, S.; Furui, H. Lethal and mutagenic effects of malondialdehyde, a decomposition product of
       peroxidized lipids, on *Escherichia coli* with different DNA-repair capacities. *Mutat. Res.*, **1981**, *88*(1),
       23-32.
       [http://dx.doi.org/10.1016/0165-1218(81)90086-0] [PMID: 7010145]

[17]   Garrison, W.M.; Jayko, M.E.; Bennett, W. Radiation-induced oxidation of protein in aqueous solution.
       Radiat. Res., **1962**, *16*, 483-502.
       [http://dx.doi.org/10.2307/3571084] [PMID: 13897079]

[18] Garrison, W.M. Reaction-mechanisms in the radiolysis of peptides, polypeptides, and proteins. *Chem. Rev.,* **1987**, *87*(2), 381-398.
[http://dx.doi.org/10.1021/cr00078a006]

[19] Levine, R.L. Carbonyl modified proteins in cellular regulation, aging, and disease. *Free Radic. Biol. Med.,* **2002**, *32*(9), 790-796.
[http://dx.doi.org/10.1016/S0891-5849(02)00765-7] [PMID: 11978480]

[20] Wiseman, H.; Kaur, H.; Halliwell, B. DNA damage and cancer: measurement and mechanism. *Cancer Lett.,* **1995**, *93*(1), 113-120.
[http://dx.doi.org/10.1016/0304-3835(95)03792-U] [PMID: 7600538]

[21] Cadet, J.; Delatour, T.; Douki, T.; Gasparutto, D.; Pouget, J.P.; Ravanat, J.L.; Sauvaigo, S. Hydroxyl radicals and DNA base damage. *Mutat. Res.,* **1999**, *424*(1-2), 9-21.
[http://dx.doi.org/10.1016/S0027-5107(99)00004-4] [PMID: 10064846]

[22] Halliwell, B. Oxygen and nitrogen are pro-carcinogens. Damage to DNA by reactive oxygen, chlorine and nitrogen species: measurement, mechanism and the effects of nutrition. *Mutat. Res.,* **1999**, *443*(1-2), 37-52.
[http://dx.doi.org/10.1016/S1383-5742(99)00009-5] [PMID: 10415430]

[23] Chatgilialoglu, C.; O'Neill, P. Free radicals associated with DNA damage. *Exp. Gerontol.,* **2001**, *36*(9), 1459-1471.
[http://dx.doi.org/10.1016/S0531-5565(01)00132-2] [PMID: 11525869]

[24] Barreiros, A.L.B.S.; David, J.M.; David, J.P. Estresse oxidativo: relação entre geração de espécies reativas e defesa do organismo. *Quim. Nova,* **2006**, *29*(1), 113-123.
[http://dx.doi.org/10.1590/S0100-40422006000100021]

[25] Berger, P.; Leitner, N.K.V.; Doré, M.; Legube, B. Ozone and hydroxyl radicals induced oxidation of glycine. *Water Res.,* **1999**, *33*(2), 433-441.
[http://dx.doi.org/10.1016/S0043-1354(98)00230-9]

[26] Blair, I.A. Lipid hydroperoxide-mediated DNA damage. *Exp. Gerontol.,* **2001**, *36*(9), 1473-1481.
[http://dx.doi.org/10.1016/S0531-5565(01)00133-4] [PMID: 11525870]

[27] Halliwell, B.; Aeschbach, R.; Löliger, J.; Aruoma, O.I. The characterization of antioxidants. *Food Chem. Toxicol.,* **1995**, *33*(7), 601-617.
[http://dx.doi.org/10.1016/0278-6915(95)00024-V] [PMID: 7628797]

[28] Pietta, P.G. Flavonoids as antioxidants. *J. Nat. Prod.,* **2000**, *63*(7), 1035-1042.
[http://dx.doi.org/10.1021/np9904509] [PMID: 10924197]

[29] Finkel, T.; Holbrook, N.J. Oxidants, oxidative stress and the biology of ageing. *Nature,* **2000**, *408*(6809), 239-247.
[http://dx.doi.org/10.1038/35041687] [PMID: 11089981]

[30] Husain, S.R.; Cillard, J.; Cillard, P. Hydroxyl radical scavenging activity of flavonoids. *Phytochemistry,* **1987**, *26*(9), 2489-2491.
[http://dx.doi.org/10.1016/S0031-9422(00)83860-1]

[31] Okuno, E. Efeitos biológicos das radiações ionizantes: acidente radiológico de Goiânia. *Estud. Av.,* **2013**, *27*, 77.
[http://dx.doi.org/10.1590/S0103-40142013000100014]

[32] Dowd, S.B.; Tilson, E.R. *Practical Radiation Protection and Applied Radiobiology,* 2nd ed; Saunders: Philadelphia, PA, **1999**, pp. 118-120.

[33] Dörr, H.; Meineke, V. Acute radiation syndrome caused by accidental radiation exposure - therapeutic principles. *BMC Med.,* **2011**, *9*, 126.
[http://dx.doi.org/10.1186/1741-7015-9-126] [PMID: 22114866]

[34] Dainiak, N.; Waselenko, J.K.; Armitage, J.O.; MacVittie, T.J.; Farese, A.M. The hematologist and

radiation casualties. *Hematology (Am. Soc. Hematol. Educ. Program),* **2003**, *1,* 473-496.
[http://dx.doi.org/10.1182/asheducation-2003.1.473] [PMID: 14633795]

[35] Hall, E.J.; Giaccia, A.J. *Radiobiology for the Radiologist,* 6th ed; Lippincott Williams & Wilkins, **2006**, p. 656.

[36] Arora, R.; Chawla, R. Bioprospection for radioprotective molecules from indigenous flora. In: *Recent Progress in Medicinal Plants*; Govil, J.N.; Singh, V.K.; Bhardwaj, R., Eds.; Studium Press, LLC.: USA, **2006**; 16, pp. 179-219.

[37] Arora, R.; Chawla, R.; Singh, S.; Sagar, R.K.; Kumar, R.; Sharma, A.K.; Singh, S.; Prasad, J.; Sharma, R.K.; Tripathi, R.P. Radioprotection by Himalayan high–altitude region plants. In: *Herbal Drugs: A Twenty First Century Perspective*; Sharma, R.K.; Arora, R., Eds.; Jaypee Brothers Medical Publishers Private Ltd.: Delhi, India, **2006**; pp. 301-325.

[38] Sharma, R.K.; Arora, R. *Herbal drugs: a twenty first century perspective*; Jaypee Brothers Medical Publishers Private Ltd.: Delhi, India, **2006**, p. 688.
[http://dx.doi.org/10.5005/jp/books/10352]

[39] Stone, H.B.; Moulder, J.E.; Coleman, C.N.; Ang, K.K.; Anscher, M.S.; Barcellos-Hoff, M.H.; Dynan, W.S.; Fike, J.R.; Grdina, D.J.; Greenberger, J.S.; Hauer-Jensen, M.; Hill, R.P.; Kolesnick, R.N.; Macvittie, T.J.; Marks, C.; McBride, W.H.; Metting, N.; Pellmar, T.; Purucker, M.; Robbins, M.E.; Schiestl, R.H.; Seed, T.M.; Tomaszewski, J.E.; Travis, E.L.; Wallner, P.E.; Wolpert, M.; Zaharevitz, D. Models for evaluating agents intended for the prophylaxis, mitigation and treatment of radiation injuries. Report of an NCI Workshop, December 3-4, 2003. *Radiat. Res.,* **2004**, *162*(6), 711-728.https://doi-org.ez393.periodicos.capes.gov.br/10.1667/RR3276
[http://dx.doi.org/10.1667/RR3276] [PMID: 15548121]

[40] Dowlath, M.J.H.; Karuppannan, S.K.; Sinha, P.; Dowlath, N.S.; Arunachalam, K.D.; Ravindran, B.; Chang, S.W.; Nguyen-Tri, P.; Nguyen, D.D. Effects of radiation and role of plants in radioprotection: A critical review. *Sci. Total Environ.,* **2021**, *779,* 146431.
[http://dx.doi.org/10.1016/j.scitotenv.2021.146431] [PMID: 34030282]

[41] Urtasun, R.C. Chemical modifiers of radiation. In: *Text Book of Radiation Oncology*; Lieberl, S.A.; Phillips, T.L., Eds.; WB Saunders Company, Philadelphia: USA, **1998**; pp. 42-52.

[42] Bump, E.A.; Hoffman, S.J.; Foye, W.O. Radiosensitizers and radio-protective agents. In: *Burger's Medicinal Chemistry and Drug Discovery*; Abraham, D.J., Ed.; Chemotherapeutic Drugs. John Wiley and Sons. Inc: USA, **2003**; 5, pp. 151-211.

[43] Gong, L.; Zhang, Y.; Liu, C.; Zhang, M.; Han, S. Application of Radiosensitizers in Cancer Radiotherapy. *Int. J. Nanomedicine,* **2021**, *16,* 1083-1102.
[http://dx.doi.org/10.2147/IJN.S290438] [PMID: 33603370]

[44] Arora, R.; Gupta, D.; Chawla, R.; Sagar, R.; Sharma, A.; Kumar, R.; Prasad, J.; Singh, S.; Samanta, N.; Sharma, R.K. Radioprotection by plant products: present status and future prospects. *Phytother. Res.,* **2005**, *19*(1), 1-22.
[http://dx.doi.org/10.1002/ptr.1605] [PMID: 15799007]

[45] Arora, R.; Kumar, R.; Sharma, A.; Tripathi, R.P. *Herbals for Radiomodulation (Radioprotection/Radiosensitization): An Overview. In: Herbal Radiomodulators: Applications in Medicine, Homeland Defence and Space*; Arora, R. CABI Publishing: Wallingford, Oxon, UK, **2008**, pp. 1-22.

[46] Jaffee, E.M.; Dang, C.V.; Agus, D.B.; Alexander, B.M.; Anderson, K.C.; Ashworth, A.; Barker, A.D.; Bastani, R.; Bhatia, S.; Bluestone, J.A.; Brawley, O.; Butte, A.J.; Coit, D.G.; Davidson, N.E.; Davis, M.; DePinho, R.A.; Diasio, R.B.; Draetta, G.; Frazier, A.L.; Futreal, A.; Gambhir, S.S.; Ganz, P.A.; Garraway, L.; Gerson, S.; Gupta, S.; Heath, J.; Hoffman, R.I.; Hudis, C.; Hughes-Halbert, C.; Ibrahim, R.; Jadvar, H.; Kavanagh, B.; Kittles, R.; Le, Q.T.; Lippman, S.M.; Mankoff, D.; Mardis, E.R.; Mayer, D.K.; McMasters, K.; Meropol, N.J.; Mitchell, B.; Naredi, P.; Ornish, D.; Pawlik, T.M.; Peppercorn, J.; Pomper, M.G.; Raghavan, D.; Ritchie, C.; Schwarz, S.W.; Sullivan, R.; Wahl, R.; Wolchok, J.D.;

Wong, S.L.; Yung, A. Future cancer research priorities in the USA: a Lancet Oncology Commission. *Lancet Oncol.,* **2017**, *18*(11), e653-e706.
[http://dx.doi.org/10.1016/S1470-2045(17)30698-8] [PMID: 29208398]

[47]   Klement, A.W. *Handbook of Environmental Radiation*; CRC Press, **2019**.
[http://dx.doi.org/10.1201/9781351073028]

[48]   Patt, H.M.; Tyree, E.B.; Straube, R.L.; Smith, D.E. Cysteine protection against X-irradiation. *Science,* **1949**, *110*(2852), 213-214.
[http://dx.doi.org/10.1126/science.110.2852.213] [PMID: 17811258]

[49]   Bump, E.A.; Malaker, K. *Radioprotectors: Chemical, Biological and Clinical Perspective*; CRC Press: Boca Raton, Florida, **1998**.

[50]   Nair, C.K.K.; Parida, D.K.; Nomura, T. Radioprotectors in radiotherapy. *J. Radiat. Res. (Tokyo),* **2001**, *42*(1), 21-37.
[http://dx.doi.org/10.1269/jrr.42.21] [PMID: 11393887]

[51]   Coleman, C.N.; Blakely, W.F.; Fike, J.R.; MacVittie, T.J.; Metting, N.F.; Mitchell, J.B.; Moulder, J.E.; Preston, R.J.; Seed, T.M.; Stone, H.B.; Tofilon, P.J.; Wong, R.S.L. Molecular and cellular biology of moderate-dose (1-10 Gy) radiation and potential mechanisms of radiation protection: report of a workshop at Bethesda, Maryland, December 17-18, 2001. *Radiat. Res.,* **2003**, *159*(6), 812-834.
[http://dx.doi.org/10.1667/RR3021] [PMID: 12751965]

[52]   Arora, R. Biological Radioprotection: A Phytochemical Perspective. *Proceedings of the Continuing Education Programme on Phytochemistry,* **2007**, , pp. 19-37.

[53]   Sweeney, T.R. *A Survey of Compounds from the Antiradiation Drug Development Program of the US Army Medical Research and Development Command*; Walter Reed Army Institute of Research: Washington, DC, USA, **1979**.

[54]   Giambarresi, L.; Jacobs, A.J. Radioprotectants. In: *Military Radiobiology*; Conklin, J.J.; Walker, R.I., Eds.; Academic Press, Inc: London, **1987**; pp. 265-301.

[55]   Weiss, J.F.; Simic, M.G. Introduction: Perspectives in radioprotection. *Pharmacol. Ther.,* **1988**, *39*(1-3), 1-2.
[http://dx.doi.org/10.1016/0163-7258(88)90031-9] [PMID: 3200882]

[56]   Capizzi, R.L.; Oster, W. Protection of normal tissue from the cytotoxic effects of chemotherapy and radiation by amifostine: clinical experiences. *Eur. J. Cancer,* **1995**, *31A*(1) Suppl. 1, S8-S13.
[http://dx.doi.org/10.1016/0959-8049(95)00144-8] [PMID: 7577096]

[57]   Jeong, M.H.; Park, Y.S.; Jeong, D.H.; Lee, C.G.; Kim, J.S.; Oh, S.J.; Jeong, S.K.; Yang, K.; Jo, W.S. *In vitro* evaluation of Cordyceps militaris as a potential radioprotective agent. *Int. J. Mol. Med.,* **2014**, *34*(5), 1349-1357.
[http://dx.doi.org/10.3892/ijmm.2014.1901] [PMID: 25176413]

[58]   Barlas, A.M.; Sadic, M.; Atilgan, H.I.; Bag, Y.M.; Onalan, A.K.; Yumusak, N.; Senes, M.; Fidanci, V.; Pekcici, M.R.; Korkmaz, M.; Kismet, K.; Koca, G. Melatonin: a hepatoprotective agent against radioiodine toxicity in rats. *Bratisl. Lek Listy,* **2017**, *118*(2), 95-100.
[http://dx.doi.org/10.4149/BLL_2017_020] [PMID: 28814090]

[59]   Kadivar, F.; Haddadi, G.; Mosleh-Shirazi, M.A.; Khajeh, F.; Tavasoli, A. Protection effect of cerium oxide nanoparticles against radiation-induced acute lung injuries in rats. *Rep. Pract. Oncol. Radiother.,* **2020**, *25*(2), 206-211.
[http://dx.doi.org/10.1016/j.rpor.2019.12.023] [PMID: 32194345]

[60]   Vesna, J.; Danica, J.; Kamil, K.; Viktorija, D-S.; Silva, D.; Sanja, T.; Ivana, B.; Zoran, S.; Zoran, M.; Dubravko, B.; Aleksandar, D. Effects of fullerenol nanoparticles and amifostine on radiation-induced tissue damages: histopathological analysis. *J. Appl. Biomed.,* **2016**, *14*(4), 285-297.
[http://dx.doi.org/10.1016/j.jab.2016.05.004]

[61]   Xie, J.; Wang, C.; Zhao, F.; Gu, Z.; Zhao, Y. *Application of multifunctional nanomaterials in*

radioprotection of healthy tissues; Wiley Online Library, **2018**.
[http://dx.doi.org/10.1002/adhm.201800421]

[62]   Aalapati, S.; Ganapathy, S.; Manapuram, S.; Anumolu, G.; Prakya, B.M. Toxicity and bio-accumulation of inhaled cerium oxide nanoparticles in CD1 mice. *Nanotoxicology,* **2014**, *8*(7), 786-798.
[http://dx.doi.org/10.3109/17435390.2013.829877] [PMID: 23914771]

[63]   Rice, K.M.; Nalabotu, S.K.; Manne, N.D.P.K.; Kolli, M.B.; Nandyala, G.; Arvapalli, R.; Ma, J.Y.; Blough, E.R. Exposure to cerium oxide nanoparticles is associated with activation of mitogen-activated protein kinases signaling and apoptosis in rat lungs. *J. Prev. Med. Public Health,* **2015**, *48*(3), 132-141.
[http://dx.doi.org/10.3961/jpmph.15.006] [PMID: 26081650]

[64]   Cheki, M.; Mihandoost, E.; Shirazi, A.; Mahmoudzadeh, A. Prophylactic role of some plants and phytochemicals against radio-genotoxicity in human lymphocytes. *J. Cancer Res. Ther.,* **2016**, *12*(4), 1234-1242.
[http://dx.doi.org/10.4103/0973-1482.172131] [PMID: 28169233]

[65]   Wang, C.Z.; Calway, T.; Yuan, C.S. Herbal medicines as adjuvants for cancer therapeutics. *Am. J. Chin. Med.,* **2012**, *40*(4), 657-669.
[http://dx.doi.org/10.1142/S0192415X12500498] [PMID: 22809022]

[66]   Oyebode, O.; Kandala, N.B.; Chilton, P.J.; Lilford, R.J. Use of traditional medicine in middle-income countries: a WHO-SAGE study. *Health Policy Plan.,* **2016**, *31*(8), 984-991.
[http://dx.doi.org/10.1093/heapol/czw022] [PMID: 27033366]

[67]   Karupannan, S.K.; Dowlath, M.J.H.; Arunachalam, K.D. Phytonanotechnology: Challenges and future perspectives. In: *Phytonanotechnology Challenges and Prospects*; Thajuddin, N.; Mathew, S., Eds.; Elsevier Science Publishing Co Inc, **2020**; p. 354.

[68]   Emerit, I.; Oganesian, N.; Sarkisian, T.; Arutyunyan, R.; Pogosian, A.; Asrian, K.; Levy, A.; Cernjavski, L. Clastogenic factors in the plasma of Chernobyl accident recovery workers: anticlastogenic effect of Ginkgo biloba extract. *Radiat. Res.,* **1995**, *144*(2), 198-205.
[http://dx.doi.org/10.2307/3579259] [PMID: 7480646]

[69]   Emerit, I.; Oganesian, N.; Arutyunian, R.; Pogossian, A.; Sarkisian, T.; Cernjavski, L.; Levy, A.; Feingold, J. Oxidative stress-related clastogenic factors in plasma from Chernobyl liquidators: protective effects of antioxidant plant phenols, vitamins and oligoelements. *Mutat. Res.,* **1997**, *377*(2), 239-246.
[http://dx.doi.org/10.1016/S0027-5107(97)00080-8] [PMID: 9247620]

[70]   Nagano, J.; Kono, S.; Preston, D.L.; Moriwaki, H.; Sharp, G.B.; Koyama, K.; Mabuchi, K. Bladder-cancer incidence in relation to vegetable and fruit consumption: a prospective study of atomic-bomb survivors. *Int. J. Cancer,* **2000**, *86*, 132-138.
[http://dx.doi.org/10.1002/(SICI)1097-0215(20000401)86:1<132::AID-IJC21>3.0.CO;2-M]

[71]   Atanasov, A.G.; Waltenberger, B.; Pferschy-Wenzig, E-M.; Linder, T.; Wawrosch, C.; Uhrin, P.; Temml, V.; Wang, L.; Schwaiger, S.; Heiss, E.H.; Rollinger, J.M.; Schuster, D.; Breuss, J.M.; Bochkov, V.; Mihovilovic, M.D.; Kopp, B.; Bauer, R.; Dirsch, V.M.; Stuppner, H. Discovery and resupply of pharmacologically active plant-derived natural products: A review. *Biotechnol. Adv.,* **2015**, *33*(8), 1582-1614.
[http://dx.doi.org/10.1016/j.biotechadv.2015.08.001] [PMID: 26281720]

[72]   Srinivasan, M.; Rajendra Prasad, N.; Menon, V.P.; Menon, V.P. Protective effect of curcumin on γ-radiation induced DNA damage and lipid peroxidation in cultured human lymphocytes. *Mutat. Res.,* **2006**, *611*(1-2), 96-103.
[http://dx.doi.org/10.1016/j.mrgentox.2006.07.002] [PMID: 16973408]

[73]   Zhou, Z.; Huang, Y.; Liang, J.; Ou, M.; Chen, J.; Li, G. Extraction, purification and anti-radiation activity of persimmon tannin from *Diospyros kaki* L.f. *J. Environ. Radioact.,* **2016**, *162-163*, 182-188.

[http://dx.doi.org/10.1016/j.jenvrad.2016.05.034] [PMID: 27267156]

[74] Kim, H.G.; Jang, S.S.; Lee, J.S.; Kim, H.S.; Son, C.G. *Panax ginseng* Meyer prevents radiation-induced liver injury via modulation of oxidative stress and apoptosis. *J. Ginseng Res.,* **2017**, *41*(2), 159-168.
[http://dx.doi.org/10.1016/j.jgr.2016.02.006] [PMID: 28413320]

[75] Sinha, P.; Arunachalam, K.D.; Annamalai, S.K. Radio-protective dosimetry of Pangasius sutchi as a biomarker, against gamma radiation dosages perceived by genotoxic assays. *Ecotoxicol. Environ. Saf.,* **2018**, *164*, 629-640.
[http://dx.doi.org/10.1016/j.ecoenv.2018.08.071] [PMID: 30165340]

[76] Sayed, D.F.; Nada, A.S.; Abd El Hameed Mohamed, M.; Ibrahim, M.T. Modulatory effects of Chrysophyllum cainito L. extract on gamma radiation induced oxidative stress in rats. *Biomed. Pharmacother.,* **2019**, *111*, 613-623.
[http://dx.doi.org/10.1016/j.biopha.2018.12.137] [PMID: 30611985]

[77] Rafati, M.; Ghasemi, A.; Saeedi, M.; Habibi, E.; Salehifar, E.; Mosazadeh, M.; Maham, M. Nigella sativa L. for prevention of acute radiation dermatitis in breast cancer: A randomized, double-blind, placebo-controlled, clinical trial. *Complement. Ther. Med.,* **2019**, *47*, 102205.
[http://dx.doi.org/10.1016/j.ctim.2019.102205] [PMID: 31780017]

[78] Victório, C.P.; Lage, C.L.S. Uso de plantas medicinais. Revista Arquivos FOG – Saúde, Sociedade. *Gestão e Meio Ambiente,* **2008**, *5*(1), 33-41.

[79] Heinrich, M. Ethnopharmacology: quo vadis? Challenges for the future. *Rev. Bras. Farmacogn.,* **2014**, *24*, 99-102.
[http://dx.doi.org/10.1016/j.bjp.2013.11.019]

[80] Gottlieb, O.R. Ethnopharmacology versus chemosystematics in the search for biologically active principles in plants. *J. Ethnopharmacol.,* **1982**, *6*(2), 227-238.
[http://dx.doi.org/10.1016/0378-8741(82)90005-8] [PMID: 6127441]

[81] Zidorn, C. Plant chemophenetics - A new term for plant chemosystematics/plant chemotaxonomy in the macro-molecular era. *Phytochemistry,* **2019**, *163*, 147-148.
[http://dx.doi.org/10.1016/j.phytochem.2019.02.013] [PMID: 30846237]

[82] Zappi, D.C. Growing knowledge: an overview of Seed Plant diversity in Brazil. *Rodriguésia,* **2015**, *66*(4), 1085-1113.
[http://dx.doi.org/10.1590/2175-7860201566411]

[83] Chang, H-M.; But, P.P-H. *Pharmacology and Applications of Chinese Materia Medica*; Word Scientific Publ: Singapore, **1987**, p. 2, 740.
[http://dx.doi.org/10.1142/0284]

[84] Lin, Y.; Lou, K.; Wu, G.; Wu, X.; Zhou, X.; Feng, Y.; Zhang, H.; Yu, P. Bioactive metabolites in of *Ginkgo biloba* leaves: variations by seasonal, meteorological and soil. *Braz. J. Biol.,* **2020**, *80*(4), 790-797.
[http://dx.doi.org/10.1590/1519-6984.220519] [PMID: 31800764]

[85] Okumus, S.; Taysi, S.; Orkmez, M.; Saricicek, E.; Demir, E.; Adli, M.; Al, B. The effects of oral *Ginkgo biloba* supplementation on radiation-induced oxidative injury in the lens of rat. *Pharmacogn. Mag.,* **2011**, *7*(26), 141-145.
[http://dx.doi.org/10.4103/0973-1296.80673] [PMID: 21716624]

[86] Baliga, M.S.; Jimmy, R.; Thilakchand, K.R.; Sunitha, V.; Bhat, N.R.; Saldanha, E.; Rao, S.; Rao, P.; Arora, R.; Palatty, P.L. *Ocimum sanctum* L (Holy Basil or Tulsi) and its phytochemicals in the prevention and treatment of cancer. *Nutr. Cancer,* **2013**, *65* Suppl. 1, 26-35.
[http://dx.doi.org/10.1080/01635581.2013.785010] [PMID: 23682780]

[87] Kma, L. Plant extracts and plant-derived compounds: promising players in a countermeasure strategy against radiological exposure. *Asian Pac. J. Cancer Prev.,* **2014**, *15*(6), 2405-2425.

[http://dx.doi.org/10.7314/APJCP.2014.15.6.2405] [PMID: 24761841]

[88] Mahendran, G.; Rahman, L.U. Ethnomedicinal, phytochemical and pharmacological updates on Peppermint (Mentha × piperita L.)-A review. *Phytother. Res., 2020, 34*(9), 2088-2139.
[http://dx.doi.org/10.1002/ptr.6664] [PMID: 32173933]

[89] Boix, Y.F.; Victório, C.P.; Defaveri, A.C.A.; Arruda, R.C.O.; Sato, A.; Lage, C.L.S. Glandular trichomes of *Rosmarinus officinalis* L.: anatomical and phytochemical analyses of leaf volatiles. *Plant Biosyst., 2011, 145*(4), 1-9.
[http://dx.doi.org/10.1080/11263504.2011.584075]

[90] Hajdari, A.; Mustafa, B.; Hyseni, L.; Bajrami, A.; Mustafa, G.; Quave, C.L.; Nebija, D. Phytochemical study of eight medicinal plants of the Lamiaceae family traditionally used as tea in the sharri mountains region of the Balkans. *ScientificWorldJournal, 2020, 2020*, 4182064.
[http://dx.doi.org/10.1155/2020/4182064] [PMID: 32148465]

[91] Baliga, M.S.; Haniadka, R.; Pereira, M.M.; Thilakchand, K.R.; Rao, S.; Arora, R. Radioprotective effects of *Zingiber officinale* Roscoe (ginger): past, present and future. *Food Funct., 2012, 3*(7), 714-723.
[http://dx.doi.org/10.1039/c2fo10225k] [PMID: 22596078]

[92] Pancharoen, O.; Prawat, U.; Tuntiwachwuttikul, P. Phytochemistry of the zingiberaceae. *Studies in Natural Products Chemistry, 2000, 2000*, 797-865.
[http://dx.doi.org/10.1016/S1572-5995(00)80142-8]

[93] Victório, C.P. Therapeutic value of the genus *Alpinia*, Zingiberaceae. *Brazilian Journal of Pharmacognosy, 2011, 21*(1), 194-201.
[http://dx.doi.org/10.1590/S0102-695X2011005000025]

[94] Samarth, R.M.; Samarth, M.; Matsumoto, Y. Medicinally important aromatic plants with radioprotective activity. *Future Sci. OA, 2017, 3*(4), FSO247.
[http://dx.doi.org/10.4155/fsoa-2017-0061] [PMID: 29134131]

[95] Kariuki, J.M.; Horemans, N.; Saenen, E.; Van Hees, M.; Verhoeven, M.; Nauts, R.; Van Gompel, A.; Wannijn, J.; Cuypers, A. The responses and recovery after gamma irradiation are highly dependent on leaf age at the time of exposure in rice (*Oryza sativa* L.). *Environ. Exp. Bot., 2019, 162*, 157-167.
[http://dx.doi.org/10.1016/j.envexpbot.2019.02.020]

[96] Jamil, M.; Anwar, F. Properties, health benefits and medicinal uses of *Oryza sativa. European Journal of Biological Sciences, 2016, 8*(4), 136-141.

[97] Ghasemzadeh, A.; Karbalaii, MT; Jaafar, HZE; Rahmat, A. Phytochemical constituents, antioxidant activity, and antiproliferative properties of black, red, and brown rice bran. *Chem Cent J, 2018, 17;12*(1), 17.
[http://dx.doi.org/10.1186/s13065-018-0382-9]

[98] Baliga, M.S.; Meera, S.; Mathai, B.; Rai, M.P.; Pawar, V.; Palatty, P.L. Scientific validation of the ethnomedicinal properties of the Ayurvedic drug Triphala: a review. *Chin. J. Integr. Med., 2012, 18*(12), 946-954.
[http://dx.doi.org/10.1007/s11655-012-1299-x] [PMID: 23239004]

[99] Canuto, G.A.B. da Costa JL, da Cruz PLR, de Souza ARL, Faccio AT, Klassen A, Rodrigues KT, Tavares MFM. Metabolômica: definições, estado-da-arte e aplicações representativas. *Quim. Nova, 2018, 41*(1), 75-91.
[http://dx.doi.org/10.21577/0100-4042.20170134]

[100] Mun, G.I.; Kim, S.; Choi, E.; Kim, C.S.; Lee, Y.S. Pharmacology of natural radioprotectors. *Arch. Pharm. Res., 2018, 41*(11), 1033-1050.
[http://dx.doi.org/10.1007/s12272-018-1083-6] [PMID: 30361949]

[101] Madan, R. Radiosensitizers and radioprotectors. , *2020*.
[http://dx.doi.org/10.1007/978-981-15-0073-2_29]

[102] Singh, V.K.; Seed, T.M. The efficacy and safety of amifostine for the acute radiation syndrome. *Expert Opin. Drug Saf.,* **2019**, *18*(11), 1077-1090.
[http://dx.doi.org/10.1080/14740338.2019.1666104] [PMID: 31526195]

[103] Tiwari, D.K.; Deen, B. Prepration and storage of blended ready-to-serve beverage from bael and Aloe vera. *Bioscan,* **2015**, *10*(1), 113-116.

[104] Lapornik, B.; Prosek, M.; Wondra, A.G. Comparison of extracts prepared from plant by-products using different solvents and extraction time. *Journal of Food Engineering, Essex,* **2005**, *2*(71), 214-222.
[http://dx.doi.org/10.1016/j.jfoodeng.2004.10.036]

[105] Angelo, P.M.; Jorge, N. Antioxidantes na turais: técnicas de extração. *B.CEPPA,* **2006**, *24*(2), 319-336.

[106] Pokorny, J.; Korczak, J. Preparation of Natural antioxidants. In: *Yanishlieva, N.; Gordon, M. Antioxidants in food: practical applications*; Pokorny, J., Ed.; CRC Press: New York, **2001**; pp. 311-330.
[http://dx.doi.org/10.1016/9781855736160.4.311]

[107] Angelo, P.M.; Jorge, N. Compostos fenólicos em alimentos – Uma breve revisão. *Rev. Inst. Adolfo Lutz,* **2007**, *66*(1), 1-9.

[108] Vongsak, B.; Sithisarna, P.; Mangmool, S.; Thongpraditchotec, S.; Wongkrajangc, Y.; Gritsanapana, W. Maximizing total phenolics, total flavonoids contents and antioxidant activity of Moringa oleifera leaf extract by the appropriate extraction method. *Ind. Crops Prod.,* **2013**, *44*, 566-571.
[http://dx.doi.org/10.1016/j.indcrop.2012.09.021]

[109] Oliveira, V.B.; Zuchetto, M.; Oliveira, C.F.; Paula, C.S.; Duarte, A.F.S.; Miguel, M.D.; Miguel, O.G. Efeito de diferentes técnicas extrativas no rendimento, atividade antioxidante, doseamentos totais e no perfil por CLAE-DAD de dicksonia sellowiana (presl.). Hook, dicksoniaceae. *Revista Brasileira. Pl. Med,* **2016**, *18*(1) Suppl. I, 230-239.

[110] Terci, D.B.L. *Aplicações analíticas e didáticas de antocianinas extraídas de frutas*; 224f. PHD Thesis: Universidade Estadual de Campinas, Campinas, São Paulo, **2004**.

[111] Casanova, L.M.; Costa, S.S. Interações Sinérgicas em Produtos Naturais: Potencial Terapêutico e Desafios. *Rev. Virtual Quimica,* **2017**, *9*(2), 575-595.
[http://dx.doi.org/10.21577/1984-6835.20170034]

[112] Randhir, R.; Lin, Y.; Shetty, K. Stimulation of phenolics, antioxidant and antimicrobial activities in dark germinated mung bean sprouts in response to peptide and phytochemical elicitors. *Process Biochem.,* **2004**, *39*(5), 637-646.
[http://dx.doi.org/10.1016/S0032-9592(03)00197-3]

[113] Shaidi, F.; Naczk, M. *Food phenolics: sources, chemistry, effects and applications*; Technomic Publishing: Lancaster, **1995**, pp. 281-319.

[114] Soares, S.E. Ácidos fenólicos como antioxidantes. *Rev. Nutr.,* **2002**, *15*(1), 71-81.
[http://dx.doi.org/10.1590/S1415-52732002000100008]

[115] King, A.; Young, G. Characteristics and occurrence of phenolic phytochemicals. *J. Am. Diet. Assoc.,* **1999**, *99*(2), 213-218.
[http://dx.doi.org/10.1016/S0002-8223(99)00051-6] [PMID: 9972191]

[116] Walton, M.C. *Berry Fruit.,* **2006**.

[117] Imran, M.; Ghorat, F.; Ul-Haq, I.; Ur-Rehman, H.; Aslam, F.; Heydari, M.; Shariati, M.A.; Okuskhanova, E.; Yessimbekov, Z.; Thiruvengadam, M.; Hashempur, M.H.; Rebezov, M. Lycopene as a Natural Antioxidant Used to Prevent Human Health Disorders. *Antioxidants,* **2020**, *9*(8), 706.
[http://dx.doi.org/10.3390/antiox9080706] [PMID: 32759751]

[118] Santiago, M.C.P. A. *Avaliação de processos para obtenção de produtos ricos em antocianinas*

utilizando suco de romã (Punica granatum L.); PhD Thesis.: Universidade Federal do rio de Janeiro, Escola de Quimica, Rio de Janeiro, **2014**.

[119] He, J.; Giusti, M.M. Anthocyanins: natural colorants with health-promoting properties. *Annu. Rev. Food Sci. Technol.*, **2010**, *1*, 163-187.
[http://dx.doi.org/10.1146/annurev.food.080708.100754] [PMID: 22129334]

[120] Ingold, K.U. *Inhibition of autoxidation.in Oxidation of Organic Compounds*; American chemical society, ACS Publications: New Orleans, LA, **1999**, pp. 22-26.

[121] Gordon, M.H. The mechanism of antioxidant action *in vitro*. In: *Food antioxidants*; Hudson, B.J.F., Ed.; Elsevier Applied Science: London, **1990**; pp. 1-18.

[122] Rojita, M.; Bisht, S.S. Antioxidants and their charecterization. *J. Pharm. Res.*, **2011**, *4*(8), 2744-2746.

[123] Heim, K.E.; Tagliaferro, A.R.; Bobilya, D.J. Flavonoid antioxidants: chemistry, metabolism and structure-activity relationships. *J. Nutr. Biochem.*, **2002**, *13*(10), 572-584.
[http://dx.doi.org/10.1016/S0955-2863(02)00208-5] [PMID: 12550068]

[124] Haenen, G.R.; Paquay, J.B.; Korthouwer, R.E.; Bast, A. Peroxynitrite scavenging by flavonoids. *Biochem. Biophys. Res. Commun.*, **1997**, *236*(3), 591-593.
[http://dx.doi.org/10.1006/bbrc.1997.7016] [PMID: 9245694]

[125] Rice-Evans, C.A.; Miller, N.J.; Paganga, G. Structure-antioxidant activity relationships of flavonoids and phenolic acids. *Free Radic. Biol. Med.*, **1996**, *20*(7), 933-956.
[http://dx.doi.org/10.1016/0891-5849(95)02227-9] [PMID: 8743980]

[126] Gouvêa. Quantificação das antocianinas majoritárias do açaí por cromatografia líquida de alta eficiência. In: *Dissertation*; Universidade Federal Rural do Rio de Janeiro: Seropédica, **2010**.

[127] Lien, E.J.; Ren, S.; Bui, H.H.; Wang, R. Quantitative structure-activity relationship analysis of phenolic antioxidants. *Free Radic. Biol. Med.*, **1999**, *26*(3-4), 285-294.
[http://dx.doi.org/10.1016/S0891-5849(98)00190-7] [PMID: 9895218]

[128] Sroka, Z.; Cisowski, W. Hydrogen peroxide scavenging, antioxidant and anti-radical activity of some phenolic acids. *Food Chem. Toxicol.*, **2003**, *41*(6), 753-758.
[http://dx.doi.org/10.1016/S0278-6915(02)00329-0] [PMID: 12738180]

[129] Correia, H.S.N. Agrimonia eupatoria L. e Equisetum telmateia Ehrh. In: *Perfil Polifenólico e Capacidade de Captação de Espécies Reactivas de Oxigénio. Dissertation*; Coimbra University: Coimbra, **2005**.

[130] Sichel, G.; Corsaro, C.; Scalia, M.; Di Bilio, A.J.; Bonomo, R.P. *In vitro* scavenger activity of some flavonoids and melanins against O2-(.). *Free Radic. Biol. Med.*, **1991**, *11*(1), 1-8.
[http://dx.doi.org/10.1016/0891-5849(91)90181-2] [PMID: 1657731]

[131] Ferreira, M.K.A.; Fontenelle, R.O.S.; Magalhães, F.E.A.; Bandeira, P.N. S.; Menezes, J. E. S. A.; Dos Santos, H. Potencial Farmacológico de Chalconas: Uma Breve Revisão. *Rev. Virtual Quimica*, **2018**, *10*, 1455-1473.

[132] Harborne, J.B.; Williams, C.A. Advances in flavonoid research since 1992. *Phytochemistry*, **2000**, *55*(6), 481-504.
[http://dx.doi.org/10.1016/S0031-9422(00)00235-1] [PMID: 11130659]

[133] Richter, C. Biophysical consequences of lipid peroxidation in membranes. *Chem. Phys. Lipids*, **1987**, *44*(2-4), 175-189.
[http://dx.doi.org/10.1016/0009-3084(87)90049-1] [PMID: 3311416]

[134] Ratty, A.K.; Das, N.P. Efeitos dos flavonóides na peroxidação lipídica não enzimática: relação estrutura-atividade. *Biochem Med Metab Biol*, 1988, 39, 69 – 79. 135. 135. Fukumoto, L R.; Mazza, G. Assessing antioxidant and prooxidant activities of phenolic compounds. *J. Agric. Food Chem.*, **2000**, *8*(48), 3597-3604.

[136] Fernandes, I.; de Freitas, V.; Reis, C.; Mateus, N. A new approach on the gastric absorption of

anthocyanins. *Food Funct.,* **2012**, *3*(5), 508-516.
[http://dx.doi.org/10.1039/c2fo10295a] [PMID: 22391951]

[137] Bors, W.; Heller, W. MICHEL, C.; SARAN, M. Flavonóides como antioxidantes: determinação das eficiências de eliminação de radicais. *Methods Enzymol.,* **1990**, *186*, 343-355.
[http://dx.doi.org/10.1016/0076-6879(90)86128-I] [PMID: 2172711]

CHAPTER 5

Chemical Perspective and Drawbacks in Flavonoid Estimation Assays

Denni Mammen[1,*]

[1] *Division of Chemistry, School of Science, Navrachana University, Vasana-Bhayli Road, Vadodara, India*

Abstract: Colorimetric or spectrophotometric methods have been used over the past few decades for rapid and convenient estimation of certain classes of flavonoids in fruits, vegetables, grains, raw herbal material, herbal formulations, and nutraceuticals. This has resulted in a surge in the numbers of research articles discussing the use of these methods for comparison between numbers of samples of the same kind, such as analysis to find differences between various tea samples, food articles, raw drug powders, *etc*. However, these methods are not selective since several factors influence color development. Also, the reagents used to form the colored complex are not specific to a certain class of compounds. There are studies performed where all compounds belonging to a particular class do not react uniformly to the reagents used in the method. Chelation using $AlCl_3$ was used to develop deep yellow-colored complexes of the flavonoids and absorbance was subsequently measured at 420 nm, using quercetin as the standard. In a modification, potassium acetate was added after the addition of $AlCl_3$, and the absorbance was measured at 415 nm, again against standard quercetin solutions, wherein only flavones and flavonols were estimated. A study conducted by our team proves that all flavonoids do not form complexes that absorb at 420 nm, and each flavonoid shows variation in absorption maxima. Only flavonoids with *o*-dihydroxy systems show good results, while others absorb at either higher or lower wavelengths. This research work has been one of the top 20 most downloaded articles in flavonoid chemistry since its date of publication. Catechins, flavanones, and anthocyanins cannot be estimated using this method, due to either inability to bind with $AlCl_3$ in an appropriate manner or due to differences in absorption maxima of the complex formed. Flavanones like naringenin, naringin, and hesperidin have been estimated using the 2,4-dinitrophenyl hydrazine method. The method does not work for flavonols and flavones. Estimation of catechins in tea samples has been described where caffeine is removed from solution using extraction by chloroform, and the absorbance of the aqueous phase is taken at 274 nm. The technique however is flawed since the aqueous extract will also contain phenolic acids like gallic, protocatechuic, and syringic acids, and a good amount of flavonols such as quercetin and kaempferol, which also absorb around 274 nm. These phenolic acids and

---

[*] **Corresponding author Denni Mammen:** Division of Chemistry, School of Science, Navrachana University, Vasana-Bhayli Road, Vadodara, India; Tel: +91-8980294648; E-mail: drdenni.mammen@gmail.com

Atta-ur-Rahman (Ed.)

flavonols need to be removed before the estimation of catechins. The reaction of flavanols like catechin and epicatechin with vanillin in presence of H_2SO_4 yields red-colored complexes that show absorptions around 500 nm, but certain matrices interferences of proanthocyanins. Many flavonoid compounds occur in the form of glycosides, where the presence of sugar molecules like glucose, rhamnose, galactose, *etc.* can hamper complex formation responsible for color development. The effect of hydrolysis can yield better results to remove the sugar moieties, and the aglycones can be estimated. Another widely used method is the Folin-Ciocalteu method for estimation of phenolics, developed by Folin and Denis in 1915, and modified by Singleton and Rossi in 1965, where a blue-colored complex due to reduction of molybdenum by phenolate ions formed in a basic medium. One major drawback of this method is that the absorption maxima of the complex formed varies between 620 and 765 nm. Studies also confirm that this assay is not specific to only phenolics, but can also react to interferences of ascorbic acid, reducing sugars, certain metals, amino acids, and reducing agents like $NaHSO_3$. Most results published in thousands of research papers worldwide are erroneous due to a lack of knowledge of the actual chemical reactions taking place in the estimation methods, and how the flavonoids react with the reagents.

Keywords: $AlCl_3$ chelation, Anthocyanins, Flavones, Flavonols, Flavanols, Flavanones, Folin-Ciocalteau, UV-Vis Spectrophotometry.

INTRODUCTION

Plant pigments derived from benzo-γ-pyran are collectively known as flavonoids, which are synthesized using the phenylpropanoid pathway. The first flavonoid was isolated from oranges in 1930 but was initially considered a new class of vitamins, and later identified as the flavonoid rutin [1]. Biosynthesis of flavonoids can take place in most plant cells, with the amino acid phenylalanine as the precursor. The C_6-C_3 system arises due to de-amination of the phenylalanine precursor, in the phenylpropanoid pathway. These phenylpropanoids are key agents that help in interaction with microbes and insects, attracting pollinators, defense against infection, induction of root nodulation by rhizobia leading to symbiotic nitrogen fixation [2]. Flavonoids have a wide spectrum of functions such as protection from UV light, plant defense, as well as the coloration of flowers, fruits, and other plant parts [3]. Since they are pigments, representing all colors of the spectrum, their electronic properties are correlated with the capture and transfer of energy in plants. These properties are also said to have notable roles in their selectivity in biological systems [4]. The fluorescent property of flavonoids can also help in transferring energy to activate light-sensitive pigments which are associated with light-sensitive genes [5].

Flavonoids are categorized into six major subclasses based on their chemical structures, namely, flavones, flavonols, anthocyanins, flavanones, flavanols, and isoflavones (Fig. **1**). They are synthesized through the phenylpropanoid pathway, where phenyl alanine is initially converted into 4-coumaroyl CoA, which then, in turn, gains entry into the biosynthesis pathway [6]. Chalcone synthase is the first enzyme that works in this pathway to produce a chalcone skeleton, from which all types of flavonoids are derived with the help of several enzymes such as reductases, isomerases, hydroxylases, *etc* [7]. Transferases help in attaching methyl, acyl, and sugar moieties to the flavonoid rings to modify their reactivity, solubility, and interaction with receptor sites [2 - 8].

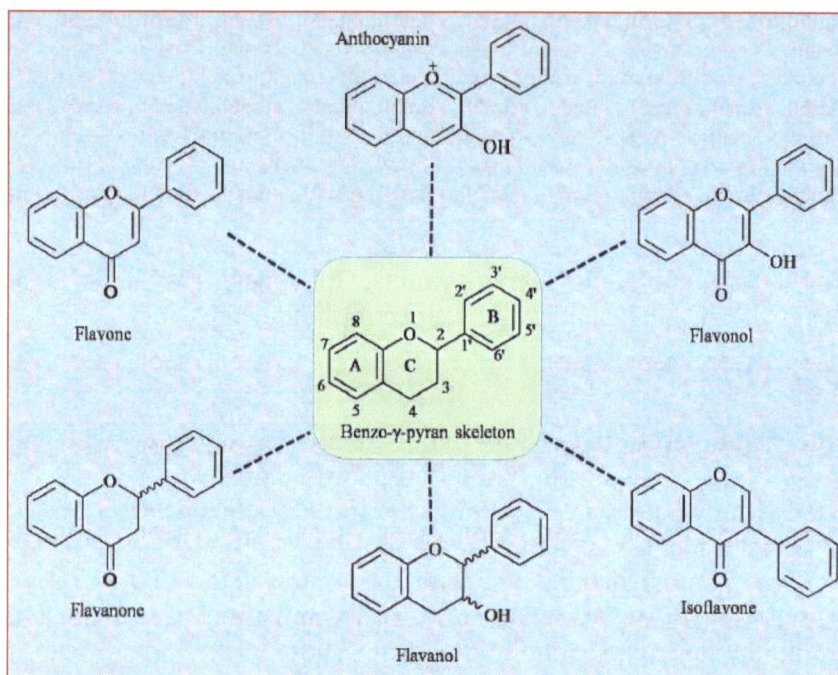

Fig. (1). General structures of various flavonoid subclasses.

The chemistry of these flavonoids also depends on various factors such as the number and position of hydroxyl groups, type of substitutions, degree of polymerization, and conjugation [9]. Being important components of fruits, vegetables, grain, and tea, they are proven to show profound antioxidant activity in both *in vitro* and *in vivo* systems. Flavonoids such as quercetin, myricetin, luteolin, taxifolin, eriodictyol and fusetin show high scavenging power against peroxide radicals. Single hydroxylation at position C-5 does not contribute to antioxidant activity, while *o*-dihydroxy substitution at positions C-3' and C-4' shows very high peroxide scavenging power. Glycosylation and *O*-methylation both result in decrease in antioxidant power. Scavenging activities of flavones and flavonols against hydroxyl radicals were found to be almost half as compared to the activities of flavanones. In presence of copper ions, and the absence of H_2O_2, the flavonoids showed high pro-oxidant activity instead of antioxidant activity, causing oxidative stress. The flavonoids such as quercetin, myricetin, taxifolin, and eriodictyol having more hydroxyl groups were found to be more pro-oxidant as compared to kaempferol containing lesser hydroxyl groups. The presence of *O*-methylated groups caused a further decrease in the pro-oxidant potential of the flavonoids [10]. Flavonols and flavan-3-ols are planar due to the hydroxyl group at C-3, assisting in conjugation and movement of electrons. This increases the stability of the phenoxy radical of the flavonoid. Flavones and flavanes, devoid of the C-3 hydroxyl group, show lesser antioxidant activities. Also, glycosylation at position 3 decreases the antioxidant potential in comparison to the flavonoid aglycones [11, 12]. Flavonoids also act as protective agents in plants, animals, and cell cultures in case of poisoning or oxidative stress caused by metal ions [13]. Plants do not contain flavonoid aglycones commonly, but they can be formed during processing. Sugars are attached to the flavonoid nucleus *via* β-glycosidic bonds. About 80 types of sugars have been established to be linked to flavonoids in the form of mono-, di-, tri-, and tetrasaccharides [14]. Aglycones were considered to be easy to absorb as compared to their glycosides. Studies on rats have revealed that the flavonoid glycosides are converted into the aglycones, based on analysis of their fecal matter [15].

The enzymes required for hydrolysis of the glycosides are present in the colon, and not in the gut or intestines. However, these enzymes can also metabolize the flavonoid structure [16 - 18]. Studies have shown that the absorption of quercetin glycosides is higher than quercetin alone. The absorption of quercetin glucosides from onions has shown 52% absorption, as compared to quercetin which showed absorption of 24% [19].

Flavonoids such as rutin, quercetin, apigenin, naringenin, and catechin have been proven to show hepatoprotective action, both *in vivo* using CCl_4 induced injury in hepatocytes in neonatal rats [20], and *in vitro* using chemically induced hepatotoxicity in HepG2 cells [21].

Apigenin, luteolin, baicalin, kaempferol, and quercetin show activity against SARS, dengue, herpes simplex, hepatitis C, chikungunya, and influenza viruses, by inhibition of replication of viruses, and destruction of genetic material and capsids of virus nuclei [22]. The isoflavone eriodictyol, and the flavonol myricetin are active against SARS-CoV-2 virus [23]. Apigenin is active against picrona virus and African swine flu virus [24], inhibits enterovirus-71 [25], and inhibits replication of hepatitis C virus [26]. Luteolin acts against Japanese encephalitis virus [27], rotavirus [28], chikungunya virus [29], HIV-I virus [30], coxsackievirus [31], and SARS-CoV-2 virus [32]. Baicalin is effective in inhibiting dengue virus, hepatitis C virus [33], SARS-CoV-2 virus [34], a*vian* influenza virus, and influenza A virus [35, 36]. Daidzein and kaempferol are effective against the Japanese encephalitis virus [37]. Rhamnoside containing derivatives of kaempferol are found to act against hepatitis C virus [38], corona virus [39], and influenza a virus [40]. The flavonol quercetin attenuates hepatitis C virus [41, 42], arrests pathogenesis of rhinovirus [43], and works in synergy with vitamin C against SARS-CoV-2 virus [44].

Total Flavonoid Content (TPC) is one of the most widely used methods to estimate the content of flavonoids in a sample, whose results are expressed as Quercetin Equivalents (QE). There are many modifications and critical evaluations of these methods. One method involved treatment of flavonoid solution with 2% $AlCl_3$ solution, and the yellow-colored complex was estimated at 420 nm, against a calibration graph using different concentrations of quercetin reference standard [45]. Another modification of this method is the addition of 10% $AlCl_3$ solution to the test solution, followed by treatment with potassium acetate. The absorbance of the yellow-colored solution is recorded at 415 nm, and flavonoid content was estimated using a standard curve using quercetin as a reference standard [46]. Fig. (**2**) shows the possible chelation of $AlCl_3$ with the *o*-dihydroxy systems in flavonoids.

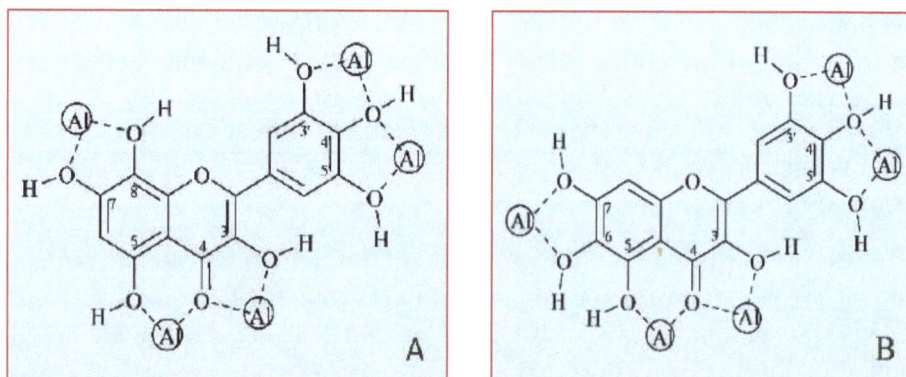

Fig. (2). Possible chelation of $AlCl_3$ with hydroxyl groups at positions. 3,4,5,7,8,3',4' and 5' (**A**) and 3,4,5, 6, 7, 3',4' and 5' (**B**).

Flavones and Flavonols

Flavones and flavonols form the largest subclass of flavonoids. Flavones are essentially 2-phenyl-chromen-4-one systems, while flavonols contain an additional hydroxyl group at position C-3, making a 3-hydroxy-2-pheyl-chromen-4-one system. They possess lighter shades so they help in dilution the strong colors of anthocyanins. They are responsible for the different hues of white, especially in flowers that bloom at night [47].

These compounds also show a wide variety of *O*-methylated derivatives showing methoxy groups at 3, 5, 6, 7, 8, 2', 3', 4', and 5' positions. Studies have shown that these derivatives are formed due to the action of *O*-methyl transferase (OMT) and their recombinant proteins [48, 49]. Though the native form of the enzyme gives majorly *O*-methylation at positions 3 and 6, the products with the recombinant proteins give a wider range of *O*-methylated derivatives. This has been attributed to the presence of the N-terminal region of the proteins [50].

Flavones and flavonols, along with their glycosylated and methylated derivatives have also been observed to form esters with sulfate groups. These esters are formed by the transfer of the sulfonate group from 3'-phosphoadenosine 5'-phosphosulfate (PAPS) by the action of soluble sulfotransferases (STs). At the molecular level, several such STs have been identified such as F3ST, F4'ST, AtST3, and BFST3 [51, 52].

The UV-B radiation that ranges from 280-315 nm is known to induce oxidative damage to the photosystem II reaction center, apart from damage to proteins and DNA. Flavones and flavonols act as sunscreens that absorb this UV-B radiation [53]. The UV-B radiation induces more levels of hydroxylation in flavonols, which affects their antioxidant capacity.

Flavones

Flavones occur in cell vacuoles as well as heartwood in the form of *O*- or *C*-glycosides. There are almost 400 flavone aglycones in nature. The *O*-glycosylated forms are more than 500 in number and can have sugars attached to the C-3, C-7, and C-4' positions, with some rare occurrences at the C-5 position. The *C*-glycosidic forms have sugars attached directly to the ring system at C-6 and C-8 positions. There are almost 300 such *C*- glycosides where either of the two or both positions can be linked to sugars [54]. Flavone aglycones have been identified in several species such as *Betula, Prunus, Primula, Alnus, Ostrya, Cheilanthes, Pityrogramma,* and *Notholaena*. The *O*- and *C*-glycosides of flavones are widespread from bryophytes to higher plants. Fig. (**3**) shows structures of some common flavones.

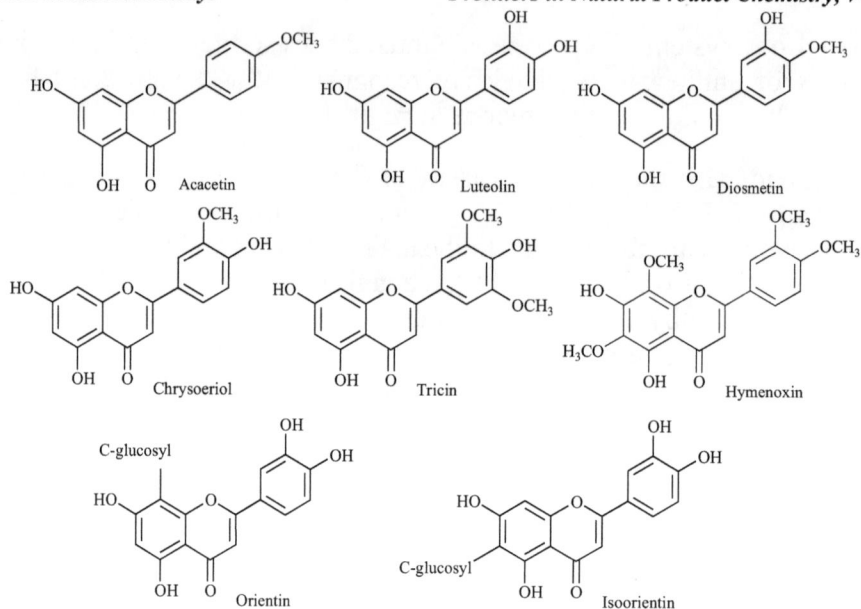

Fig. (3). Structures of some common flavones.

Flavones behave as co-pigments of anthocyanins such as delphinidin to impart blue color to flowers, which is the color preferred by bees. This helps in increasing the chances of pollination [55]. Flavones act as a deterrent to feeding by herbivores as well as shows inhibition to feeding by larvae [56]. The mortality of tobacco armyworm larvae has been related to the presence of flavonols quercetin along with its glycoside rutin [57]. Feeding experiments have shown a positive correlation between larval mortality and flavonol content in plants. Flavones are proved to exhibit inhibitory effects against bacteria [58], fungi [59, 60], mollusks [61], oomycetes [61, 62], and even other plants [63, 64]. Flavones and flavonols are proven to be powerful antioxidants that scavenge reactive oxygen species (ROS). The presence of the hydroxyl group at the C-3 position on the C-ring enhances the antioxidant power. Thus flavonols show higher antioxidant activities as compared to flavones. If the C-3 position is glycosylated as in rutin, there is a stark decrease in its activity, as compared to quercetin which has a free hydroxyl group at that position. If the B-ring has three hydroxyl groups (pyrogallol type), its activity is higher than that of those having two hydroxyl groups (catechol type). Thus myricetin shows greater radical scavenging activity than quercetin [65]. The compounds are antiviral, anti-inflammatory, anticancer, antiallergic, and provide protective action against cardiovascular, liver, and cataract related diseases [66].

Flavones have been known to show Wessely-Moser rearrangement, especially if there is the presence of an unprotected –OH group at the C-5 position [67]. This rearrangement is possible in presence of acid or base. This rearrangement can also take place during acid hydrolysis when the aglycone of the flavone can give rise to two isomers that could be detected during further analysis. This due to this rearrangement the analysis of plant extract can show the presence of isovitexin along with vitexin, and iso-orientin along with orientin.

Apigenin is a flavone that has low toxicity, and many biological actions. It is sourced from chocolate, basil leaf, dil weed, oregano, peppermint, rosemary, sage, celery, parsley, thyme, olive oil, apples, apricots, avocadoes, bananas, blackberries, blueberries, cherries, currants, dates, figs, guava, lemon juice, melons, *etc* [68]. Apigenin exists in various glycosidic forms such as apigenin-8-*C*-glucoside (vitexin), apigenin-6-*C*-glucoside (isovitexin), apigenin-7-*O*-glucoside, apigenin-6-*C*-glucoside-8-*C*-arabinoside (schafoside), and apigenin-7-*O*-neohesperidoside (rhoifolin) [69, 70]. Apigenin shows good anti-oxidant, anticancer, anti-proliferative, anti-progression, anti-mutagenic, and anti-inflammatory activities [71]. It exhibited synergistic effects in enhancing the efficacy of known anticancer drugs such as 5-fluorouracil, paclitaxel, and N-(--hydroxyphenyl) retinamide. Apigenin and its derivatives are active against bacteria such as *H. Pylori, E. coli, P. aeruginosa, B. subtilis* and *S. aureus* [72]. It is active against several viruses such as hepatitis C virus, influenza virus, enterovirus 71 (EV71), herpes simplex virus HSV-1 and HSV-2, African swine fever virus, as well as hand, foot, and mouth disease virus, and, but is not active against coxsackievirus A16 [25]. Studies on mice models revealed that apigenin reduces blood glucose levels by increasing serum insulin and sensitivity of pyruvate kinase [73]. It is found to be hypolipidemic and anti-oxidant when tested on mice models [74].

Luteolin is another common flavone that can be sourced from basil, cashew nut, coffee, tomatoes, apricots, apple, pumpkin, radish, soybean, apricots, thyme, spinach, oregano, and so on. The compound is anti-inflammatory, anti-tumor, and anti-oxidant. Studies *in vitro* and *in vivo* showed that luteolin is cardioprotective [75]. Luteolin helps in reducing secondary effects of diabetes such as damage to the retina [76]. Luteolin-7-glucoside showed good proliferative and anti-inflammatory activity on *in vitro* epithelial cell cultures [77].

Vitexin is sourced from green gram, bamboo, hawthorn, passionflower, *etc* [78]. The compound has some derivatives such as isovitexin, methylvitexin (isoembigenin), rhamnopyranosyl-vitexin, vitexin-2-*O*-xyloside, and vitexin-2-*O*-rhamnoside [79]. Vitexin shows good neuroprotective action when studied on rat pups [80]. Pretreatment of vitexin on cell line cultures shows good anti-oxidant and anti-apoptotic effects [81]. Vitexin also reduces pain caused due to inflammation and also shows antinociceptive activity [82]. Vitexin and isovitexin show good radical scavenging activities against DPPH, FRAP, and ABTS [83]. Vitexin-2-*O*-xyloside is found to show anti-cancer activities against bladder cancer cell lines [84]. Vitexin also induces apoptosis in lung cancer cell lines [85]. It also shows good activity against colorectal cancer cells [86]. The compound is also antibacterial, antiviral, and neuroprotective [87].

The absorption maxima and spectral shifts in commonly occurring flavones and flavonols on chelation with AlCl$_3$ have been shown in Table **1**.

Table 1. Spectral shifts observed in the absorption bands of flavones and flavonols on chelation with aluminum chloride [47].

Name of flavonoid	Absorption maxima in methanol (nm)	Absorption maxima on chelation with AlCl$_3$ (nm)	Name of flavonoid	Absorption maxima in methanol (nm)	Absorption maxima on chelation with AlCl$_3$ (nm)
Flavones			*Flavonols*		
Apigenin	283, 346	285, 337	Kaempferol	266, 367	269, 423
Luteolin	255, 348	273, 404	Quercetin	255, 370	267, 426
Vitexin	270, 336	277, 350	Myricetin	255, 375	268, 423
Orientin	255, 347	270, 411	Galangin	267, 359	273, 413
Isoorientin	255, 349	278, 429	Fisetin	248, 362	281, 458
Chrysoeriol	241, 269	274, 390	Rutin	259, 359	275, 433
Acacetin	270, 326	278, 330	Gossypetin	261, 385	273, 395
Baicalein	274, 323	272, 375	Rhamnetin	256, 371	273,451
Saponarin	271, 336	277, 352	Isorhamnetin	253, 370	264, 431
Scoparin	270, 345	274, 392	Morin	264, 370	268, 421
Diosmetin	252, 344	273, 390	Penduletin	271, 340	280, 369
Tricin	245, 350	245, 350	Jacein	257, 352	270, 387

AlCl$_3$ binds with the flavonoid molecule through the carbonyl group at position C-4 as well as the –OH groups in the near vicinity (preferably C-5 position) to form a chelate. Thus flavones will show one chelation of AlCl$_3$ with the carbonyl oxygen at C-4 and the –OH group at C-5. The presence of the *o*-dihydroxy groups alters the spectrum even more by causing a higher bathochromic shift due to chelation with AlCl$_3$. The spectrophotometric method for the determination of flavonoids mainly employs the recording of absorbance at 415 nm or 420 nm. The flavonoid-AlCl$_3$ complex must show good absorbance above 400nm to contribute to the reading. Previous studies reported by our team show that only flavones luteolin, orientin, and isoorientin show absorption maxima between 400-430 nm as shown in Fig. (**4**), and can contribute to the spectrophotometric reading [88]. This is due to the presence of –OH groups at positions C-3' and C-4', which provides an additional site for AlCl$_3$ to chelate. Chrysoeriol and diosmetin are the mono-*O*-methylated derivatives of luteolin. Chrysoeriol has a methoxy group at position C-3', while diosmetin has a methoxy group at C-4', which hampers the chelation with AlCl$_3$. The absorption maxima for both the compounds is 390 nm.

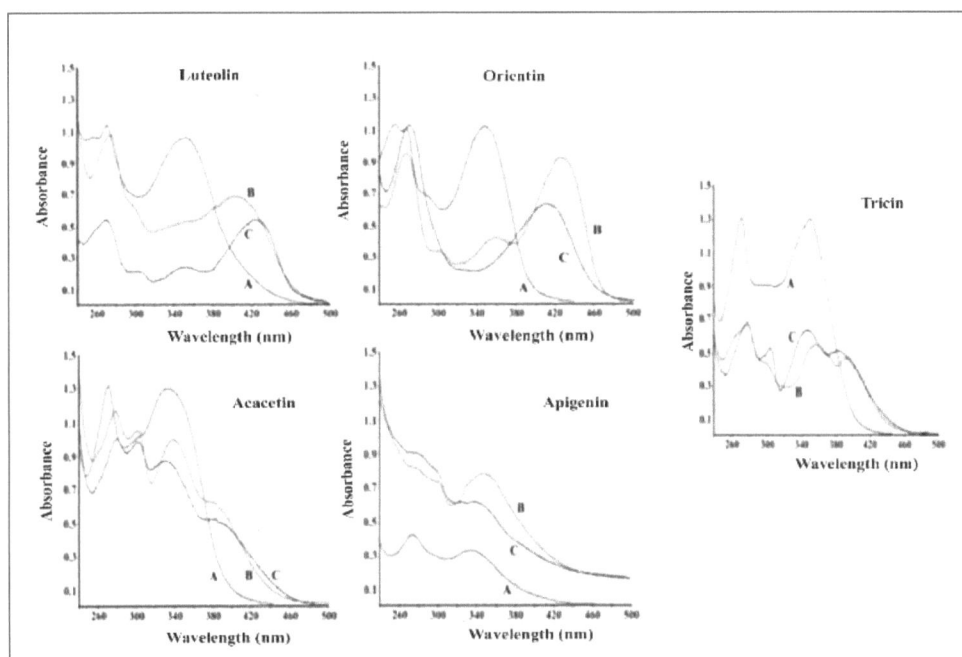

Fig. (4). Spectral shifts exhibited by various flavones on the addition of 10% AlCl$_3$(**B**), and further shift observed on addition of potassium acetate solution (**C**), as compared to spectra in neat ethanol (**A**) (*Reprinted with permission from Elsevier [88]*).

The absorption maxima observed in hymenoxin is even less (365nm) due to both C-3' and C-4' positions being occupied by methoxy groups. Similarly, tricin shows an –OH group at C-4' flanked by two methoxy groups on both C-3' and C-5' positions due to which AlCl$_3$ does not react (Fig. **5**) and the absorption maxima is observed to be 350 nm.

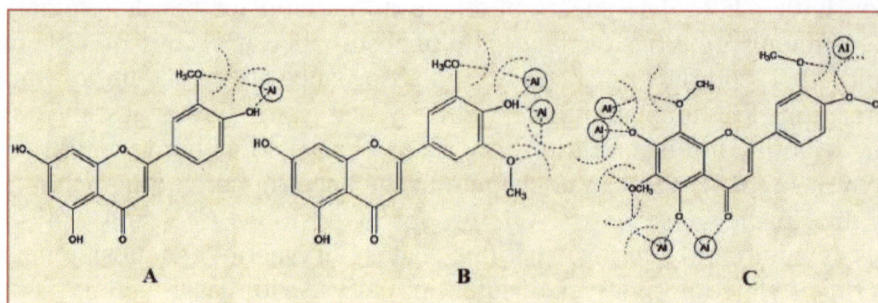

Fig. (5). Chelation of AlCl₃ hampered due to presence of methoxy groups at C-3' as in case of chrysoeriol (**A**), at C-3' and C-5' in tricin (**B**), and at C-3', C-4', C-6, and C-8 in hymenoxin (**C**).

Flavonols

About 450 flavonol aglycones have been reported, apart from 900 types of *O*-glycosides with glycosidic linkages at C-3, C-7, C-3', and C-4' positions. The 6-C-glycosides of flavonols have also been reported. Sugars attached to are generally glucose, along with rhamnose, mannose, galactose, xylose, and arabinose. Galactouronic and glucouronic acids have also been identified in such glycosides [3]. Flavonols in free, methylated, and glycosylated forms have been reported in many plants as well as fungi like *Aspergillus candidus* [89, 90]. Structures of commonly occurring flavonols are given in Fig. (**6**).

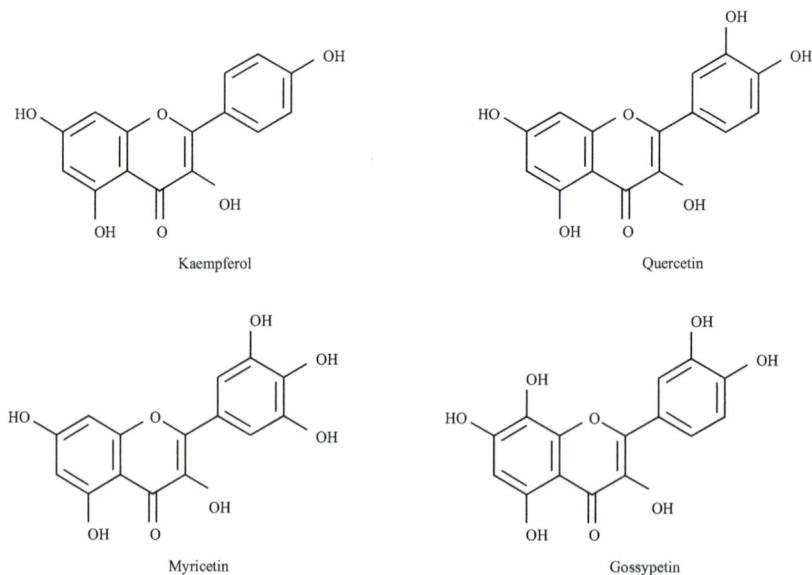

Fig. (6). Structures of some common flavonols.

Flavonols show high anti-inflammatory and anticancer action due to their pro-oxidant nature and reaction with biomolecules *via* electrophilic conjugation. The flavonols are oxidized into *o*- and *p*-quinones, which in turn form adducts with nucleophilic thiol groups, glutathione, and amino groups of proteins [11]. Structure requisite for good anti-inflammatory and anticancer activities is the presence of a double bond between C-2 and C-3, presence of hydroxyl groups at C-5, C-7, and C-4'. The presence of –OH group at position C-3' causes reduction of activity, while that at position C-5' induces total inactivity [91].

Quercetin is found in tea, fruits like apples and berries, and vegetables like onion. The highest content of quercetin is reported in onion (almost 1.5 g/kg), where it exists in two glycosidic forms. One form is quercetin-4'-glucoside and the other is quercetin-3,4'-glucoside. Tea contains quercetin-4'-rhamnoglucoside, while apple contains quercetin-4'-galactoside, quercetin-4'-glucoside, quercetin-4'--arabinoside and quercetin-4'-rhamnoside. Black currant contains quercetin-4'--rhamnoglucoside, quercetin-4'-rhamnoside, and quercetin-4'-galactoside [92].

Quercetin acts against asthma and allergy by behaving as an antihistamine agent. It prevents cataract formation and can improve the strength of blood vessels. It reduces cardiac problems by decreasing levels of Low Density Lipoprotein (LDL) and cholesterol. Human trials have also shown that it has a good vasodilating effect [93]. Quercetin is found to be a strong anti-oxidant, which is attributed to its ability to chelate metals [94, 95], scavenge radicals [96, 97], inhibit enzyme action [98, 99], and induce expression of protective enzymes [100]. Quercetin and its six derivatives showed good anti-inflammatory activity [101].

Kaempferol is found in tea, fruits like strawberries, grapes, and apples, and vegetables like tomatoes, beans, and broccoli [102]. It is found to be less toxic than many anticancer drugs but is found to induce apoptosis in cancer cell lines [103]. It has also shown impairment of cancer angiogenesis by inhibition of vascular endothelial growth factor (VEGF) in cancer cells, as confirmed by both *in vitro* as well as *in vivo* studies [104, 105]. Kaempferol is also proven to show good anti-inflammatory activity [106, 107]. Nicotiflorin, which is a derivative of kaempferol, showed very good hepatoprotective activity in mice [108]. Seven rhamnosides of kaempferol showed good antimicrobial and anti-oxidant activities [109]. Kaempferol also shows good cardioprotective action in rats [110].

Myricetin is sourced from tea, tomatoes, berries, nuts, grapes, and oranges. It is a powerful anti-oxidant that can scavenge several free radicals [111]. It exhibits good activity against the herpes simplex virus [112], African swine flu virus [113], and HIV virus [114]. The compound is anti-inflammatory [115] and antidiabetic [116].

In the case of flavonols, there is an additional –OH group at C-3 which creates one more site where AlCl₃ can chelate. Thus one chelate can be formed using the carbonyl oxygen at C-4 and -OH at C-3, while another chelate can be formed by carbonyl at C-4 and the hydroxyl group at C-5. Thus many flavonols do not show good absorbance around the required wavelength of 415 or 420 nm, as compared to flavones that are devoid of the hydroxyl group at C-3. Any additional *o*-dihydroxy systems, especially in the B-ring, cause higher bathochromic shifts in the spectra, on reaction with AlCl₃. Common flavonols such as kaempferol, quercetin, myricetin, rutin, *etc.* show absorption maxima around 420nm, which makes them good contributors to the reading taken for the flavonoid estimation at that wavelength (Fig. **7**). This has been supported by our previously reported work [88].

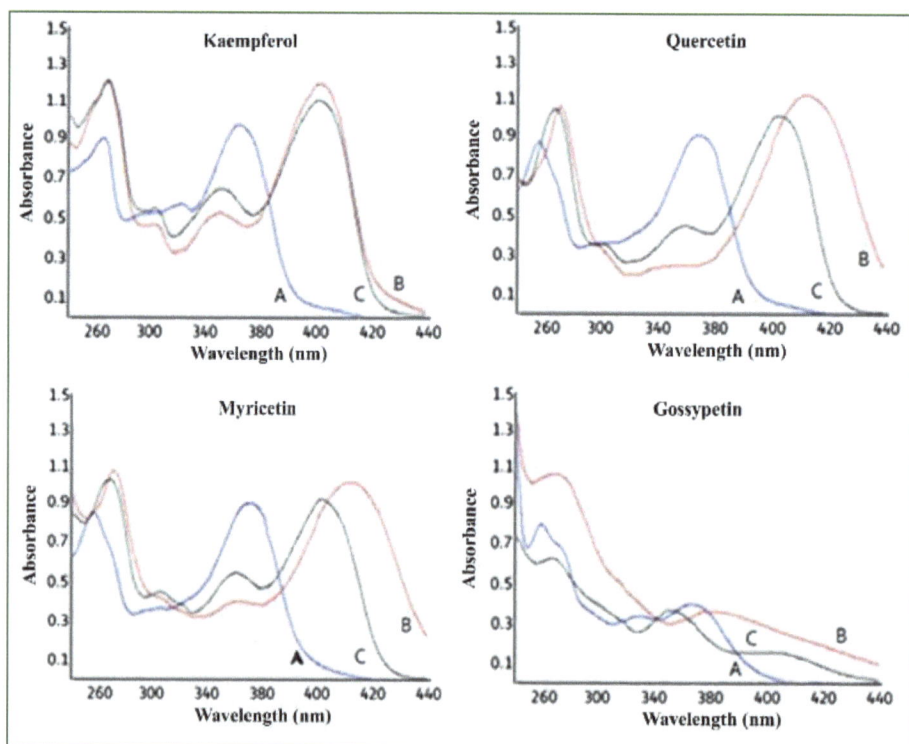

Fig. (7). Spectral shifts exhibited by various flavonols on the addition of 10% AlCl₃(**B**), and further shift observed on addition of potassium acetate solution (**C**), as compared to spectra in neat ethanol (**A**)*(Reprinted with permission from Elsevier [88]).*

Rhamnetin shows high absorption maxima since its methoxy group is at C-7 position which anyways does not hamper chelation with AlCl₃. However, its isomer isorhamnetin shows a methoxy group at C-3', which prevents chelation so the absorption maximum decreases by 20 nm. The presence of the methoxy group prevents $AlCl_3$ chelation is further proved by the fact that if the –OH group at C-3 is replaced by –OCH_3 group, there is a stark decrease in absorption maxima (below 400nm), as observed in the case of penduletin and jacein. Gossypetin shows very high absorption maxima (492 nm) due to the presence of hydroxyl groups at C-3, C-5, C-7, C-8, C-3', and C-4'. There are 4 interactions possible with the $AlCl_3$ (C-3—C-4, C-4—C-5, C-7—C-8, and C-3'—C-4'), but it shows an additional peak near 401nm, which can contribute to the flavonoid content during estimation. As observed in Table 1 not all flavonols contribute uniformly to the absorbance when estimated using $AlCl_3$ assays.

Anthocyanins

Anthocyanins are a subclass of flavonoids that are glucosides of 2-phenyl benzopyrilium salts. The major structural difference of anthocyanins from other flavonoids is that they possess a flavylium cation in the C-ring, and the carbonyl group at C-4 is absent. Derived from Greek words 'anthos' which means flower, and 'kiano' which stands for blue, that impart pink, red, purple, and blue colors to flowers, fruits, stem, roots, and leaves. They provide a wide spectrum of colors and are thus projected as potential candidates for food colorants. There are more than 700 kinds of anthocyanins reported in the literature [117]. Major sources of anthocyanins are red grapes, plums, red currants, onions, grapefruit, strawberry, peach, and so on. Anthocyanins contain sugar moieties such as glucose, rhamnose, galactose, *etc.*, either monosaccharide or disaccharide forms, while their aglycones are referred to as 'anthocyanidins'. They can also have sinapic, coumaric, succinic, ferulic, caffeic, and malonic acids attached to the rings. Most of the anthocyanins have benzoic or cinnamic acid derivatives which are esterified to sugars. Methoxylation or glycosylation influences the hue of anthocyanins. An increase in –OH or sugar moieties causes blue coloration, while an increase in –OCH_3 groups causes red coloration. The reddish colors are stable in an acidic medium but change to a blue color when the medium turns alkaline due to its conversion into quinonoid form [47]. In some plants, anthocyanins appear as anthocyanoplasts, while in most plants they accumulate in the vacuoles. Content of anthocyanins can vary from 0.1-1% in the plant parts, with permissible intake between 180-225mg [118]. Being very powerful anti-oxidants, anthocyanins are proven to show very good activities against microbes, diabetes, inflammation, cancer, and obesity. They are also known to improve neurological and visual ailments, as well as the prevention of cardiovascular diseases [119 - 121]. Anthocyanins have been characterized mainly using techniques such as UV-Visible spectroscopy, mass spectrometry, and HPLC. Structures of the most commonly occurring anthocyanidins have been depicted in Fig. (8).

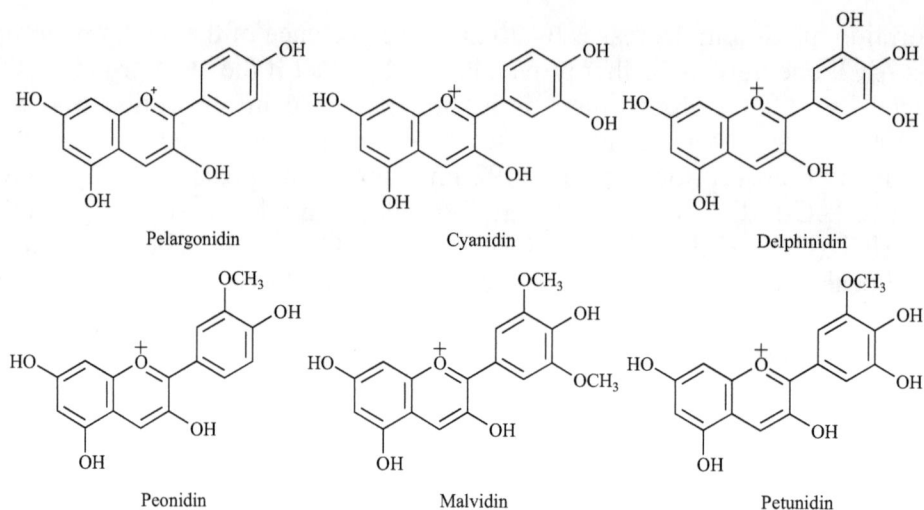

Fig. (8). Structures of some commonly occurring anthocyanins.

The nonacylated derivatives pelargonidin, cyanidin, and delphinidin show absorption maxima 520 nm, 535nm, and 546 respectively. Mono and di-acylated derivatives peonidin, petunidin, and malvidin show absorption maxima 532 nm, 543nm, and 542nm respectively. Since all anthocyanins have absorption maxima above 500nm, their complexes with $AlCl_3$ will not absorb in the 415-420nm range. Thus anthocyanins will have no contribution in the readings taken using $AlCl_3$ chelation methods for estimation of Total Flavonoid Content in samples.

The spectrophotometric method for the determination of Total Anthocyanin Content was proposed by Lees and Francis [122] and further validated by Lee, Durst, and Wrolstad [123]. The method is quick and inexpensive and can be used to estimate anthocyanin levels without the use of expensive analytical standards of anthocyanins. The method has been used to estimate the content of anthocyanidins and proanthocyanidins in several food samples and plant extracts. The test sample is treated separately with KCl solution (pH 1), and sodium acetate solution (pH 4.5). At pH 1, where the solution is red due to the presence of the flavylium cation, and pH 4.5 where the cation is converted into colorless pseudocarbinol species. The absorbance of the test solutions is recorded first at 520 nm. For food samples containing pulp, skin, yeast, *etc.* the correction for the haze of the solution is performed by also recording the absorbance of the solutions at 700 nm, at both the pH levels. The anthocyanin content is then calculated using the following formula.

Total Monomeric Anthocyanin Content (mg/L) = $\dfrac{A \times MW \times DF \times 1000}{\epsilon \times L}$

where A= $(A_{520} - A_{700})$ pH$_1$ - $(A_{520} - A_{700})$ pH$_{4.5}$, MW represents the molecular weight of the most abundant anthocyanin in the sample, DF is the dilution factor of the solution, ϵ is the molar extinction coefficient of the most abundant anthocyanin in the sample, L being the volume of the solution.

Flavanones and Flavanols

Flavanones consist of 2-phenyl-3,4-dihydro-2H-chromene skeleton, while flavanols are 2-phenyl-3,4-dihydro-2H-chromen-3-ol systems, containing a hydroxyl group at position C-3. These colorless compounds have complete saturation in the B ring of the C_6-C_3-C_6 system, are widely distributed in higher plants, but may escape detection due to their low concentrations. They remain stable in an acidic medium but on reaction with bases, they get converted in chalcones. Since the bond between carbons C-2 and C-3 is saturated, the compound loses its planarity and the C-2 carbon becomes chiral. They are optically active, mostly existing in the levorotatory forms.

Flavanones

The flavanones naringenin and eriodictyol are similar to apigenin and luteolin respectively, except for the fact that the latter have unsaturation in the C_3 ring system. Similarly, the flavanol counterpart of quercetin is taxifolin, with two phenolic groups at C-3' and C-4' positions. Another important flavanolol is hesperidin, which has a methoxy group in the 4'-position, and a phenolic group at the 3'-position. Both naringenin and hesperidin are responsible for the bitter taste in the peel and juice of citrus fruits. Comprehensive work using 1-D and 2-D HPLC studies have been conducted to determine naringin, hesperidin, narirutin, didymin, and eriocitrin in different citrus fruits [124].

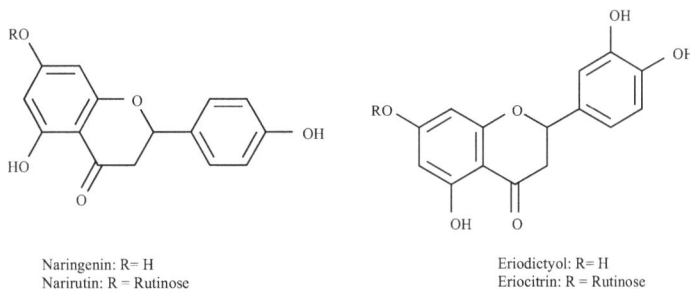

Naringenin: R= H
Narirutin: R = Rutinose

Eriodictyol: R= H
Eriocitrin: R = Rutinose

(Fig. 9) contd.....

Hesperedin   Taxifolin   Didymin

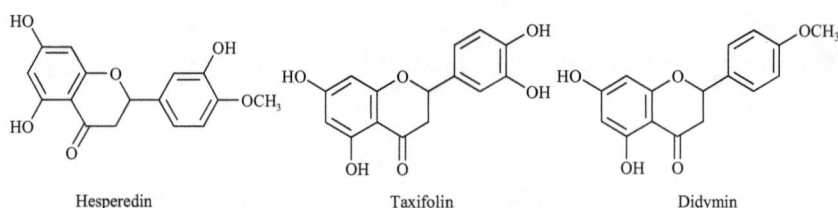

Fig. (9). Structures of some commonly occurring flavanones.

Dose dependent studies have shown that naringenin is effective against dengue virus [125], chikungunya virus [126], and hepatitis C virus [127]. It shows the ability to repair DNA, which is being attributed as the factor responsible for its anticancer properties. Peels of *Citrus sinensis, Citrus unshiu,* and *Citrus aurantium* are good sources from which hesperidin can be isolated in high amounts [128]. The compound shows good anticarcinogenic, anti-inflammatory, antihypercholesterolemic, and anti-oxidant properties [129]. Neuronal damage induced by rotenone induced by pesticide rotenone on human neuroblastoma SK-N-SH cells has been reduced by hesperidin, showing good signs of reduction of oxidative stress, apoptosis, and dysfunction of mitochondria [130]. Sorghum and millets are known to contain high amounts of flavanones such as hesperidin and naringenin. Reports claim that millets contain very high amounts of flavanones as compared to citrus fruits [131, 132].

Estimation of flavanones employing $AlCl_3$ chelation does not yield proper readings, as depicted in Table **2**.

Table 2. Spectral shifts observed in the absorption bands of flavanones and flavanols on chelation with aluminum chloride [47].

Name of flavonoid	Absorption maxima in methanol (nm)	Absorption maxima on chelation with $AlCl_3$ (nm)	Name of flavonoid	Absorption maxima in methanol (nm)	Absorption maxima on chelation with $AlCl_3$ (nm)
Flavonones			*Flavanols*		
Naringenin	289	375	Catechin	276	277
Taxifolin	290	312	Epicatechin	278	278
Eriodictyol	289	310	EGC	270	-*
Hesperidin	283	308	EGCG	276	322
Garbanzol	276	309	ECG	276	-*
Sakuranin	280	280	-	-	-
Astilbin	292	316	-	-	-

*Data not available

This inability of flavanones to chelate with $AlCl_3$ is also evident from the spectra which does not show absorbance above 400nm, as shown in Fig. (**10**).

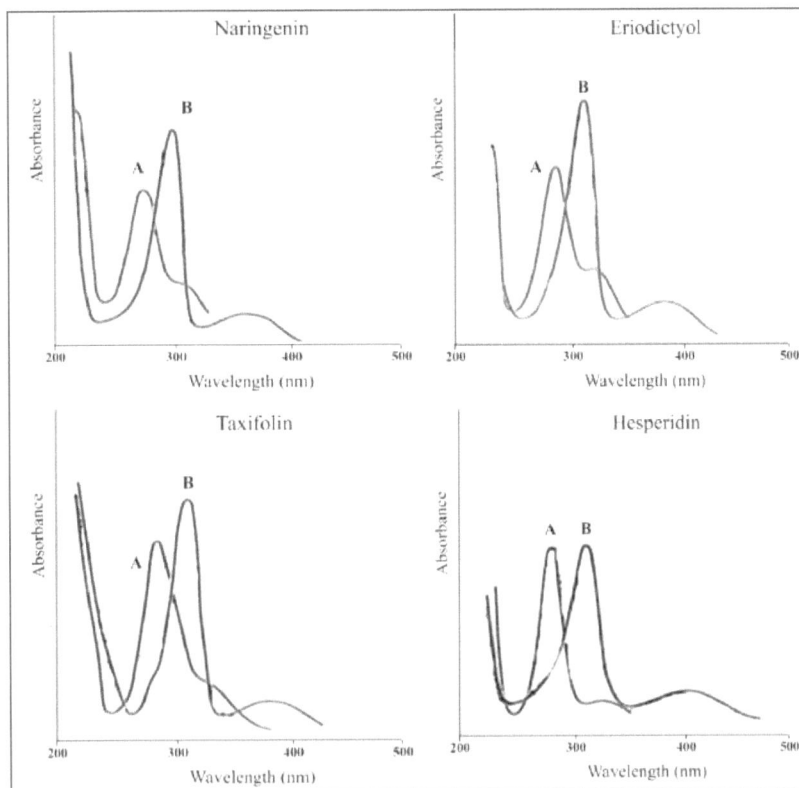

Fig. (10). UV spectra of some flavanones in neat methanol (**A**)and their spectral shifts after chelation with $AlCl_3$(**B**).

There is another method reported for estimation of flavanones, which employs a reaction of 2,4-dinitrophenyl hydrazine the ketone at C-4, to form a phenyl hydrazone. The method involved treatment of the test solution with 1% phenyl hydrazine solution at 50°C for 50 minutes, allowed to cool to room temperature, and then treated with a hydroalcoholic solution of KOH. Methanol is added and the solution is centrifuged. The supernatant is then diluted to the appropriate volume and absorbance is recorded at 495 nm [46]. The method was tested for flavanones naringin, its aglycone naringenin, and hesperidin. This colorimetric method, however, was selective only to flavanones and did not form phenyl hydrazones with flavones, flavonols, and isoflavones. Also, the response of all flavanones to this method is yet to be ascertained.

Flavanols

Flavan-3-ols or simply flavanols, commonly known as catechins are abundant in tea. They are also found in fruits like apples, apricots, cherries, strawberries, and green grapes. Red and green algae, as well as vegetables like beans and lemon, are sources of catechins [133, 134]. Almost 70% of the flavonoids in green tea consist of catechins. Catechins in tea are responsible for the anti-oxidant, antimicrobial, anti-aging, and anti-radiation potentials of tea [135]. Catechins are stable in acidic conditions at pH less than 4 but degrade rapidly in alkaline conditions at pH greater than 8 in solution [136]. They are also sensitive to degradation by heat and enzymes [137]. They get easily oxidized to radicals of quinone and semiquinone by losing hydrogens [138]. These catechins have been investigated to show profound biological activities against cancer [139], bacterial growth, mutagenicity [140], obesity [141], lipid deposition [142], inflammation [143, 144], diabetes [145], and so on. These compounds also show very good anti-oxidant properties due to profound radical scavenging potential caused by the reductive nature of the phenolic groups [146].

Major catechins found are (-)-epicatechin (EC), (-)-epicatechingallate (ECG), (-)-epigallocatechin (EGC), (-)-epigallocatechingallate (EGCG) and (+)-catechin (Fig. **11**). The structure of catechins, especially EGCG, helps in proper binding with proteins and nucleic acids, which can help to target key factors causing carcinogenesis [147]. Studies have shown that EGCG shows even better anti-oxidant activity than vitamin E and vitamin C [148].

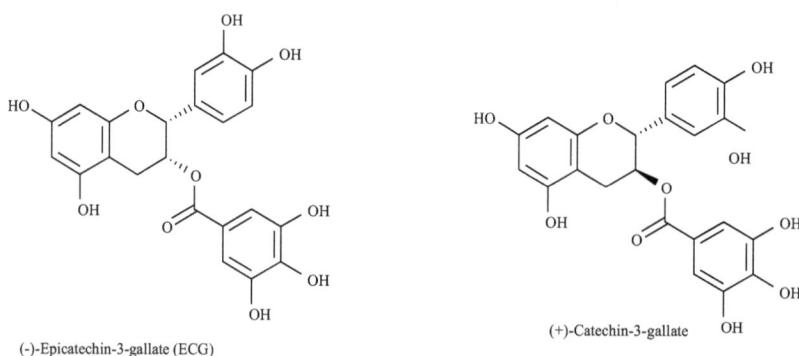

(-)-Epicatechin-3-gallate (ECG)

(+)-Catechin-3-gallate

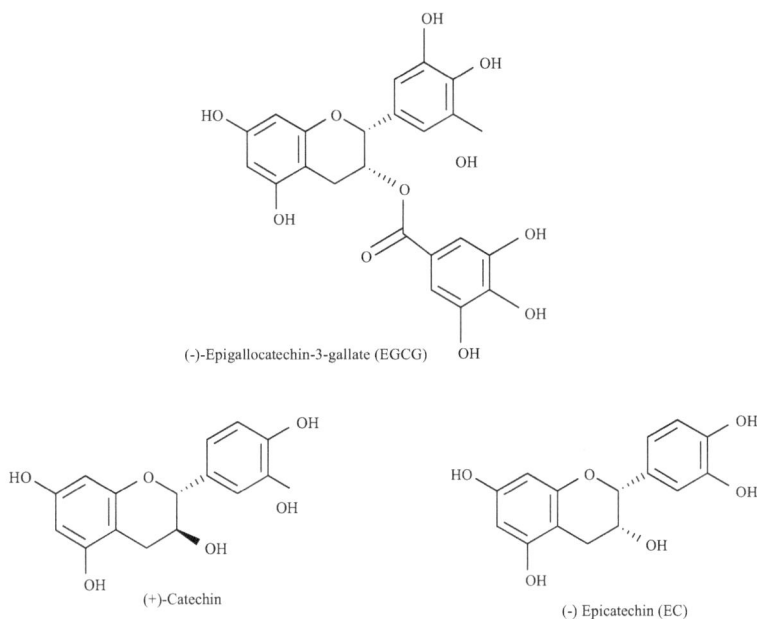

Fig. (11). Structures of some common flavan-3-ols (catechins).

Catechins do not show any significant change in absorption maxima, even when reacted with $AlCl_3$ (**Table 2**). Thus catechins also do not contribute to the reading taken for Total Flavonoid Content using $AlCl_3$ chelation methods. There are, however, other methods reported for the estimation of catechins, which are as follows.

1. Vanillin-HCl/ vanillin-H_2SO_4 method [149]:

This method involves reaction with vanillin in presence of HCl or H_2SO_4. The method is specific for catechins since it requires a single bond to be present between C-2 and C-3, as well as free –OH groups at meta-position in the B-ring. Experiments also show that the method does not work for flavones, flavonols, isoflavones, and gallotannins. Vanillin is protonated using strong mineral acid (pH close to 1), forming a carbocation that acts as a weak electrophile. This electrophile on reaction with catechins forms a red colored complex, whose absorbance is recorded at 500 nm. Parameters of the method were studied in detail by Sun, Ricardo-da-Silva, and Spranger, who suggested that reaction with H_2SO_4 gave better and precise results as compared to HCl. The presence of ascorbic acid and its salts, chlorophyll, and anthocyanins in the plant matrix, can interfere in the test results [150].

2. Butanol-HCl-Fe(II) Assay:

Initially devised by Swain and Hillis, the method involved the conversion of proanthocyanidins to anthocyanidins using an acid-alcohol combination of HCl-butanol. The method was modified to involve complexation with Fe (II) ion, by adding ferrous sulfate. This method is now widely used for quantitative analysis of flavanols [151]. The flavanol test solution is reacted with a solution of $FeSO_4$·$7H_2O$ dissolved in a mixture of n-butanol and HCl (3:2 v/v), at 90°C for 25 minutes, followed by recording absorbance of the solution at 540 nm. Catechin or epicatechin can be used as reference standards to prepare calibration curves.

3. *p*-dimethylaminocinnamaldehyde (DMAC) Assay:

This method developed by Delcour and de Varebeke uses DMAC as the chromogen that develops color with flavanols [152]. First proposed to analyze catechins in beer, it has been since then used for assessment of flavanols in many food products [153, 154]. The test solution is reacted with 0.1% of *p*-dimethylaminocinnamaldehyde dissolved in HCl, incubated for 10 minutes, and absorbance read at 640 nm. Calibration curves could be prepared using catechin or epicatechin reference standards.

Isoflavones

Isoflavones are 3-phenyl chromones, which are isomeric with flavones. They are different from flavones due to the position of the phenyl ring at the C-3 position, instead of the C-2 position. The patterns of their hydroxylation are similar to that of flavones. More than 50 isoflavones have been isolated so far [47]. They are polyphenolic compounds that possess estrogen-agonist as well as estrogen-antagonist properties. They are found abundantly in legumes such as soybean, beans, chickpeas, black bean, and other plants such as red clover, alfalfa, nuts, currants, coffee, and cereals [155 - 157]. Naturally isoflavones are found as inactive glycosides such as 7-*O*-glycosides, 6"-*O*-acetyl-7-*O*-glycosides, and 6"-*O*-malonyl-7-*O*-glycosides. They are absorbed by systemic circulation post hydrolysis into their aglycones by the mucosa of the intestine and action of gut microbiota [158]. Soybean contains genistin, daidzin, and glycitin in good amounts, which are converted into their aglycones genistein, daidzein, and glycitein respectively. Structures of commonly occurring isoflavones have been given in Fig. (**12**).

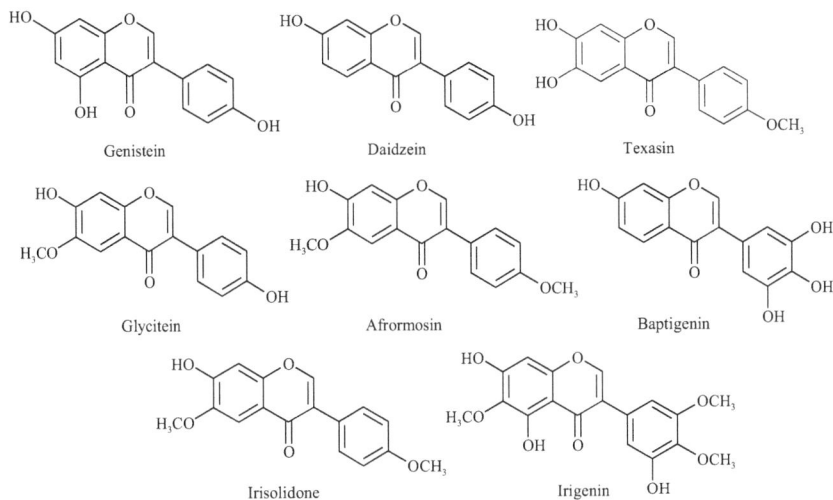

Fig. (12). Structures of some commonly occurring isoflavones.

Legumes also contain other isoflavone glycosides such as sissotrin and ononin, which are converted into their aglycones biochanin and formononetin in the body. The amount of isoflavones produced in the plant depends on temperature, water content, soil fertility, as well as growth and harvesting conditions. Stress conditions like pathogen attack, low humidity, and disease increase the synthesis of isoflavones in the plant [159]. Sprouting can induce the biosynthesis of isoflavones. Studies have shown that sprouted chickpeas develop higher contents of biochanin A and B, as compared to pre-sprouted grains [160]. Sprouted green gram has been found to contain good amounts of daidzein, genistein, and isorhamnetin [161]. Concentrations of glycosides of biochanin A and B have also been found to increase in dark beans when sprouted [162].

Isoflavones show good antibacterial, antiviral, antifungal, and anti-oxidant activities [163]. These compounds play pivotal roles in legume-rhizobium symbiosis, as well as other defense responses [164]. As far as biological activities in humans are concerned, they are known to help in the treatment of several disorders caused by hormonal imbalances. Isoflavones are active against osteoporosis [165], cardiovascular diseases [166, 167], menopausal problems [168, 169], along with prostrate [170], and breast cancers [171, 172].

Spectra of isoflavones on reaction with $AlCl_3$ for commonly occurring isoflavones has been depicted in has been depicted (Fig. **13**). The spectral shifts in absorption maxima of the isoflavones on chelation with $AlCl_3$ have been shown in Table **1**.

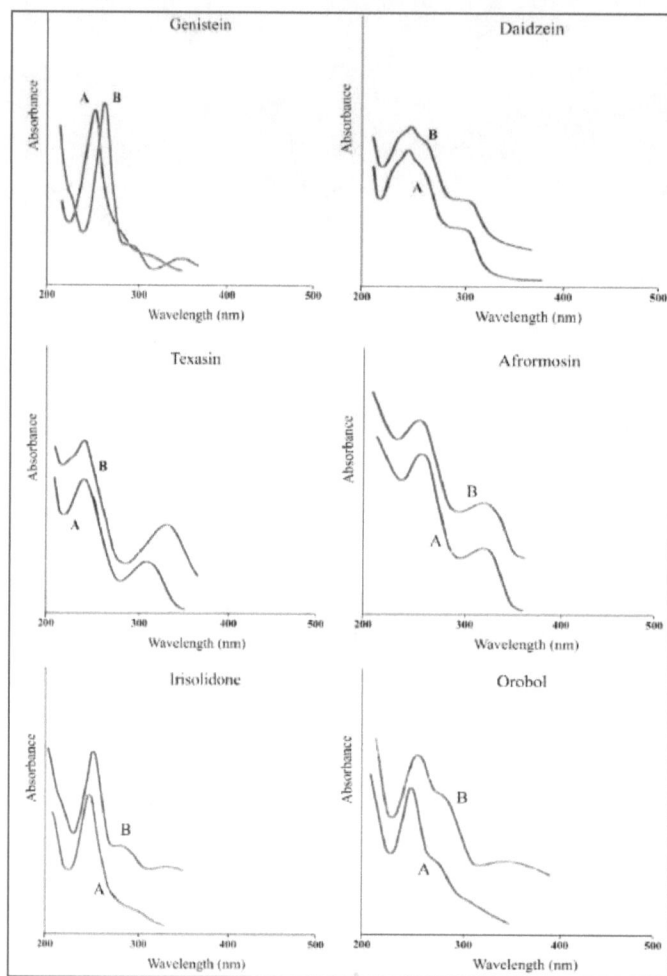

Fig. (13). UV spectra of some isoflavones in neat methanol (A)and their spectral shifts after chelation with AlCl₃ (B).

Table 3. Spectral shifts observed in the absorption bands of isoflavones on chelation with aluminum chloride.

Name of flavonoid	Absorption maxima in methanol (nm)	Absorption maxima on chelation with AlCl₃ (nm)	Name of flavonoid	Absorption maxima in methanol (nm)	Absorption maxima on chelation with AlCl₃ (nm)
Genistein	261, 328	272, 372	Formonetin	248, 311	248, 301

(Table 3) cont.....

Name of flavonoid	Absorption maxima in methanol (nm)	Absorption maxima on chelation with AlCl₃ (nm)	Name of flavonoid	Absorption maxima in methanol (nm)	Absorption maxima on chelation with AlCl₃ (nm)
Daidzein	249, 303	249, 300	Prunetin	262, 327	273, 374
Texasin	255, 325	251, 344	Tectoridin	266, 331	277, 380
Afrormosin	258, 320	255, 319	Irigenin	268, 336	275, 371
Baptigenin	249, 265	238, 283	Pinocembrin	289, 325	311, 375
Irisolidone	265, 335	276, 378	Pratensein	262, 330	272, 371
Orobol	262, 338	270, 365	Iridin	268, 331	277, 382

As observed in the Table **3**, none of the isoflavones show absorption maxima beyond 380 nm on treatment with $AlCl_3$. Here even the presence of *o*-dihydroxy systems such as baptigenin seems to be insufficient to complex with $AlCl_3$. Since there is no absorbance at wavelengths close to 415/420 nm, isoflavones do not contribute to the reading taken when $AlCl_3$ chelation methods for flavonoid quantitation are employed.

Total Phenolic Content (TPC)

The method for estimation of phenolics was initially developed as the Folin-Denis method to analyze urine samples using a reaction of tyrosine with a phosphotungstate-molybdate reagent which resulted in the development of a blue colored complex [173]. This method had to be modified later due to the inference of white precipitates that formed during the reaction [174]. The specificity of the method was then increased by more modifications in reagents using both cuvettes as well as 96 well plates [175]. The method known as the Folin-Ciocalteu method employs a phosphotungstic-phosphomolybdic reagent prepared by refluxing a mixture of sodium tungstate and sodium molybdate with concentrated hydrochloric and 85% phosphoric acids for 10 hours. Lithium sulfate is added on cooling, followed by treatment of bromine liquid or 30% hydrogen peroxide solution. The reagent is yellow and can be stored indefinitely if protected from reducing agents. The solution containing phenolics is treated with a basic solution (pH 10-12) containing sodium carbonate, whereby the phenolic groups are converted into their respective phenolate anions. A redox reaction between the phenolate ions and the Folin-Ciocalteu reagent causes reduction of the molybdenum, which is manifested by the development of blue color of solution due to formation of $[PMoW_{11}O_4)^{4-}]$ complex. There are, however, many studies that indicate the flaws in the method. The reagent is not specific to just phenolics but also reacts with ascorbic acid, sodium bisulfite, reducing sugars, amino acids like tyrosine, and tryptophan, which skews the actual value of the Total Phenolic

Content of the sample [176]. Aromatic amines, organic acids, sulfur dioxide, ascorbic acid, *etc*. can also interfere with the readings [177]. Reference standards such as gallic acid or catechin used in the method are unstable at higher pH [178]. Also, the accuracy of the results depends on several factors such as the order of addition of reagents, reference standard used, alkalinity of the solution, and wavelength of detection [179].

CONCLUDING REMARKS

Though the basic scaffold is identical, the various classes of flavonoids show several variations based on the presence or absence of different functionalities. Anthocyanins and flavanols are devoid of the carbonyl group at C-4, which is an important functional group in flavones, flavonols, flavanones, and isoflavones. The unsaturation between C-2 and C-3 is absent in the case of flavanones and flavonols. This double bond is an important characteristic for flavones, flavonols, and isoflavones, giving rise to a different extent of absorption of UV light as evident from their spectral data. The formation of flavylium cation on the C-ring of the anthocyanins, makes them a separate entity showing very different characteristics in terms of the various hues they impart to the plant parts, especially in the floral systems. The benzenoid character of all three rings gives absorption in the visible region owing to the extended conjugation in the molecule. The presence, number, and position of methyl, hydroxyl, and glycosyl derivatives also contribute significantly to the spectral and chemical differences among the flavonoid classes. Thus the interaction of different flavonoids with various reagents has no uniformity and thus gives rise to incomplete and erroneous results. The aluminium chloride chelation methods are credible to some extent flavones and flavonols, mainly those containing *o*-dihydroxy systems. Flavanols, flavanones, and anthocyanins cannot be estimated using this method, due to either inability to bind with $AlCl_3$ in an appropriate manner or due to differences in absorption maxima of the complex formed. Flavanols are estimated using the vanillin-HCl/vanillin H_2SO_4 method, *p*-dimethylaminocinnamaldehyde (DMAC) assay, or the butanol-HCl-Fe (II) assay. Flavanones like naringenin and hesperidin have been estimated using hydrazine formation at the C-4 carbonyl group by reaction with 2,4-dinitrophenyl hydrazine. However other flavonoids like flavones, flavonols, and isoflavones possessing a similar carbonyl group do not react likewise with 2,4-dinitrophenyl hydrazine. This makes the assay using reaction with 2,4-dinitrophenyl hydrazine another unsuitable candidate for estimation of total flavonoids in samples. Anthocyanin pigments need to be estimated using the pH differential method, which cannot be used for the estimation of any other subclass of flavonoids.

None of the above mentioned methods employed for the estimation of flavonoids show uniform results since each class of flavonoids behave differently towards the reagents used to develop color reactions. There is no universal method that can be used to estimate all the subclasses of flavonoids at the same time. Therefore, the term 'Total Flavonoid Content' using the $AlCl_3$ chelation method is not acceptable and cannot be used as a parameter indicating the total amount of flavonoids in the samples, as stated in thousands of research articles. The method needs to be referred to as simply 'Flavonoid Content'. The method can however be used only for comparison of flavonoid content among various samples of the same type, such as comparing different varieties of fruits, vegetables, cereals, *etc*. The method can also be for comparison between species of the same genus, or different varieties of plants. One can also use flavonoid content as an important parameter that can be investigated during the processing of food and beverages, or while studying effects of changes in pH, temperature, and enzyme activity in food products or plant extracts.

Estimation of Total Phenolic Content is another routinely used method using a color reaction with phenolic compounds in solution, including flavonoids. The method has been used worldwide to assess TPC in fruits, beverages, juices, *etc*. This method has its flaws such as inference from reducing agents such as certain amino acids, sugars, $NaHSO_3$, organic acids, *etc*.

The unscrupulous use of colorimetric methods for flavonoids has resulted in thousands of research articles being published each year, without the basic knowledge and understanding of the chemistry involved in them. The results of these colorimetric methods should not be used as the final values. There are flaws and drawbacks in each method and they should rightly be used only for comparative studies among similar samples, or to follow the variation in samples caused as a result of storage or processing conditions. The purpose and validity of each reported colorimetric method need a thorough study before presenting data before the world. This fact has been unfortunately neglected and requires a thorough study to come up with corrective measures or alternative methods of estimation of flavonoids need to be developed.

CONSENT FOR PUBLICATION

Not Applicable

CONFLICT OF INTEREST

The author declares no conflict of interest, financial or otherwise.

ACKNOWLEDGEMENTS

Declared none.

REFERENCES

[1]   Gattuso, G.; Barreca, D.; Gargiulli, C.; Leuzzi, U.; Caristi, C. Flavonoid composition of Citrus juices. *Molecules,* **2007**, *12*(8), 1641-1673.
        [http://dx.doi.org/10.3390/12081641] [PMID: 17960080]

[2]   Ferrer, J.L.; Austin, M.B.; Stewart, C., Jr; Noel, J.P. Structure and function of enzymes involved in the biosynthesis of phenylpropanoids. *Plant Physiol. Biochem.,* **2008**, *46*(3), 356-370.https://doi.org/https://doi.org/10.1016/j.plaphy.2007.12.009
        [http://dx.doi.org/10.1016/j.plaphy.2007.12.009] [PMID: 18272377]

[3]   Zhang, Q.; Zhao, X.; Qiu, H. Flavones and flavonols: Phytochemistry and Biochemistry. In: *In Natural Products: Phytochemistry, Botany and Metabolism of Alkaloids, Phenolics and Terpenes*; Springer: Verlag Berlin Heidelberg, **2013**; pp. 1821-1847.
        [http://dx.doi.org/10.1007/978-3-642-22144-6]

[4]   Havsteen, B.H. The biochemistry and medical significance of the flavonoids. *Pharmacol. Ther.,* **2002**, *96*(2-3), 67-202.
        [http://dx.doi.org/10.1016/S0163-7258(02)00298-X]

[5]   Kirby, L.T.; Styles, E.D. Flavonoids associated with specific gene action in maize aleurone, and the role of light in substituting for the action of a gene. *Can. J. Genet. Cytol.,* **1970**, *12*(4), 934-940.
        [http://dx.doi.org/10.1139/g70-117]

[6]   Falcone Ferreyra, M.L.; Rius, S.P.; Casati, P. Flavonoids: biosynthesis, biological functions, and biotechnological applications. *Front. Plant Sci.,* **2012**, *3*, 222.
        [http://dx.doi.org/10.3389/fpls.2012.00222] [PMID: 23060891]

[7]   Martens, S.; Preuß, A.; Matern, U. Multifunctional flavonoid dioxygenases: Flavonol and anthocyanin biosynthesis in *Arabidopsis thaliana* L. *Phytochemistry,* **2010**, *71*(10), 1040-1049.
        [http://dx.doi.org/10.1016/j.phytochem.2010.04.016] [PMID: 20457455]

[8]   Bowles, D.; Isayenkova, J.; Lim, E.K.; Poppenberger, B. Glycosyltransferases: managers of small molecules. *Curr. Opin. Plant Biol.,* **2005**, *8*(3), 254-263.
        [http://dx.doi.org/10.1016/j.pbi.2005.03.007] [PMID: 15860422]

[9]   Heim, K.E.; Tagliaferro, A.R.; Bobilya, D.J. Flavonoid antioxidants: chemistry, metabolism and structure-activity relationships. *J. Nutr. Biochem.,* **2002**, *13*(10), 572-584.
        [http://dx.doi.org/10.1016/S0955-2863(02)00208-5] [PMID: 12550068]

[10]   Cao, G.; Sofic, E.; Prior, R.L. Antioxidant and prooxidant behavior of flavonoids: structure-activity relationships. *Free Radic. Biol. Med.,* **1997**, *22*(5), 749-760.
        [http://dx.doi.org/10.1016/S0891-5849(96)00351-6] [PMID: 9119242]

[11]   Sharma, A.; Sharma, P.; Singh Tuli, H.; Sharma, A.K. Phytochemical and pharmacological properties of flavonols. In: *eLS*; No. January, **2018**; pp. 1-12.
        [http://dx.doi.org/10.1002/9780470015902.a0027666]

[12]   Chang, H.; Mi, M.; Ling, W.; Zhu, J.; Zhang, Q.; Wei, N.; Zhou, Y.; Tang, Y.; Yu, X.; Zhang, T.; Wang, J.; Yuan, J. Structurally related anticancer activity of flavonoids: involvement of reactive oxygen species generation. *J. Food Biochem.,* **2010**, *34* Suppl. 1, 1-14.
        [http://dx.doi.org/10.1111/j.1745-4514.2009.00282.x]

[13]   Kasprzak, M.M.; Erxleben, A.; Ochocki, J. Properties and applications of flavonoid metal complexes. *RSC Advances,* **2015**, *5*(57), 45853-45877.
        [http://dx.doi.org/10.1039/C5RA05069C]

[14] Hollman, P.C.H.; Arts, I.C.W. Flavonols, flavones and flavanols - nature, occurrence and dietary burden. *J. Sci. Food Agric.,* **2000**, *80*(7), 1081-1093.
      [http://dx.doi.org/10.1002/(SICI)1097-0010(20000515)80:7<1081::AID-JSFA566>3.0.CO;2-G]

[15] Griffiths, L.A.; Barrow, A. Metabolism of flavonoid compounds in germ-free rats. *Biochem. J.,* **1972**, *130*(4), 1161-1162.
      [http://dx.doi.org/10.1042/bj1301161] [PMID: 4656801]

[16] Griffiths, L.A.; Smith, G.E. Metabolism of myricetin and related compounds in the rat. Metabolite formation *in vivo* and by the intestinal microflora *in vitro. Biochem. J.,* **1972**, *130*(1), 141-151.
      [http://dx.doi.org/10.1042/bj1300141] [PMID: 4655415]

[17] Scheline, R.R. Drug metabolism by intestinal microorganisms. *J. Pharm. Sci.,* **1968**, *57*(12), 2021-2037.
      [http://dx.doi.org/10.1002/jps.2600571202] [PMID: 4974346]

[18] Griffiths, L.A.; Smith, G.E. Metabolism of apigenin and related compounds in the rat. Metabolite formation *in vivo* and by the intestinal microflora *in vitro. Biochem. J.,* **1972**, *128*(4), 901-911.
      [http://dx.doi.org/10.1042/bj1280901] [PMID: 4638796]

[19] Hollman, P.C.; de Vries, J.H.; van Leeuwen, S.D.; Mengelers, M.J.; Katan, M.B. Absorption of dietary quercetin glycosides and quercetin in healthy ileostomy volunteers. *Am. J. Clin. Nutr.,* **1995**, *62*(6), 1276-1282.
      [http://dx.doi.org/10.1093/ajcn/62.6.1276] [PMID: 7491892]

[20] Wu, Y.; Wang, F.; Zheng, Q.; Lu, L.; Yao, H.; Zhou, C.; Wu, X.; Zhao, Y. Hepatoprotective effect of total flavonoids from *Laggera alata* against carbon tetrachloride-induced injury in primary cultured neonatal rat hepatocytes and in rats with hepatic damage. *J. Biomed. Sci.,* **2006**, *13*(4), 569-578.
      [http://dx.doi.org/10.1007/s11373-006-9081-y] [PMID: 16547767]

[21] Kim, S.M.; Kang, K.; Jho, E.H.; Jung, Y.J.; Nho, C.W.; Um, B.H.; Pan, C.H. Hepatoprotective effect of flavonoid glycosides from *Lespedeza cuneata* against oxidative stress induced by tert-butyl hyperoxide. *Phytother. Res.,* **2011**, *25*(7), 1011-1017.
      [http://dx.doi.org/10.1002/ptr.3387] [PMID: 21226126]

[22] Dhama, K.; Karthik, K.; Khandia, R.; Munjal, A.; Tiwari, R.; Rana, R.; Khurana, S.K.; Sana Ullah, ; Khan, R.U.; Alagawany, M.; Farag, M.R.; Dadar, M.; Joshi, S.K. Karthik, K.; Khandia, R.; Munjal, A.; Tiwari, R.; Rana, R.; Khurana, S. K.; Ullah, S.; Khan, R. U.; Alagawany, M.; Farag, M. R.; Joshi, M. D. and S. K. Medicinal and therapeutic potential of herbs and plant metabolites / extracts countering viral pathogens - current knowledge and future prospects. *Curr. Drug Metab.,* **2018**, *19*(3), 236-263.https://doi.org/http://dx.doi.org/10.2174/1389200219666180129145252
      [http://dx.doi.org/10.2174/1389200219666180129145252] [PMID: 29380697]

[23] Tahir ul Qamar, M.; Alqahtani, S.M.; Alamri, M.A.; Chen, L.L. Structural basis of SARS-CoV-2 3CL[pro] and anti-COVID-19 drug discovery from medicinal plants. *J. Pharm. Anal.,* **2020**, *10*(4), 313-319.https://doi.org/https://doi.org/10.1016/j.jpha.2020.03.009
      [http://dx.doi.org/10.1016/j.jpha.2020.03.009] [PMID: 32296570]

[24] Hakobyan, A.; Arabyan, E.; Avetisyan, A.; Abroyan, L.; Hakobyan, L.; Zakaryan, H. Apigenin inhibits African swine fever virus infection *in vitro. Arch. Virol.,* **2016**, *161*(12), 3445-3453.
      [http://dx.doi.org/10.1007/s00705-016-3061-y] [PMID: 27638776]

[25] Lv, X.; Qiu, M.; Chen, D.; Zheng, N.; Jin, Y.; Wu, Z. Apigenin inhibits enterovirus 71 replication through suppressing viral IRES activity and modulating cellular JNK pathway. *Antiviral Res.,* **2014**, *109*, 30-41.
      [http://dx.doi.org/10.1016/j.antiviral.2014.06.004] [PMID: 24971492]

[26] Shibata, C.; Ohno, M.; Otsuka, M.; Kishikawa, T.; Goto, K.; Muroyama, R.; Kato, N.; Yoshikawa, T.; Takata, A.; Koike, K. The flavonoid apigenin inhibits hepatitis C virus replication by decreasing mature microRNA122 levels. *Virology,* **2014**, *462–463*, 42-48.
      [http://dx.doi.org/10.1016/j.virol.2014.05.024]

[27]   Fan, W.; Qian, S.; Qian, P.; Li, X. Antiviral activity of luteolin against Japanese encephalitis virus. *Virus Res.,* **2016**, *220,* 112-116.
[http://dx.doi.org/10.1016/j.virusres.2016.04.021] [PMID: 27126774]

[28]   Knipping, K.; Garssen, J.; van't Land, B. An evaluation of the inhibitory effects against rotavirus infection of edible plant extracts. *Virol. J.,* **2012**, *9*(1), 137.
[http://dx.doi.org/10.1186/1743-422X-9-137] [PMID: 22834653]

[29]   Murali, K.S.; Sivasubramanian, S.; Vincent, S.; Murugan, S.B.; Giridaran, B.; Dinesh, S.; Gunasekaran, P.; Krishnasamy, K.; Sathishkumar, R. Anti—chikungunya activity of luteolin and apigenin rich fraction from *Cynodon dactylon. Asian Pac. J. Trop. Med.,* **2015**, *8*(5), 352-358.https://doi.org/https://doi.org/10.1016/S1995-7645(14)60343-6
[http://dx.doi.org/10.1016/S1995-7645(14)60343-6] [PMID: 26003593]

[30]   Mehla, R.; Bivalkar-Mehla, S.; Chauhan, A. A flavonoid, luteolin, cripples HIV-1 by abrogation of tat function. *PLoS One,* **2011**, *6*(11), e27915.
[http://dx.doi.org/10.1371/journal.pone.0027915] [PMID: 22140483]

[31]   Xu, L.; Su, W.; Jin, J.; Chen, J.; Li, X.; Zhang, X.; Sun, M.; Sun, S.; Fan, P.; An, D.; Zhang, H.; Zhang, X.; Kong, W.; Ma, T.; Jiang, C. Identification of luteolin as enterovirus 71 and coxsackievirus A16 inhibitors through reporter viruses and cell *via*bility-based screening. *Viruses,* **2014**, *6*(7), 2778-2795.
[http://dx.doi.org/10.3390/v6072778] [PMID: 25036464]

[32]   Shen, L.; Niu, J.; Wang, C.; Huang, B.; Wang, W.; Zhu, N.; Deng, Y.; Wang, H.; Ye, F.; Cen, S.; Tan, W. High-throughput screening and identification of potent broad-spectrum inhibitors of coronaviruses. *J. Virol.,* **2019**, *93*(12), e00023-19.
[http://dx.doi.org/10.1128/JVI.00023-19] [PMID: 30918074]

[33]   Huang, H.; Zhou, W.; Zhu, H.; Zhou, P.; Shi, X. Baicalin benefits the anti-HBV therapy *via* inhibiting HBV viral RNAs. *Toxicol. Appl. Pharmacol.,* **2017**, *323,* 36-43.
[http://dx.doi.org/10.1016/j.taap.2017.03.016] [PMID: 28322895]

[34]   Su, H.; Yao, S.; Zhao, W.; Li, M.; Liu, J.; Shang, W.; Xie, H.; Ke, C.; Gao, M.; Yu, K.; Liu, H.; Shen, J.; Tang, W.; Zhang, L.; Zuo, J.; Jiang, H.; Bai, F.; Wu, Y.; Ye, Y.; Xu, Y. Discovery of baicalin and baicalein as novel, natural product inhibitors of SARS-CoV-2 3CL protease *in vitro. bioRxiv,* **2020**.
[http://dx.doi.org/10.1101/2020.04.13.038687]

[35]   Sithisarn, P.; Michaelis, M.; Schubert-Zsilavecz, M.; Cinatl, J., Jr Differential antiviral and anti-inflammatory mechanisms of the flavonoids biochanin A and baicalein in H5N1 influenza A virus-infected cells. *Antiviral Res.,* **2013**, *97*(1), 41-48.
[http://dx.doi.org/10.1016/j.antiviral.2012.10.004] [PMID: 23098745]

[36]   Chu, M.; Xu, L.; Zhang, M.; Chu, Z.; Wang, Y. Role of baicalin in anti-influenza virus A as a potent inducer of IFN-Gamma. *BioMed Res. Int.,* **2015**, *2015,* 1-11.
[http://dx.doi.org/10.1155/2015/263630] [PMID: 26783516]

[37]   Zhang, T.; Wu, Z.; Du, J.; Hu, Y.; Liu, L.; Yang, F.; Jin, Q. Anti-Japanese-encephalitis-viral effects of kaempferol and daidzin and their RNA-binding characteristics. *PLoS One,* **2012**, *7*(1), e30259.
[http://dx.doi.org/10.1371/journal.pone.0030259] [PMID: 22276167]

[38]   Yang, L.; Lin, J.; Zhou, B.; Liu, Y.; Zhu, B. Activity of compounds from *Taxillus sutchuenensis* as inhibitors of HCV NS3 serine protease. *Nat. Prod. Res.,* **2017**, *31*(4), 487-491.
[http://dx.doi.org/10.1080/14786419.2016.1190719] [PMID: 27295355]

[39]   Schwarz, S.; Sauter, D.; Wang, K.; Zhang, R.; Sun, B.; Karioti, A.; Bilia, A. R.; Efferth, T.; Schwarz, W. Kaempferol derivatives as antiviral drugs against the 3a channel protein of coronavirus. *Planta Med,* **2014**, *80*(02/03), 177-182.

[40]   Jeong, H.J.; Ryu, Y.B.; Park, S.J.; Kim, J.H.; Kwon, H.J.; Kim, J.H.; Park, K.H.; Rho, M.C.; Lee, W.S. Neuraminidase inhibitory activities of flavonols isolated from *Rhodiola rosea* roots and their *in*

vitro anti-influenza viral activities. *Bioorg. Med. Chem.*, **2009**, *17*(19), 6816-6823.
[http://dx.doi.org/10.1016/j.bmc.2009.08.036] [PMID: 19729316]

[41]   Gonzalez, O.; Fontanes, V.; Raychaudhuri, S.; Loo, R.; Loo, J.; Arumugaswami, V.; Sun, R.; Dasgupta, A.; French, S.W. The heat shock protein inhibitor Quercetin attenuates hepatitis C virus production. *Hepatology,* **2009**, *50*(6), 1756-1764.https://doi.org/https://doi.org/10.1002/hep.23232
[http://dx.doi.org/10.1002/hep.23232] [PMID: 19839005]

[42]   Bachmetov, L.; Gal-Tanamy, M.; Shapira, A.; Vorobeychik, M.; Giterman-Galam, T.; Sathiyamoorthy, P.; Golan-Goldhirsh, A.; Benhar, I.; Tur-Kaspa, R.; Zemel, R. Suppression of hepatitis C virus by the flavonoid quercetin is mediated by inhibition of NS3 protease activity. *J. Viral Hepat.*, **2012**, *19*(2), e81-e88.https://doi.org/https://doi.org/10.1111/j.1365-2893.2011.01507.x
[http://dx.doi.org/10.1111/j.1365-2893.2011.01507.x] [PMID: 22239530]

[43]   Ganesan, S.; Faris, A.N.; Comstock, A.T.; Wang, Q.; Nanua, S.; Hershenson, M.B.; Sajjan, U.S. Quercetin inhibits rhinovirus replication *in vitro* and *in vivo*. *Antiviral Res.,* **2012**, *94*(3), 258-271.https://doi.org/https://doi.org/10.1016/j.antiviral.2012.03.005
[http://dx.doi.org/10.1016/j.antiviral.2012.03.005] [PMID: 22465313]

[44]   Colunga Biancatelli, R.M.L.; Berrill, M.; Catravas, J.D.; Marik, P.E. Quercetin and vitamin C: An experimental, synergistic therapy for the prevention and treatment of SARS-CoV-2 related disease (COVID-19). *Front. Immunol.,* **2020**, *11*, 1451.
[http://dx.doi.org/10.3389/fimmu.2020.01451] [PMID: 32636851]

[45]   Woisky, R.G.; Salatino, A. Analysis of propolis: some parameters and procedures for chemical quality control. *J. Apic. Res.,* **1998**, *37*(2), 99-105.
[http://dx.doi.org/10.1080/00218839.1998.11100961]

[46]   Chang, C.C.; Yang, M.H.; Wen, H.M.; Chern, J.C. Estimation of total flavonoid content in propolis by two complementary colometric methods. *Yao Wu Shi Pin Fen Xi,* **2020**, *10*(3), 178-182.
[http://dx.doi.org/10.38212/2224-6614.2748]

[47]   Daniel, M. *D. M. Analytical Methods for Medicinal Plants and Economic Botany*; Scientific Publishers: New Delhi, **2016**.

[48]   Gauthier, A.; Gulick, P.J.; Ibrahim, R.K. Characterization of two cDNA clones which encode O-methyltransferases for the methylation of both flavonoid and phenylpropanoid compounds. *Arch. Biochem. Biophys.,* **1998**, *351*(2), 243-249.
[http://dx.doi.org/10.1006/abbi.1997.0554] [PMID: 9514654]

[49]   Cacace, S.; Schröder, G.; Wehinger, E.; Strack, D.; Schmidt, J.; Schröder, J. A flavonol O-methyltransferase from *Catharanthus roseus* performing two sequential methylations. *Phytochemistry,* **2003**, *62*(2), 127-137.
[http://dx.doi.org/10.1016/S0031-9422(02)00483-1] [PMID: 12482447]

[50]   Vogt, T. Regiospecificity and kinetic properties of a plant natural product *O* -methyltransferase are determined by its N-terminal domain. *FEBS Lett.,* **2004**, *561*(1-3), 159-162.
[http://dx.doi.org/10.1016/S0014-5793(04)00163-2] [PMID: 15013769]

[51]   Ananvoranich, S.; Varin, L.; Culick, P.; Ibrahim, R. *Cloning and regulation of flavonol 3-sulfotransferase in Ce II suspension cultures of*; Haveria Bidentis, **1994**, pp. 485-491.

[52]   Varin, L.; DeLuca, V.; Ibrahim, R.K.; Brisson, N. Molecular characterization of two plant flavonol sulfotransferases. *Proc. Natl. Acad. Sci. USA,* **1992**, *89*(4), 1286-1290.
[http://dx.doi.org/10.1073/pnas.89.4.1286] [PMID: 1741382]

[53]   Wilson, M.I.; Greenberg, B.M. Protection of the D1 photosystem II reaction center protein from degradation in ultraviolet radiation following adaptation of *Brassica napus* l. to growth in ultraviolet☐B. *Photochem. Photobiol.,* **1993**, *57*(3), 556-563.
[http://dx.doi.org/10.1111/j.1751-1097.1993.tb02333.x]

[54]   Markham, K.R.; Porter, L.J. Flavonoids of the primitive liverwort Takakia and their taxonomic and

phylogenetic significance. *Phytochemistry,* **1979**, *18*(4), 611-615.
[http://dx.doi.org/10.1016/S0031-9422(00)84270-3]

[55] Harborne, J.B.; Williams, C.A. Advances in flavonoid research since 1992. *Phytochemistry,* **2000**, *55*(6), 481-504.
[http://dx.doi.org/10.1016/S0031-9422(00)00235-1] [PMID: 11130659]

[56] Simmonds, M.S.J. Flavonoid–insect interactions: recent advances in our knowledge. *Phytochemistry,* **2003**, *64*(1), 21-30.
[http://dx.doi.org/10.1016/S0031-9422(03)00293-0] [PMID: 12946403]

[57] Mallikarjuna, N.; Kranthi, K.R.; Jadhav, D.R.; Kranthi, S.; Chandra, S. Influence of foliar chemical compounds on the development of *Spodoptera litura* (Fab.) in interspecific derivatives of groundnut. *J. Appl. Entomol.,* **2004**, *128*(5), 321-328.
[http://dx.doi.org/10.1111/j.1439-0418.2004.00834.x]

[58] Xu, H.X.; Lee, S.F. Activity of plant flavonoids against antibiotic-resistant bacteria. *Phytother. Res.,* **2001**, *15*(1), 39-43.
[http://dx.doi.org/10.1002/1099-1573(200102)15:1<39::AID-PTR684>3.0.CO;2-R]   [PMID: 11180521]

[59] Del Río, J.A.; Arcas, M.C.; Benavente-García, O.; Ortuño, A. Citrus polymethoxylated flavones can confer resistance against *Phytophthora citrophthora, Penicillium digitatum*, and *Geotrichum* species. *J. Agric. Food Chem.,* **1998**, *46*(10), 4423-4428.
[http://dx.doi.org/10.1021/jf980229m]

[60] Weidenbörner, M.; Jha, H.C. Antifungal spectrum of flavone and flavanone tested against 34 different fungi. *Mycol. Res.,* **1997**, *101*(6), 733-736.
[http://dx.doi.org/10.1017/S0953756296003322]

[61] Lahlou, M. Study of the molluscicidal activity of some phenolic compounds: Structure-Activity Relationship. *Pharm. Biol.,* **2004**, *42*(3), 258-261.
[http://dx.doi.org/10.1080/13880200490514195]

[62] Kong, C.; Liang, W.; Hu, F.; Xu, X.; Wang, P.; Jiang, Y.; Xing, B. Allelochemicals and their transformations in the *Ageratum conyzoides* intercropped citrus orchard soils. *Plant Soil,* **2004**, *264*(1/2), 149-157.
[http://dx.doi.org/10.1023/B:PLSO.0000047759.65133.fa]

[63] Beninger, C.W.; Hall, J.C. Allelopathic activity of luteolin 7-O-β-glucuronide isolated from *Chrysanthemum morifolium* L. *Biochem. Syst. Ecol.,* **2005**, *33*(2), 103-111.
[http://dx.doi.org/10.1016/j.bse.2004.06.016]

[64] Basile, A.; Sorbo, S.; López-Sáez, J.A.; Castaldo Cobianchi, R. Effects of seven pure flavonoids from mosses on germination and growth of Tortula muralis HEDW. (Bryophyta) and Raphanus sativus L. (Magnoliophyta). *Phytochemistry,* **2003**, *62*(7), 1145-1151.
[http://dx.doi.org/10.1016/S0031-9422(02)00659-3] [PMID: 12591270]

[65] Bors, W.; Heller, W.; Michel, C.; Saran, M. Flavonoids as antioxidants: Determination of radical-scavenging efficiencies. *Methods Enzymol.,* **1990**, *186*(C), 343-355.
[http://dx.doi.org/10.1016/0076-6879(90)86128-I] [PMID: 2172711]

[66] Halliwell, B. Free radicals, antioxidants, and human disease: curiosity, cause, or consequence? *Lancet,* **1994**, *344*(8924), 721-724.
[http://dx.doi.org/10.1016/S0140-6736(94)92211-X] [PMID: 7915779]

[67] Wessely, F.; Moser, G.H. Synthese und konstitution des skutellareins. *Monatsh. Chem.,* **1930**, *56*(1), 97-105.
[http://dx.doi.org/10.1007/BF02716040]

[68] Bhagwat, S.; Haytowitz, D.B.; Holden, J.M. *USDA Database for the flavonoid content of selected foods Release 3*; U.S. Dep. Argiculture, **2011**, pp. 1-156.

[69] Simirgiotis, M.; Schmeda-Hirschmann, G.; Bórquez, J.; Kennelly, E. The *Passiflora tripartita* (Banana Passion) fruit: a source of bioactive flavonoid C-glycosides isolated by HSCCC and characterized by HPLC–DAD–ESI/MS/MS. *Molecules,* **2013**, *18*(2), 1672-1692.
[http://dx.doi.org/10.3390/molecules18021672] [PMID: 23358325]

[70] Tang, D.; Chen, K.; Huang, L.; Li, J. Pharmacokinetic properties and drug interactions of apigenin, a natural flavone. *Expert Opin. Drug Metab. Toxicol.,* **2017**, *13*(3), 323-330.
[http://dx.doi.org/10.1080/17425255.2017.1251903] [PMID: 27766890]

[71] Patel, D.; Shukla, S.; Gupta, S. Apigenin and cancer chemoprevention: Progress, potential and promise (Review). *Int. J. Oncol.,* **2007**, *30*(1), 233-245.
[http://dx.doi.org/10.3892/ijo.30.1.233] [PMID: 17143534]

[72] Liu, R.; Zhang, H.; Yuan, M.; Zhou, J.; Tu, Q.; Liu, J.J.; Wang, J. Synthesis and biological evaluation of apigenin derivatives as antibacterial and antiproliferative agents. *Molecules,* **2013**, *18*(9), 11496-11511.
[http://dx.doi.org/10.3390/molecules180911496] [PMID: 24048283]

[73] Zhou, Y.; Wang, Z.; Xu, L.; Tang, H.; Wang, D.; Meng, Q. 39 Studies on the antidiabetic activity of apigenin in mice with streptozotocin-induced diabetes. *J. Investig. Med.,* **2016**, *64* Suppl. 8, A14-A14.
[http://dx.doi.org/10.1136/jim-2016-000328.39]

[74] Al-rawi, M.I.; Almzaien, A.K.; Almzaien, K.A. Hypolipidemic and antioxidant efficacy of apigenin in hydrogen peroxide induced oxidative stress in adult male rats. *Med.-Leg. Update,* **2021**, *21*(1), 1473-1480.
[http://dx.doi.org/10.37506/mlu.v21i1.2530]

[75] Luo, Y.; Shang, P.; Li, D. Luteolin: A flavonoid that has multiple cardio-protective effects and its molecular mechanisms. *Front. Pharmacol.,* **2017**, *8*, 692.
[http://dx.doi.org/10.3389/fphar.2017.00692] [PMID: 29056912]

[76] Lu, H.; Chen, Y.; Sun, X.B.; Tong, B.; Fan, X.H. Effects of luteolin on retinal oxidative stress and inflammation in diabetes. *RSC Advances,* **2015**, *5*(7), 4898-4904.
[http://dx.doi.org/10.1039/C4RA10756J]

[77] De Stefano, A.; Caporali, S.; Di Daniele, N.; Rovella, V.; Cardillo, C.; Schinzari, F.; Minieri, M.; Pieri, M.; Candi, E.; Bernardini, S.; Tesauro, M.; Terrinoni, A. Anti-inflammatory and proliferative properties of luteolin-7-O-glucoside. *Int. J. Mol. Sci.,* **2021**, *22*(3), 1321.
[http://dx.doi.org/10.3390/ijms22031321] [PMID: 33525692]

[78] Babaei, F.; Moafizad, A.; Darvishvand, Z.; Mirzababaei, M.; Hosseinzadeh, H.; Nassiri-Asl, M. Review of the effects of vitexin in oxidative stress-related diseases. *Food Sci. \& Nutr.,* **2020**, *8*(6), 2569-2580.https://doi.org/https://doi.org/10.1002/fsn3.1567

[79] Ninfali, P.; Angelino, D. Nutritional and functional potential of Beta vulgaris cicla and rubra. *Fitoterapia,* **2013**, *89*, 188-199.
[http://dx.doi.org/10.1016/j.fitote.2013.06.004] [PMID: 23751216]

[80] Malar, D.S.; Suryanarayanan, V.; Prasanth, M.I.; Singh, S.K.; Balamurugan, K.; Devi, K.P. Vitexin inhibits $A\beta_{25-35}$ induced toxicity in Neuro-2a cells by augmenting Nrf-2/HO-1 dependent antioxidant pathway and regulating lipid homeostasis by the activation of LXR-α. *Toxicol. In Vitro,* **2018**, *50*, 160-171.
[http://dx.doi.org/10.1016/j.tiv.2018.03.003] [PMID: 29545167]

[81] Malar, D.S.; Prasanth, M.I.; Shafreen, R.B.; Balamurugan, K.; Devi, K.P. *Grewia tiliaefolia* and its active compound vitexin regulate the expression of glutamate transporters and protect Neuro-2a cells from glutamate toxicity. *Life Sci.,* **2018**, *203*, 233-241.
[http://dx.doi.org/10.1016/j.lfs.2018.04.047] [PMID: 29704481]

[82] Borghi, S.M.; Carvalho, T.T.; Staurengo-Ferrari, L.; Hohmann, M.S.N.; Pinge-Filho, P.; Casagrande, R.; Verri, W.A., Jr Vitexin inhibits inflammatory pain in mice by targeting TRPV1, oxidative stress,

and cytokines. *J. Nat. Prod.*, **2013**, *76*(6), 1141-1149.
[http://dx.doi.org/10.1021/np400222v] [PMID: 23742617]

[83]   Li, H.; Cao, D.; Yi, J.; Cao, J.; Jiang, W. Identification of the flavonoids in mungbean (*Phaseolus radiatus* L.) soup and their antioxidant activities. *Food Chem.*, **2012**, *135*(4), 2942-2946.
[http://dx.doi.org/10.1016/j.foodchem.2012.07.048] [PMID: 22980894]

[84]   Scarpa, E.S.; Emanuelli, M.; Frati, A.; Pozzi, V.; Antonini, E.; Diamantini, G.; Di Ruscio, G.; Sartini, D.; Armeni, T.; Palma, F.; Ninfali, P. Betacyanins enhance vitexin-2-O-xyloside mediated inhibition of proliferation of T24 bladder cancer cells. *Food Funct.*, **2016**, *7*(12), 4772-4780.
[http://dx.doi.org/10.1039/C6FO01130F] [PMID: 27812566]

[85]   Liu, X.; Jiang, Q.; Liu, H.; Luo, S. Vitexin induces apoptosis through mitochondrial pathway and PI3K/Akt/mTOR signaling in human non-small cell lung cancer A549 cells. *Biol. Res.*, **2019**, *52*(1), 7.
[http://dx.doi.org/10.1186/s40659-019-0214-y] [PMID: 30797236]

[86]   Bhardwaj, M.; Paul, S.; Jakhar, R.; Kang, S.C. Potential role of vitexin in alle*via*ting heat stress-induced cytotoxicity: Regulatory effect of Hsp90 on ER stress-mediated autophagy. *Life Sci.*, **2015**, *142*, 36-48.
[http://dx.doi.org/10.1016/j.lfs.2015.10.012] [PMID: 26475763]

[87]   Peng, Y.; Gan, R.; Li, H.; Yang, M.; McClements, D.J.; Gao, R.; Sun, Q. Absorption, metabolism, and bioactivity of vitexin: recent advances in understanding the efficacy of an important nutraceutical. *Crit. Rev. Food Sci. Nutr.*, **2021**, *61*(6), 1049-1064.
[http://dx.doi.org/10.1080/10408398.2020.1753165] [PMID: 32292045]

[88]   Mammen, D.; Daniel, M. A critical evaluation on the reliability of two aluminum chloride chelation methods for quantification of flavonoids. *Food Chem.*, **2012**, *135*(3), 1365-1368.
[http://dx.doi.org/10.1016/j.foodchem.2012.05.109] [PMID: 22953867]

[89]   Shilin, Y.; Roberts, M.F.; Phillipson, J.D. Methoxylated flavones and coumarins from *Artemisia annua*. *Phytochemistry*, **1989**, *28*(5), 1509-1511.
[http://dx.doi.org/10.1016/S0031-9422(00)97776-8]

[90]   Marchelli, R.; Vining, L.C. The biosynthetic origin of chlorflavonin, a flavonoid antibiotic from *Aspergillus candidus*. *Can. J. Biochem.*, **1973**, *51*(12), 1624-1629.
[http://dx.doi.org/10.1139/o73-218] [PMID: 4775434]

[91]   Lago, J.; Toledo-Arruda, A.; Mernak, M.; Barrosa, K.; Martins, M.; Tibério, I.; Prado, C. Structure-activity association of flavonoids in lung diseases. *Molecules*, **2014**, *19*(3), 3570-3595.
[http://dx.doi.org/10.3390/molecules19033570] [PMID: 24662074]

[92]   Erlund, I. Review of the flavonoids quercetin, hesperetin, and naringenin. Dietary sources, bioactivities, bioavailability, and epidemiology. *Nutr. Res.*, **2004**, *24*(10), 851-874.
[http://dx.doi.org/10.1016/j.nutres.2004.07.005]

[93]   Perez, A.; Gonzalez-Manzano, S.; Jimenez, R.; Perez-Abud, R.; Haro, J.M.; Osuna, A.; Santos-Buelga, C.; Duarte, J.; Perez-Vizcaino, F. The flavonoid quercetin induces acute vasodilator effects in healthy volunteers: Correlation with beta-glucuronidase activity. *Pharmacol. Res.*, **2014**, *89*, 11-18.
[http://dx.doi.org/10.1016/j.phrs.2014.07.005] [PMID: 25076013]

[94]   Ferrali, M.; Signorini, C.; Caciotti, B.; Sugherini, L.; Ciccoli, L.; Giachetti, D.; Comporti, M. Protection against oxidative damage of erythrocyte membrane by the flavonoid quercetin and its relation to iron chelating activity. *FEBS Lett.*, **1997**, *416*(2), 123-129.
[http://dx.doi.org/10.1016/S0014-5793(97)01182-4] [PMID: 9369196]

[95]   Sestili, P.; Guidarelli, A.; Dachà, M.; Cantoni, O. Quercetin prevents DNA single strand breakage and cytotoxicity caused by tert-butylhydroperoxide: free radical scavenging *versus* iron chelating mechanism. *Free Radic. Biol. Med.*, **1998**, *25*(2), 196-200.
[http://dx.doi.org/10.1016/S0891-5849(98)00040-9] [PMID: 9667496]

[96]   Huk, I.; Brovkovych, V.; Nanobash Vili, J.; Weigel, G.; Neumayer, C.; Partyka, L.; Patton, S.;

Malinski, T. Bioflavonoid quercetin scavenges superoxide and increases nitric oxide concentration in ischaemia–reperfusion injury: an experimental study. *Br. J. Surg.,* **2003**, *85*(8), 1080-1085.
[http://dx.doi.org/10.1046/j.1365-2168.1998.00787.x] [PMID: 9718001]

[97]   Aherne, S.A.; O'Brien, N.M. Mechanism of protection by the flavonoids, quercetin and rutin, against tert-butylhydroperoxide- and menadione-induced DNA single strand breaks in Caco-2 cells. *Free Radic. Biol. Med.,* **2000**, *29*(6), 507-514.
[http://dx.doi.org/10.1016/S0891-5849(00)00360-9] [PMID: 11025194]

[98]   da Silva, E.L.; Tsushida, T.; Terao, J. Inhibition of mammalian 15-lipoxygenase-dependent lipid peroxidation in low-density lipoprotein by quercetin and quercetin monoglucosides. *Arch. Biochem. Biophys.,* **1998**, *349*(2), 313-320.
[http://dx.doi.org/10.1006/abbi.1997.0455] [PMID: 9448720]

[99]   Nagao, A.; Seki, M.; Kobayashi, H. Inhibition of xanthine oxidase by flavonoids. *Biosci. Biotechnol. Biochem.,* **1999**, *63*(10), 1787-1790.
[http://dx.doi.org/10.1271/bbb.63.1787] [PMID: 10671036]

[100]   Myhrstad, M.C.W.; Carlsen, H.; Nordström, O.; Blomhoff, R.; Moskaug, J.Ø. Flavonoids increase the intracellular glutathione level by transactivation of the γ-glutamylcysteine synthetase catalytical subunit promoter. *Free Radic. Biol. Med.,* **2002**, *32*(5), 386-393.
[http://dx.doi.org/10.1016/S0891-5849(01)00812-7] [PMID: 11864778]

[101]   Lesjak, M.; Beara, I.; Simin, N.; Pintać, D.; Majkić, T.; Bekvalac, K.; Orčić, D.; Mimica-Dukić, N. Antioxidant and anti-inflammatory activities of quercetin and its derivatives. *J. Funct. Foods,* **2018**, *40*, 68-75.https://doi.org/https://doi.org/10.1016/j.jff.2017.10.047
[http://dx.doi.org/10.1016/j.jff.2017.10.047]

[102]   Somerset, S.M.; Johannot, L. Dietary flavonoid sources in Australian adults. *Nutr. Cancer,* **2008**, *60*(4), 442-449.
[http://dx.doi.org/10.1080/01635580802143836] [PMID: 18584477]

[103]   Kim, B.W.; Lee, E.R.; Min, H.M.; Jeong, H.S.; Ahn, J.Y.; Kim, J.H.; Choi, H.Y.; Choi, H.; Kim, E.Y.; Park, S.P.; Cho, S.G. Sustained ERK activation is involved in the kaempferol-induced apoptosis of breast cancer cells and is more evident under 3-D culture condition. *Cancer Biol. Ther.,* **2008**, *7*(7), 1080-1089.
[http://dx.doi.org/10.4161/cbt.7.7.6164] [PMID: 18443432]

[104]   Luo, H.; Rankin, G.O.; Juliano, N.; Jiang, B.H.; Chen, Y.C. Kaempferol inhibits VEGF expression and *in vitro* angiogenesis through a novel ERK-NFκB-cMyc-p21 pathway. *Food Chem.,* **2012**, *130*(2), 321-328.
[http://dx.doi.org/10.1016/j.foodchem.2011.07.045] [PMID: 21927533]

[105]   Luo, H.; Rankin, G.O.; Liu, L.; Daddysman, M.K.; Jiang, B.H.; Chen, Y.C. Kaempferol inhibits angiogenesis and VEGF expression through both HIF dependent and independent pathways in human ovarian cancer cells. *Nutr. Cancer,* **2009**, *61*(4), 554-563.
[http://dx.doi.org/10.1080/01635580802666281] [PMID: 19838928]

[106]   Lee, S.H.; Kim, Y.J.; Kwon, S.H.; Lee, Y.H.; Choi, S.Y.; Park, J.S.; Kwon, H.J. Inhibitory effects of flavonoids on TNF-α-induced IL-8 gene expression in HEK 293 cells. *BMB Rep.,* **2009**, *42*(5), 265-270.
[http://dx.doi.org/10.5483/BMBRep.2009.42.5.265] [PMID: 19470239]

[107]   Qazi, B.S.; Tang, K.; Qazi, A. Recent advances in underlying pathologies provide insight into interleukin-8 expression-mediated inflammation and angiogenesis. *Int. J. Inflamm.,* **2011**, *2011*, 1-13.
[http://dx.doi.org/10.4061/2011/908468] [PMID: 22235381]

[108]   Zhao, J.; Zhang, S.; You, S.; Liu, T.; Xu, F.; Ji, T.; Gu, Z. Hepatoprotective effects of nicotiflorin from *Nymphaea candida* against concanavalin A-induced and D-galactosamine-induced liver injury in mice. *Int. J. Mol. Sci.,* **2017**, *18*(3), 587.
[http://dx.doi.org/10.3390/ijms18030587] [PMID: 28282879]

[109] Tatsimo, S.J.N.; Tamokou, J.D.; Havyarimana, L.; Csupor, D.; Forgo, P.; Hohmann, J.; Kuiate, J.R.; Tane, P. Antimicrobial and antioxidant activity of kaempferol rhamnoside derivatives from *Bryophyllum pinnatum. BMC Res. Notes,* **2012**, *5*(1), 158.
[http://dx.doi.org/10.1186/1756-0500-5-158] [PMID: 22433844]

[110] Zhou, M.; Ren, H.; Han, J.; Wang, W.; Zheng, Q.; Wang, D. Protective effects of kaempferol against myocardial ischemia/reperfusion injury in isolated rat heart *via* antioxidant activity and inhibition of glycogen synthase kinase. *Oxid. Med. Cell. Longev.,* **2015**, *2015*, 1-8.
[http://dx.doi.org/10.1155/2015/481405] [PMID: 26265983]

[111] Semwal, D.; Semwal, R.; Combrinck, S.; Viljoen, A. Myricetin: A dietary molecule with diverse biological activities. *Nutrients,* **2016**, *8*(2), 90.
[http://dx.doi.org/10.3390/nu8020090] [PMID: 26891321]

[112] Li, W.; Xu, C.; Hao, C.; Zhang, Y.; Wang, Z.; Wang, S.; Wang, W. Inhibition of herpes simplex virus by myricetin through targeting viral gD protein and cellular EGFR/PI3K/Akt pathway. *Antiviral Res.,* **2020**, *177*, 104714.
[http://dx.doi.org/10.1016/j.antiviral.2020.104714] [PMID: 32165083]

[113] Jo, S.; Kim, S.; Shin, D.H.; Kim, M.S. Inhibition of African swine fever virus protease by myricetin and myricitrin. *J. Enzyme Inhib. Med. Chem.,* **2020**, *35*(1), 1045-1049.
[http://dx.doi.org/10.1080/14756366.2020.1754813] [PMID: 32299265]

[114] Ortega, J.T.; Suárez, A.I.; Serrano, M.L.; Baptista, J.; Pujol, F.H.; Rangel, H.R. The role of the glycosyl moiety of myricetin derivatives in anti-HIV-1 activity *in vitro. AIDS Res. Ther.,* **2017**, *14*(1), 57.
[http://dx.doi.org/10.1186/s12981-017-0183-6] [PMID: 29025433]

[115] Cho, B.O.; Yin, H.H.; Park, S.H.; Byun, E.B.; Ha, H.Y.; Jang, S.I. Anti-inflammatory activity of myricetin from *Diospyros lotus* through suppression of NF-κB and STAT1 activation and Nrf2-mediated HO-1 induction in lipopolysaccharide-stimulated RAW264.7 macrophages. *Biosci. Biotechnol. Biochem.,* **2016**, *80*(8), 1520-1530.
[http://dx.doi.org/10.1080/09168451.2016.1171697] [PMID: 27068250]

[116] Li, Y.; Ding, Y. Minireview: Therapeutic potential of myricetin in diabetes mellitus. *Food Sci. Hum. Wellness,* **2012**, *1*(1), 19-25.https://doi.org/https://doi.org/10.1016/j.fshw.2012.08.002
[http://dx.doi.org/10.1016/j.fshw.2012.08.002]

[117] Gowd, V.; Chen, W.; Jia, Z. Anthocyanins as promising molecules and dietary bioactive components against diabetes – a review of recent advances. *Trends food Sci. &amp. Technol.,* **2017**, *68*, 1-13.
[http://dx.doi.org/10.1016/j.tifs.2017.07.015]

[118] Saha, S.; Singh, J.; Paul, A.; Sarkar, R.; Khan, Z.; Banerjee, K. Anthocyanin profiling using UV-Vis spectroscopy and liquid chromatography mass spectrometry. *J. AOAC Int.,* **2020**, *103*(1), 23-39.
[http://dx.doi.org/10.5740/jaoacint.19-0201] [PMID: 31462350]

[119] Charepalli, V.; Reddivari, L.; Vadde, R.; Walia, S.; Radhakrishnan, S.; Vanamala, J. *Eugenia jambolana* (Java plum) fruit extract exhibits anti-cancer activity against early stage human HCT-116 colon cancer cells and colon cancer stem cells. *Cancers (Basel),* **2016**, *8*(3), 29.
[http://dx.doi.org/10.3390/cancers8030029] [PMID: 26927179]

[120] Joshi, S.; Howell, A.B.; D'Souza, D.H. Blueberry proanthocyanidins against human norovirus surrogates in model foods and under simulated gastric conditions. *Food Microbiol.,* **2017**, *63*, 263-267.
[http://dx.doi.org/10.1016/j.fm.2016.11.024] [PMID: 28040178]

[121] Silva, S.; Costa, E.M.; Calhau, C.; Morais, R.M.; Pintado, M.E. Anthocyanin extraction from plant tissues: A review. *Crit. Rev. Food Sci. Nutr.,* **2017**, *57*(14), 3072-3083.
[http://dx.doi.org/10.1080/10408398.2015.1087963] [PMID: 26529399]

[122] Lees, D.H.; Francis, F.J. Quantitative methods for anthocyanins. *J. Food Sci.,* **1971**, *36*(7), 1056-1060.https://doi.org/https://doi.org/10.1111/j.1365-2621.1971.tb03345.x

[http://dx.doi.org/10.1111/j.1365-2621.1971.tb03345.x]

[123] Lee, J.; Durst, R.W.; Wrolstad, R.E. Determination of total monomeric anthocyanin pigment content of fruit juices, beverages, natural colorants, and wines by the pH differential method: collaborative study. *J. AOAC Int.,* **2005**, *88*(5), 1269-1278.
[http://dx.doi.org/10.1093/jaoac/88.5.1269] [PMID: 16385975]

[124] Russo, M.; Cacciola, F.; Bonaccorsi, I.; Dugo, P.; Mondello, L. Determination of flavanones in *Citrus* juices by means of one- and two-dimensional liquid chromatography. *J. Sep. Sci.,* **2011**, *34*(6), 681-687.
[http://dx.doi.org/10.1002/jssc.201000844] [PMID: 21328696]

[125] Frabasile, S.; Koishi, A.C.; Kuczera, D.; Silveira, G.F.; Verri, W.A., Jr; Duarte dos Santos, C.N.; Bordignon, J. The citrus flavanone naringenin impairs dengue virus replication in human cells. *Sci. Rep.,* **2017**, *7*(1), 41864.
[http://dx.doi.org/10.1038/srep41864] [PMID: 28157234]

[126] Ahmadi, A.; Hassandarvish, P.; Lani, R.; Yadollahi, P.; Jokar, A.; Bakar, S.A.; Zandi, K. Inhibition of chikungunya virus replication by hesperetin and naringenin. *RSC Advances,* **2016**, *6*(73), 69421-69430.
[http://dx.doi.org/10.1039/C6RA16640G]

[127] Wang, Q.; Yang, J.; Zhang, X.; Zhou, L.; Liao, X.; Yang, B. Practical synthesis of naringenin. *J. Chem. Res.,* **2015**, *39*(8), 455-457.
[http://dx.doi.org/10.3184/174751915X14379994045537]

[128] Crozier, A.; Jaganath, I.B.; Clifford, M.N. Dietary phenolics: chemistry, bioavailability and effects on health. *Nat. Prod. Rep.,* **2009**, *26*(8), 1001-1043.
[http://dx.doi.org/10.1039/b802662a] [PMID: 19636448]

[129] Chen, M.; Ye, Y.; Ji, G.; Liu, J. Hesperidin upregulates heme oxygenase-1 to attenuate hydrogen peroxide-induced cell damage in hepatic L02 cells. *J. Agric. Food Chem.,* **2010**, *58*(6), 3330-3335.
[http://dx.doi.org/10.1021/jf904549s] [PMID: 20170153]

[130] Tamilselvam, K.; Braidy, N.; Manivasagam, T.; Essa, M.M.; Prasad, N.R.; Karthikeyan, S.; Thenmozhi, A.J.; Selvaraju, S.; Guillemin, G.J. Neuroprotective effects of hesperidin, a plant flavanone, on rotenone-induced oxidative stress and apoptosis in a cellular model for Parkinson's disease. *Oxid. Med. Cell. Longev.,* **2013**, *2013*, 1-11.
[http://dx.doi.org/10.1155/2013/102741] [PMID: 24205431]

[131] Dykes, L.; Peterson, G.C.; Rooney, W.L.; Rooney, L.W. Flavonoid composition of lemon-yellow sorghum genotypes. *Food Chem.,* **2011**, *128*(1), 173-179.
[http://dx.doi.org/10.1016/j.foodchem.2011.03.020] [PMID: 25214345]

[132] Yang, L.; Allred, K.F.; Dykes, L.; Allred, C.D.; Awika, J.M. Enhanced action of apigenin and naringenin combination on estrogen receptor activation in non-malignant colonocytes: implications on sorghum-derived phytoestrogens. *Food Funct.,* **2015**, *6*(3), 749-755.
[http://dx.doi.org/10.1039/C4FO00300D] [PMID: 25553799]

[133] Balasundram, N.; Sundram, K.; Samman, S. Phenolic compounds in plants and agri-industrial by-products: Antioxidant activity, occurrence, and potential uses. *Food Chem.,* **2006**, *99*(1), 191-203.https://doi.org/https://doi.org/10.1016/j.foodchem.2005.07.042
[http://dx.doi.org/10.1016/j.foodchem.2005.07.042]

[134] Shukla, A.S.; Jha, A.K.; Kumari, R.; Rawat, K.; Syeda, S.; Shrivastava, A. Chapter 9 - Role of catechins in chemosensitization. *In Role of Nutraceuticals in Cancer Chemosensitization,* **2018**, *2*, 169-198.https://doi.org/https://doi.org/10.1016/B978-0-12-812373-7.00009-7

[135] Pan, X.; Niu, G.; Liu, H. Microwave-assisted extraction of tea polyphenols and tea caffeine from green tea leaves. *Chem. Eng. Process.,* **2003**, *42*(2), 129-133.https://doi.org/https://doi.org/10.1016/S0255-2701(02)00037-5
[http://dx.doi.org/10.1016/S0255-2701(02)00037-5]

[136] Zhu, Q.Y.; Zhang, A.; Tsang, D.; Huang, Y.; Chen, Z.Y. Stability of green tea catechins. *J. Agric. Food Chem.*, **1997**, *45*(12), 4624-4628.
[http://dx.doi.org/10.1021/jf9706080]

[137] Graham, H.N. Green tea composition, consumption, and polyphenol chemistry. *Prev. Med. (Baltim).*, **1992**, *21*(3), 334-350.https://doi.org/https://doi.org/10.1016/0091-7435(92)90041-F

[138] Janeiro, P.; Oliveira Brett, A.M. Catechin electrochemical oxidation mechanisms. *Anal. Chim. Acta*, **2004**, *518*(1-2), 109-115.https://doi.org/https://doi.org/10.1016/j.aca.2004.05.038
[http://dx.doi.org/10.1016/j.aca.2004.05.038]

[139] Xiang, L.P.; Wang, A.; Ye, J.H.; Zheng, X.Q.; Polito, C.; Lu, J.L.; Li, Q.S.; Liang, Y.R. Suppressive effects of tea catechins on breast cancer. *Nutrients*, **2016**, *8*(8), 458.
[http://dx.doi.org/10.3390/nu8080458] [PMID: 27483305]

[140] Geetha, T.; Garg, A.; Chopra, K.; Pal Kaur, I. Delineation of antimutagenic activity of catechin, epicatechin and green tea extract. *Mutat. Res.*, **2004**, *556*(1-2), 65-74.
[http://dx.doi.org/10.1016/j.mrfmmm.2004.07.003] [PMID: 15491633]

[141] Huang, Y.W.; Liu, Y.; Dushenkov, S.; Ho, C.T.; Huang, M.T. Anti-obesity effects of epigallocatechin-3-gallate, orange peel extract, black tea extract, caffeine and their combinations in a mouse model. *J. Funct. Foods*, **2009**, *1*(3), 304-310.
[http://dx.doi.org/10.1016/j.jff.2009.06.002]

[142] Ishikawa, T.; Suzukawa, M.; Ito, T.; Yoshida, H.; Ayaori, M.; Nishiwaki, M.; Yonemura, A.; Hara, Y.; Nakamura, H. Effect of tea flavonoid supplementation on the susceptibility of low-density lipoprotein to oxidative modification. *Am. J. Clin. Nutr.*, **1997**, *66*(2), 261-266.
[http://dx.doi.org/10.1093/ajcn/66.2.261] [PMID: 9250103]

[143] Cavet, M.E.; Harrington, K.L.; Vollmer, T.R.; Ward, K.W.; Zhang, J-Z. Anti-inflammatory and anti-oxidative effects of the green tea polyphenol epigallocatechin gallate in human corneal epithelial cells. *Mol. Vis.*, **2011**, *17*, 533-542.
[PMID: 21364905]

[144] Oz, H.S.; Chen, T.; de Villiers, W.J.S. Green tea polyphenols and sulfasalazine have parallel anti-inflammatory properties in colitis models. *Front. Immunol.*, **2013**, *4*, 132.
[http://dx.doi.org/10.3389/fimmu.2013.00132] [PMID: 23761791]

[145] Fu, Q.Y.; Li, Q.S.; Lin, X.M.; Qiao, R.Y.; Yang, R.; Li, X.M.; Dong, Z.B.; Xiang, L.P.; Zheng, X.Q.; Lu, J.L.; Yuan, C.B.; Ye, J.H.; Liang, Y.R. Antidiabetic effects of tea. *Molecules*, **2017**, *22*(5), 849.
[http://dx.doi.org/10.3390/molecules22050849] [PMID: 28531120]

[146] Teixeira, S.; Siquet, C.; Alves, C.; Boal, I.; Marques, M.P.; Borges, F.; Lima, J.L.F.C.; Reis, S. Structure–property studies on the antioxidant activity of flavonoids present in diet. *Free Radic. Biol. Med.*, **2005**, *39*(8), 1099-1108.
[http://dx.doi.org/10.1016/j.freeradbiomed.2005.05.028] [PMID: 16198236]

[147] Yang, C.S.; Wang, X.; Lu, G.; Picinich, S.C. Cancer prevention by tea: animal studies, molecular mechanisms and human relevance. *Nat. Rev. Cancer*, **2009**, *9*(6), 429-439.
[http://dx.doi.org/10.1038/nrc2641] [PMID: 19472429]

[148] Granja, A.; Frias, I.; Neves, A. R.; Pinheiro, M.; Reis, S. Therapeutic potential of epigallocatechin gallate nanodelivery systems. *Biomed. Res. Int*, **2017**.
[http://dx.doi.org/10.1155/2017/5813793]

[149] Sarkar, S.K.; Howarth, R.E. Specificity of the vanillin test for flavanols. *J. Agric. Food Chem.*, **1976**, *24*(2), 317-320.
[http://dx.doi.org/10.1021/jf60204a041] [PMID: 3530]

[150] Sun, B.; Ricardo-da-Silva, J.M.; Spranger, I. Critical factors of vanillin assay for catechins and proanthocyanidins. *J. Agric. Food Chem.*, **1998**, *46*(10), 4267-4274.
[http://dx.doi.org/10.1021/jf980366j]

[151]   Porter, L.J. 11 - Tannins. In: *Plant Phenolics*; J. B, Harborne, Ed.; Methods in Plant Biochemistry, **1989**; 1, pp. 389-419. https://doi.org/https://doi.org/10.1016/B978-0-12-461011-8.50017-2

[152]   Delcour, J.A.; Varebeke, D.J. A new colorimetric assay for flavonoids in pilsner beers. *J. Inst. Brew.,* **1985**, *91*(1), 37-40.
[http://dx.doi.org/10.1002/j.2050-0416.1985.tb04303.x]

[153]   Prior, R.L.; Fan, E.; Ji, H.; Howell, A.; Nio, C.; Payne, M.J.; Reed, J. Multi-laboratory validation of a standard method for quantifying proanthocyanidins in cranberry powders. *J. Sci. Food Agric.,* **2010**, *90*(9), 1473-1478.
[http://dx.doi.org/10.1002/jsfa.3966] [PMID: 20549799]

[154]   Balisteiro, D.M.; Alezandro, M.R.; Genovese, M.I. Characterization and effect of clarified araçá (*Psidium guineenses* Sw.) juice on postprandial glycemia in healthy subjects. *Food Sci. Technol. (Campinas),* **2013**, *33*, 66-74.
[http://dx.doi.org/10.1590/S0101-20612013000500011]

[155]   Liggins, J.; Bluck, L.J.C.; Runswick, S.; Atkinson, C.; Coward, W.A.; Bingham, S.A. Daidzein and genistein content of fruits and nuts. *J. Nutr. Biochem.,* **2000**, *11*(6), 326-331.
[http://dx.doi.org/10.1016/S0955-2863(00)00085-1] [PMID: 11002128]

[156]   Alves, R.C.; Almeida, I.M.C.; Casal, S.; Oliveira, M.B.P.P. Method development and validation for isoflavones quantification in coffee. *Food Chem.,* **2010**, *122*(3), 914-919.
[http://dx.doi.org/10.1016/j.foodchem.2010.03.061]

[157]   Liggins, J.; Mulligan, A.; Runswick, S.; Bingham, S.A. Daidzein and genistein content of cereals. *Eur. J. Clin. Nutr.,* **2002**, *56*(10), 961-966.
[http://dx.doi.org/10.1038/sj.ejcn.1601419] [PMID: 12373616]

[158]   Setchell, K.D.R.; Brown, N.M.; Zimmer-Nechemias, L.; Brashear, W.T.; Wolfe, B.E.; Kirschner, A.S.; Heubi, J.E. Evidence for lack of absorption of soy isoflavone glycosides in humans, supporting the crucial role of intestinal metabolism for bioavailability. *Am. J. Clin. Nutr.,* **2002**, *76*(2), 447-453.
[http://dx.doi.org/10.1093/ajcn/76.2.447] [PMID: 12145021]

[159]   Křížová, L.; Dadáková, K.; Kašparovská, J.; Kašparovský, T. Isoflavones. *Molecules,* **2019**, *24*(6), 1076.
[http://dx.doi.org/10.3390/molecules24061076] [PMID: 30893792]

[160]   Wu, Z.; Song, L.; Feng, S.; Liu, Y.; He, G.; Yioe, Y.; Liu, S.Q.; Huang, D. Germination dramatically increases isoflavonoid content and diversity in chickpea (*Cicer arietinum* L.) seeds. *J. Agric. Food Chem.,* **2012**, *60*(35), 8606-8615.
[http://dx.doi.org/10.1021/jf3021514] [PMID: 22816801]

[161]   Li, L.; Dong, Y.; Ren, H.; Xue, Y.; Meng, H.; Li, M. Increased antioxidant activity and polyphenol metabolites in methyl jasmonate treated mung bean (*Vigna radiata*) sprouts. *Food Sci. Technol. (Campinas),* **2017**, *37*(3), 411-417.
[http://dx.doi.org/10.1590/1678-457x.15716]

[162]   López, A.; El-Naggar, T.; Dueñas, M.; Ortega, T.; Estrella, I.; Hernández, T.; Gómez-Serranillos, M.P.; Palomino, O.M.; Carretero, M.E. Effect of cooking and germination on phenolic composition and biological properties of dark beans (Phaseolus vulgaris L.). *Food Chem.,* **2013**, *138*(1), 547-555.
[http://dx.doi.org/10.1016/j.foodchem.2012.10.107] [PMID: 23265523]

[163]   Dakora, F.D.; Phillips, D.A. Diverse functions of isoflavonoids in legumes transcend anti-microbial definitions of phytoalexins. *Physiol. Mol. Plant Pathol.,* **1996**, *49*(1), 1-20.
[http://dx.doi.org/10.1006/pmpp.1996.0035]

[164]   Rípodas, C.; Via, V.D.; Aguilar, O.M.; Zanetti, M.E.; Blanco, F.A. Knock-down of a member of the isoflavone reductase gene family impairs plant growth and nodulation in Phaseolus vulgaris. *Plant Physiol. Biochem.,* **2013**, *68*, 81-89.
[http://dx.doi.org/10.1016/j.plaphy.2013.04.003] [PMID: 23644278]

[165]   Ye, Y.B.; Tang, X.Y.; Verbruggen, M.A.; Su, Y.X. Soy isoflavones attenuate bone loss in early postmenopausal Chinese women. *Eur. J. Nutr.,* **2006**, *45*(6), 327-334.
[http://dx.doi.org/10.1007/s00394-006-0602-2] [PMID: 16763748]

[166]   Carroll, K.K. Review of clinical studies on cholesterol-lowering response to soy protein. *J. Am. Diet. Assoc.,* **1991**, *91*(7), 820-827.
[http://dx.doi.org/10.1016/S0002-8223(21)01236-0] [PMID: 2071797]

[167]   Teede, H.J.; Dalais, F.S.; Kotsopoulos, D.; Liang, Y.L.; Davis, S.; McGrath, B.P. Dietary soy has both beneficial and potentially adverse cardiovascular effects: a placebo-controlled study in men and postmenopausal women. *J. Clin. Endocrinol. Metab.,* **2001**, *86*(7), 3053-3060.
[http://dx.doi.org/10.1210/jc.86.7.3053] [PMID: 11443167]

[168]   Lethaby, A.E.; Brown, J.; Marjoribanks, J.; Kronenberg, F.; Roberts, H.; Eden, J. Phytoestrogens for vasomotor menopausal symptoms. *Cochrane Database Syst. Rev.,* **2007**, (4), CD001395.
[http://dx.doi.org/10.1002/14651858.CD001395.pub3] [PMID: 17943751]

[169]   Farquhar, C.M.; Marjoribanks, J.; Lethaby, A.; Lamberts, Q.; Suckling, J.A. Long term hormone therapy for perimenopausal and postmenopausal women. *Cochrane Database Syst. Rev.,* **2005**, (3), CD004143.
[http://dx.doi.org/10.1002/14651858.CD004143.pub2] [PMID: 16034922]

[170]   Messina, M.; Kucuk, O.; Lampe, J.W. An overview of the health effects of isoflavones with an emphasis on prostate cancer risk and prostate-specific antigen levels. *J. AOAC Int.,* **2006**, *89*(4), 1121-1134.
[http://dx.doi.org/10.1093/jaoac/89.4.1121] [PMID: 16915855]

[171]   Messina, M.; Hilakivi-Clarke, L. Early intake appears to be the key to the proposed protective effects of soy intake against breast cancer. *Nutr. Cancer,* **2009**, *61*(6), 792-798.
[http://dx.doi.org/10.1080/01635580903285015] [PMID: 20155618]

[172]   Shu, X.O.; Zheng, Y.; Cai, H.; Gu, K.; Chen, Z.; Zheng, W.; Lu, W. Soy food intake and breast cancer survival. *JAMA,* **2009**, *302*(22), 2437-2443.
[http://dx.doi.org/10.1001/jama.2009.1783] [PMID: 19996398]

[173]   Folin, O.; Denis, W. A colorimetric method for the determination of phenols (and phenol derivatives) in urine. *J. Biol. Chem.,* **1915**, *22*(2), 305-308.https://doi.org/https://doi.org/10.1016/S0021-9258(18)87648-7
[http://dx.doi.org/10.1016/S0021-9258(18)87648-7]

[174]   Singleton, V.L.; Rossi, J.A. Colorimetry of total phenolics with phosphomolybdic-phosphotungstic acid reagents. *Am. J. Enol. Vitic.,* **1965**, *16*(3), 144-158.

[175]   Singleton, V.L.; Orthofer, R.; Lamuela-Raventós, R.M. Analysis of total phenols and other oxidation substrates and antioxidants by means of folin-ciocalteu reagent. *Methods Enzymol.,* **1999**, *299*, 152-178.
[http://dx.doi.org/10.1016/S0076-6879(99)99017-1]

[176]   Chen, L.Y.; Cheng, C.W.; Liang, J.Y. Effect of esterification condensation on the Folin–Ciocalteu method for the quantitative measurement of total phenols. *Food Chem.,* **2015**, *170*, 10-15.
[http://dx.doi.org/10.1016/j.foodchem.2014.08.038] [PMID: 25306311]

[177]   Prior, R.L.; Wu, X.; Schaich, K. Standardized methods for the determination of antioxidant capacity and phenolics in foods and dietary supplements. *J. Agric. Food Chem.,* **2005**, *53*(10), 4290-4302.
[http://dx.doi.org/10.1021/jf0502698] [PMID: 15884874]

[178]   Friedman, M.; Jürgens, H.S. Effect of pH on the stability of plant phenolic compounds. *J. Agric. Food Chem.,* **2000**, *48*(6), 2101-2110.
[http://dx.doi.org/10.1021/jf990489j] [PMID: 10888506]

[179] Folin, O.; Ciocalteu, V. On Tyrosine and tryptophane determinations in proteins. *J. Biol. Chem.,* **1927,** *73*(2), 627-650.https://doi.org/https://doi.org/10.1016/S0021-9258(18)84277-6 [http://dx.doi.org/10.1016/S0021-9258(18)84277-6]

SUBJECT INDEX

A

ABA 45, 46, 47, 48, 49, 51
  biosynthesis 45
  biosynthetic pathway 49
  conjugation pathway 45
  dependent phosphorylation 51
  glycosylation pathway 48
  metabolism 46, 48
  response gene 47
  responsive element-binding factors 47
  signal transduction 46
ABA signalling 43, 44, 45, 47, 49, 50, 51, 54, 55, 56, 57, 58
  networks 57
  pathway 44, 47, 50
  proteins 49
  system 47
Abiotic 2, 43, 44, 47, 49, 57, 58, 166
  dynamics 166
  stresses 2, 43, 44, 47, 49, 57, 58
ABTS assay 30, 116
Accumulation 49, 52, 113, 122
  reduced anthocyanin 49
Acetylcholinesterase 30, 124
AChE enzyme 23
Acid(s) 23, 24, 26, 29, 43, 44, 45, 49, 52, 55,118, 136, 157, 158, 173, 174, 189, 190, 196, 199, 207, 208, 212, 213, 214
  amino 52, 190, 212, 214
  ascorbic 118, 158, 190, 208, 212, 213
  boronic 136
  chlorogenic 174
  dicaffeoyl quinic 26
  dihydrolipoic 158
  dihydrophaseic 45
  dihydrophasic 45
  ellagic 29
  fatty 55
  ferulic 174
  gallic 23, 173, 174, 213
  glucouronic 199

  hypochlorous 157
  lewis 136
  methoxy cinnamic 136
  nordihydroguaiaretic 49
  nucleic 207
  phenolic 26, 29, 49, 174, 189
  phosphoric 212
  phytohormone abscisic 43, 44
  rosmarinic 26, 174
  salicylic 45
  salvianolic 24
  shikimic 23, 174
  syringic 189
Action 169, 192, 170
  anti-inflammatory 169
  hepatoprotective 192
  mutagenic 170
Activities 54, 84, 105, 106, 107, 108, 109, 110, 115, 120, 121, 122, 123, 124, 157, 163, 164, 197
  anti-allergic 123
  anti-anoxic 115
  anti-cancer 84, 109, 110, 197
  anti-HIV-1 122
  anti-malarial 105
  antinociceptive 197
  antiparasitic 107, 108
  antiprotozoal 106
  catalase 163, 164
  cytoprotective 123
  enzymatic 54, 120, 157
  luciferase 120
  neuroprotective 123, 124
  proteasome 122
  tyrosinase 121
Acute radiation syndrome (ARS) 158
African swine flu virus 192, 200
Agapanthus africanus 89
Agents 28, 29, 159, 161, 175, 190, 212, 214
  antibiotic 161
  oxidizing 175
  reducing 29, 190, 212, 214

Atta-ur-Rahman (Ed.)

mushroom tyrosinase 121
radical scavenging 30, 116, 119
radical scavenging activity 116

B

Bacillus 106, 107, 115
    stearothermophilus 115
    subtilis 106, 107
Barks 78, 81, 82
    anti-inflammatory activity 81, 82
    antimalarial activity 78
Base-catalysed Claisen-Schmidt reaction 132
Biflavonoid glycosides 118
Biflavonoids 73, 75, 76, 77, 106, 107, 108, 109, 110, 111, 113, 114, 115, 116, 117, 119, 120, 121, 122, 125, 130
   heterocycle-based Isoflavonechalcone 130
   induced nephrotoxicity 125
Bioflavonoids 83, 125, 134, 136
Biosynthesis 54, 121, 174, 191, 210
    melanin 121
    pathway 191
Biosynthetic pathways 174
Boenninghausenia sessilicarpa 81
Bone marrow cells (BMCs) 120, 163, 165
Branches aromatase 85, 88

C

Ca^{2+}-dependent protein kinases (CDPKs) 49, 52
Calcareous soils 6, 10, 11
Campylospermum 80, 81, 82, 83, 90, 107
    excavatum 80, 81, 82, 90, 107
    flavum 80
    mannii 83
Cancer 23, 34, 154, 161, 169, 200, 202, 207
    angiogenesis 200
    bladder 161
Candida albicans 105, 108
Carcinogenesis 156, 207

Cardiac problems 200
Cardiosclerosis 34
Catabolic reactions 158
Cell homeostasis 171
Cellular proteins 157
Cephalotaxus harringtonia 78, 80, 90
Chalcone 177, 191
    isomers 177
    synthase 191
Chikungunya 192
Chilling stress 57
Choline acetyltransferase 124
Cholinergic systems 118
Cistus 8, 12, 13, 14, 18, 25, 32, 33
    albidus 12, 18, 25, 32, 33
    creticus 8, 12, 13, 14
Cistus monspeliensis 14, 32, 33
Colorimetric methods 206, 214
CPE reduction assay 108
Curcuma longa 161, 172
Cytoprotective activity 82, 123
Cytotoxic activity 14, 15, 34, 78, 79, 84, 86, 88, 89, 90, 92, 110, 112
    and anti HBV activity 86, 89
Cytotoxicity 83, 85, 88, 91, 109, 110, 111, 160, 163

D

Damage 44, 118, 154, 155, 157, 159, 161, 164, 165, 169, 194, 196
    induced testicular 118
    oxidative 118, 164, 165, 194
Deficiency-induced bone loss 120
Degradation pathways 44
Diabetes mellitus 23
Diseases 14, 15, 23, 34, 123, 154, 168, 196, 202, 210
    cardiovascular 23, 202, 210
    coronary heart 14
    neurodegenerative 23, 123
Disorders 158, 121, 210

Treatment 14, 15, 34, 55, 113, 120, 121, 124, 129, 130, 134, 166, 170, 210, 212
  isoginkgetin 113
  sugar 55
Trichome density 10
Trichosporon beigelli 107
Trolox equivalent antioxidant capacity (TEAC) 116, 117, 118, 119
Trypanosoma 105, 106
  brucei 105
  cruzi 105, 106
Tyrosinase 87, 115
  inhibitor 87
  related protein-2 115

U

UDP-glucosyltransferase 45, 48
UGT isoforms 121
UV119, 120, 190, 202
  irradiation 119, 120
  visible spectroscopy 202
  vis spectrophotometry 190

V

Vancomycin-resistant enterococci (VRE) 106
Vascular endothelial growth factor (VEGF) 200
Virtual docking 120
Virus 108, 122, 192, 193, 196, 205
  chikungunya 193, 205
  corona 193
  herpes simplex 200
  mouth disease 196
  picrona 192
  respiratory syncytial 107, 108

W

Water 156

  radiation 156
  radiolysis 156
Western blotting analysis 112

X

Xanthine oxidase (XO) 91, 122
Xyloglucan endotransglucosylase 54

www.ingramcontent.com/pod-product-compliance
Lightning Source LLC
Chambersburg PA
CBHW050827220326
41598CB00006B/329